DATE DUE

SSRIs in Depression
and Anxiety

PERSPECTIVES IN PSYCHIATRY

This series is supported by an educational grant from
GlaxoSmithKline Pharmaceuticals

Series Advisors:

O. Benkert (Germany) G.B. Cassano (Italy)
J.P. Feighner (USA) D.G. Grahame-Smith (UK)
J.J. López-Ibor (Spain) J. Mendlewicz (Belgium)
S.A. Montgomery (UK) F. Rouillon (France)

Volume 2: Diagnosis of Depression
Edited by J.P. Feighner and W.F. Boyer
ISBN 0 471 92891 7 1991 202pp

Volume 3: Long-term Treatment of Depression
Edited by S.A. Montgomery and F. Rouillon
ISBN 0 471 92892 5 1992 275pp

Volume 4: Health Economics of Depression
Edited by B. Jönsson and J. Rosenbaum
ISBN 0 471 93746 0 1993 163pp

**Volume 5: Selective Serotonin Re-Uptake Inhibitors
(Second Edition) Advances in Basic Research and
Clinical Practice**
Edited by J.P. Feighner and W.F. Boyer
ISBN 0 471 95600 7 1996 388pp

Volume 6: Depression and Physical Illness
Edited by M.M. Robertson and C.L.E. Katona
ISBN 0 471 96148 5 1997 564pp

Volume 7: SSRIs in Depression and Anxiety
Edited by S.A. Montgomery and J.A. den Boer
ISBN 0 471 97877 9 1998 194pp

PERSPECTIVES IN PSYCHIATRY VOLUME 8

SSRIs in Depression and Anxiety

Second Edition

Edited by

Stuart A. Montgomery

Imperial College London, UK

and

Johan A. den Boer

Groningen University, The Netherlands

JOHN WILEY & SONS, LTD

Chichester · New York · Weinheim · Brisbane · Singapore · Toronto

National   01243 779777
International   (+44) 1243 779777
e-mail (for orders and customer service enquiries): cs-books@wiley.co.uk
Visit our Home Page on: http://www.wiley.co.uk or http://www.wiley.com

Other Wiley Editorial Offices

John Wiley & Sons, Inc., 605 Third Avenue,
New York, NY 10158-0012, USA

WILEY-VCH Verlag GmbH, Pappelallee 3,
D-69469 Weinheim, Germany

John Wiley & Sons Australia, Ltd., 33 Park Road, Milton,
Queensland 4064, Australia

John Wiley & Sons (Asia) Pte, Ltd., 2 Clementi Loop #02-01,
Jin Xing Distripark, Singapore 129809

John Wiley & Sons (Canada), Ltd., 22 Worcester Road,
Rexdale, Ontario M9W 1L1, Canada

Library of Congress Cataloging-in-Publication Data

SSRIs in depression and anxiety / edited by Stuart A. Montgomery, Johan A. den Boer.—
2nd ed.
    p. ; cm. — (Perspectives in psychiatry ; v. 8)
Includes bibliographical references and index
ISBN 0-470-84136-2 (cased : alk. paper)
1. Depression, Mental—Chemotherapy. 2. Anxiety—Chemotherapy. 3. Serotonin uptake
inhibitors. I. Montgomery, S. A. II. Boer, Johan A. den *1953*– III. Perspectives in
psychiatry (Chichester, England) ; v. 8.
    [DNLM: 1. Depressive Disorder—drug therapy. 2. Anxiety Disorders—drug therapy. 3.
Serotonin Uptake Inhibitors—therapeutic use. WM 171 S774 2001]
RC537 .S73 2001
616.85'27061—dc21

                                                                            2001024255

British Library Cataloguing in Publication Data

A catalogue record for this book is available from the British Library

ISBN 0-470-84136-2

Typeset in 10/12pt Garamond from the author's disks by Mathematical Composition Setters Ltd, Salisbury,
Wiltshire.
Printed and bound in Great Britain by Biddles Ltd, Guildford and King's Lynn.
This book is printed on acid-free paper responsibly manufactured from sustainable forestry, in which at least
two trees are planted for each one used for paper production.

Contents

List of contributors vii

1 Epidemiology of depression and anxiety disorders
  A. Pélissolo and J.-P. Lépine 1

2 Biological aspects of anxiety disorders and depression
  J.A. den Boer, B.R. Slaap and F.J. Bosker 25

3 Comorbidity of depression and anxiety disorders
  Ronald C. Kessler 87

4 Utility of SSRIs in anxious depression
  William Boyer and John P. Feighner 107

5 SSRIs in panic disorder
  James C. Ballenger 119

6 Social anxiety disorder treatment: role of SSRIs
  R. Bruce Lydiard 129

7 SSRIs in obsessive-compulsive disorder
  Stuart A. Montgomery 151

8 Serotonin and serotonergic drugs in post-traumatic stress disorder
  Jonathan R.T. Davidson and Kathryn M. Connor 175

9 SSRIs in the treatment of generalized anxiety disorder
  David S. Baldwin 193

Index 211

Contributors

David S. Baldwin

School of Medicine, Mental Health Group, University of Southampton, Royal South Hants Hospital, Brintons Terrace, Southampton SO14 0YG, UK

James C. Ballenger

Medical University of South Carolina, 67 President Street, PO Box 250861, Charleston, SC 29425, USA

William Boyer

Veterans' Hospital, Psychiatric Department, 1670 Clairemont Drive, Decatur, Georgia, GA 30033, USA

Johan A. den Boer

Department of Biological Psychiatry, Graduate School of Behavioural and Cognitive Neuroscience, Academic Hospital Groningen, PO Box 30001, 9700 RB Groningen, The Netherlands

F.J. Bosker

Department of Biological Psychiatry, Graduate School of Behavioural and Cognitive Neuroscience, Academic Hospital Groningen, PO Box 30001, 9700 RB Groningen, The Netherlands

Kathryn M. Connor

Department of Psychiatry and Behavioral Sciences, Duke University Medical Center, Durham, NC 27710, USA

Jonathan R.T. Davidson

Department of Psychiatry and Behavioral Sciences, Duke University Medical Center, Durham, NC 27710, USA

John P. Feighner

Feighner Research Institute, 5375 Mira Sorrento Place, East Tower Building, 2nd Floor, Suite 210, San Diego, CA 92121, USA

Ronald C. Kessler

Harvard Medical School, Department of Health Care Policy, 180 Longwood Avenue, Boston, MA 02115, USA

J.-P. Lépine

Department of Psychiatry, Hospital Fernand Widal, 200 rue du Fauberg Saint Denis, 75475 Paris, Cedex 10, France

R. Bruce Lydiard

Southeast Health Consultants, LLC, 1 Poston Road, Suite 150, Charleston, SC 29407, USA

Stuart A. Montgomery

19 St Leonard's Road, London, W13 8PN, UK

A. Pélissolo

Department of Psychiatry, Hospital Fernand Widal, 200 rue du Fauberg Saint Denis, 75475 Paris, Cedex 10, France

B.R. Slaap

Department of Biological Psychiatry, Graduate School of Behavioural and Cognitive Neuroscience, Academic Hospital Groningen, PO Box 30001, 9700 RB Groningen, The Netherlands

1

Epidemiology of depression and anxiety disorders

A. Pélissolo and J.-P. Lépine

INTRODUCTION

Epidemiologic studies in psychiatry may provide fundamental information on the prevalence, distribution, comorbidity, risk factors and course of mental disorders, as well as data on quality of life, social cost and demand and use of health services associated with those disorders. These data, when obtained in community surveys, complement clinical investigation and may favour other types of research, such as genetic studies. All these issues have been extensively addressed during the last two decades in the field of anxiety and affective disorders, particularly due to the development of classifications, with explicit diagnostic criteria facilitating the definition of caseness and the utilization of standardized diagnostic interviews. These advances have been positively useful in exploring the cross-cultural epidemiology of anxiety and depression world-wide, with a relatively high agreement in rates and patterns across the majority of countries. Such surveys have also consistently demonstrated the relationship between these disorders and a significant impairment for affected subjects in the community.

We will review in this chapter epidemiologic data on major depression, bipolar disorders and other affective disorders (dysthymia, minor depression, recurrent brief depression), and on panic disorder, phobias, generalized anxiety disorder, obsessive-compulsive disorder and post-traumatic stress disorder (PTSD), with

SSRIs in Depression and Anxiety, Second Edition. Edited by S.A. Montgomery and J.A. den Boer.
© 2001 John Wiley & Sons Ltd.

special attention focused on comorbidity issues between depression and anxiety disorders.

MAJOR DEPRESSION

Prevalence rates

A growing number of surveys referring to DSM-III, and then DSM-III-R diagnostic criteria, have been conducted in various countries since the 1980s, using diagnostic interviews such as the Diagnostic Interview Schedule (DIS) or the Composite International Diagnostic Interview (CIDI). Table 1.1 shows the prevalence rates of major depression in the most important of these studies. The point prevalence per 100 ranged between 0.6 in Taiwan and 10.3 in the USA, with a majority of rates between 3 and 7%. The lifetime rates ranged between 0.9 in Taiwan and 17.1% in the USA, and mostly between 4 and 12%. Some important discrepancies between studies, for example between the Epidemiological Catchment Area (ECA) study and the National Comorbidity Survey (NCS) in the USA, could be due in part to methodological differences, such as sociodemographic differences (age, gender and marital status) and the restrained probing for an episode of major depression in the DIS used in the ECA study (Regier *et al.*, 1998). The prevalence rates for almost all psychiatric disorders were higher in the NCS than in other surveys, suggesting a higher level of detection and/or a lower level of diagnostic threshold. Conversely, very low rates of morbidity were found in Taiwan, as in other studies in Asia, for the majority of affective and

Table 1.1. Prevalence rates per 100 for DSM-III or DSM-III-R major depression in community studies

Sites	N	1 year	Lifetime	References
USA (ECA)	18 572	2.6	4.4	Eaton *et al.* (1991)
USA (NCS)	8 098	10.3	17.1	Eaton *et al.*(1994)
Canada (Edmonton)	3 258	3.2*	8.6	Bland *et al.* (1988)
Puerto Rico	1 551	3.0*	4.6	Canino *et al.* (1987)
France (Savigny)	1 746	M 3.4	M 10.7	Lepine *et al.* (1993c)
		F 6.0	F 22.4	
Italy (Florence)	1 110	5.2	—	Faravelli *et al.* (1990)
Taiwan	11 004	0.6–1.1	0.9–1.7	Hwu *et al.* (1989)
New Zealand (Christchurch)	1 498	5.3	12.6	Joyce *et al.* (1990)
Switzerland (Zurich)	4 547	7.0	—	Angst and Dobler-Mikola (1984)

* 6-Month prevalence.

anxiety disorders. Cross-cultural variations in responders' attitudes or in actual prevalence can be hypothesized, but this still remains an unresolved issue.

In addition, the recent Depression Research in European Society (DEPRES) study conducted in six European countries with the Mini-International Neuropsychiatric Interview (MINI), including 78 463 subjects, found the 6-month mean prevalence for major depression to be 6.9%, ranging from 3.8% in Germany to 9.9% in the UK (Lépine *et al.*, 1997).

The results from DEPRES II have recently been published. This study was based upon detailed interviews from a subset of DEPRES participants ($n = 1884$) who had suffered from depression and had consulted a specialist regarding their symptoms during the previous 6 months. The study findings highlighted that although many depressed patients suffered from considerable functional disability, with many aspects of normal life affected, 70% of respondents to the interview did not receive antidepressant therapy. However, of those respondents who did receive therapy, patients prescribed serotonin reuptake inhibitors (SSRIs) were significantly more likely to feel like their "normal self", compared to those prescribed tricyclic antidepressants. Furthermore, although ineffective against depression, prescription of benzodiazepines was apparently widespread (Tylee *et al.*, 1999a). Additionally, based upon cluster analysis of the DEPRES II data, six distinct categories of depressed patient were identified. Of these categories, the patient with severe depression associated with anxiety exhibited the greatest number and chronicity of symptoms, had the most functional disability, and made the heaviest demand on healthcare resources (Tylee *et al.*, 1999b).

Another cross sectional study, the ESEMeD/MHEDEA trial, is currently being conducted across six European countries. Based upon home interviews of the non-institutionalized general population, the study aims to determine the prevalence and impact of depression and anxiety disorders as well as health services use across Europe. However, data from this trial will be available later in 2001.

Risk factors

The most consistent risk factor for major depression in all studies is gender, with a female : male ratio of approximately 2 : 1, ranging in the above quoted surveys from 1.6 : 1 in Puerto Rico (Canino *et al.*, 1987) to 2.7 : 1 in the USA (Eaton *et al.*, 1991) for lifetime prevalences. These higher prevalence rates do not seem to be linked to a tendency for women to report symptoms or to seek treatment more easily than men (Weissman and Klerman, 1985) and do not concern bipolar depression (Horwath and Weissman, 1995). In addition, various observations have suggested that the increased risk found in women may reflect an increased risk of first onset of major depression rather than a higher duration of episodes or a higher frequency of recurrence (Kessler *et al.*, 1993; Simpson *et al.*, 1997).

The ECA study has shown lower prevalence rates for major depression in the elderly than in younger age groups, although a response bias for elderly subjects in such surveys has been suggested (Knauper and Wittchen, 1994). The mean age at onset for major depression ranges between 17 and 27 years (Weissman et al., 1996).

Marital status is also a risk factor for depression. In the ECA study, divorced subjects had the highest 1-year prevalence, while married and never-divorced subjects had the lowest. Compared to persons with other marital status, the risk for major depression in currently divorced or separated subjects was between two and three times higher (Regier et al., 1993). The same figures were found in most of the countries studied in the Cross-National Collaborative Group, with a two- to six-fold increased risk for major depression in separated or divorced subjects, the odds ratios being higher for men than for women (Weissman et al., 1996).

The other sociodemographic risk factors found in the epidemiology of major depression are type of residence, with higher depression rates observed in subjects living in urban areas when compared to those living in rural areas—but conflicting results have been published on this topic (Horwath and Weissman, 1995), and work status. Indeed, rates of depression were higher among unemployed persons in the ECA study, and subjects who had been unemployed at least 6 months in the last 5 years had a three-fold higher risk of major depression in the past year (Horwath and Weissman, 1995). However, the causal direction of this association remains difficult to determine.

Historical trends

Temporal changes in rates and patterns of depression have been described in several studies, showing a decrease in the age at onset of first depression, an increase of the rates of depression in cohorts born after World War II, and an increase in prevalence rates for all ages between 1960 and 1975 (Klerman and Weissman, 1989; Cross-National Collaborative Group, 1992). These secular changes may reflect period effects and/or cohort effects. Evidence also exists for a narrowing of the differential risk of depression associated with sex, with a greater increase of the risk among young men than young women (Horwath and Weissman, 1995).

Comorbidity

The comorbidity of major depression with other psychiatric disorders has been studied in seven countries by the Cross-National Collaborative Group (Weissman et al., 1996). Increased odds ratios in subjects with major depression have been found for lifetime comorbidity with alcohol abuse or dependence (2.1–3.3), drug abuse or dependence (2.6–11.9), panic disorder (4.7–19.5), and obsessive-compulsive disorder (3.2–23.8).

In the US National Comorbidity Survey, lifetime major depressive disorders were associated with at least one other DSM-III-R disorder in 74.0% of cases, and with three or more disorders in 31.9% of cases. At least one diagnosis of anxiety disorder was recognized in 58.0% of subjects with a lifetime major depressive disorder, as well as 38.6% for substance use disorder (see Table 1.2).

Table 1.2. Comorbidity of lifetime major depressive disorder in the National Comorbidity Survey.

	%	OR	95% CI
Anxiety disorders			
Generalized anxiety disorder	17.2	6.0	4.2–8.6
Agoraphobia	16.3	3.4	2.5–4.6
Simple phobia	24.3	3.1	2.5–3.8
Social phobia	27.1	2.9	2.3–3.6
Panic disorder	9.9	4.0	2.7–6.1
Post-traumatic stress disorder	19.5	4.0	3.1–5.2
Any	58.0	4.2	3.4–5.2
Substance/alcohol use disorder	38.6	1.8	1.4–2.2
Dysthymia	6.7	2.8	1.8–4.4
Conduct disorder	16.2	1.3	1.0–1.6

OR = zero-order odds ratio; 95% CI = 95% confidence interval.
From Kessler *et al.* (1996), with permission.

In a French community study, the most frequent comorbid anxiety disorders with major depression were generalized anxiety disorder and social phobia in women (odds ratios respectively 15.5 and 12.5), and generalized anxiety disorder and panic disorder in men (odds ratios respectively 5.7 and 4.1) (Lépine and Lellouch, 1994).

Public health impact

All epidemiologic studies have stressed the burden imposed on depressed subjects in terms of impairment of their working or social lives. In these surveys, a high proportion of subjects do not seek help of any kind from professionals for their symptoms. When they consult, mostly primary care physicians, most of them do not receive adequate treatment (Lepine *et al.*, 1997).

BIPOLAR DISORDER

The lifetime prevalence of bipolar disorder has been studied in seven countries by the Cross-National Collaborative Group (Weissman *et al.*, 1996), with relatively consistent rates across countries varying between 0.3% in Taiwan and 1.5% in New Zealand (Table 1.3). Prevalence rates were slightly higher in men than in women, with female:male ratios ranging from 0.3 to 1.2. Mean age at onset was 18.1 in the USA (ECA study) and overall ranged from 17.1 in Edmonton to 29.0 in West Germany. The mean ages at onset were, on average, 6 years younger than for major depression.

In the NCS, the lifetime prevalence of manic episode was 1.6% in males and 1.7% in females, and the 12-month rates respectively 1.4% and 1.3%.

Table 1.3. Lifetime rate per 100 for bipolar disorder.

	Females	Males	Total
USA	1.0	0.8	0.9
Edmonton	0.5	0.7	0.6
Puerto Rico	0.5	0.8	0.6
West Germany	1.0	<0.1	0.5
Taiwan	0.3	0.3	0.3
Korea	0.2	0.6	0.4
Christchurch (New Zealand)	1.2	1.7	1.5

From Weissman et al. (1996), with permission. Copyright 1996 American Medical Association.

OTHER DEPRESSIVE DISORDERS

Using DSM-III criteria, the ECA study found the lifetime prevalence of dysthymic disorder to be on average 3.0%, ranging from 2.1% in the site of Baltimore to 4.2% in the site of Los Angeles (Horwath and Weissman, 1995). A lifetime comorbidity pattern with major depressive disorder was found in 42% of subjects with dysthymic disorder. Other surveys have reported lifetime prevalence rates for dysthymic disorder as high as 3.7% in Edmonton (Bland et al., 1988) and 4.7% in Puerto Rico (Canino et al., 1987) but only between 0.9% and 1.5% in Taiwan (Hwu et al., 1989). This disorder is associated with an increased risk among women, with female : male ratios ranging approximately from 1.5 to 2.5 in the above-cited studies. Some data have suggested that the prevalence of dysthymic disorder tend to increase with age, namely with higher rates between 30 and 65 years of age (Horwath and Weissman, 1995). As with major depression, dysthymic disorder is more prevalent in unmarried, divorced and widowed persons than in married ones. As shown earlier, this disorder is frequently comorbid with depressive disorder, but some epidemiologic evidence has suggested that uncomplicated forms of dysthymic disorder are associated with significantly higher rates of medical and psychiatric treatment use, and suicide thoughts and attempts (Weissman et al., 1988a).

Other depressive disorders have been more recently described, based on clinical and/or epidemiologic observations, and are suggested as categories provided for further study in the DSM-IV, such as minor depressive disorder, recurrent brief depressive disorder, or mixed anxiety-depressive disorder. Among these conditions, recurrent brief depressions (RBD) have been particularly investigated in epidemiologic studies, in the community or in primary care (Montgomery et al., 1990; Angst and Hochstrasser, 1994; Weiller et al., 1994). The 1-year prevalence of RBD in the general population has been found to be about 5%, and the lifetime prevalence about 16%. This form of affective disorder, involving brief episodes of depressed mood or loss of interest lasting less than two weeks, but approximately monthly, seems to be associated with severity of symptoms, impairment, suicide attempt rates and treatment seeking equivalent to those of major depression (Angst and Hochstrasser, 1994).

PANIC DISORDER

The NCS has studied the prevalence of panic symptoms in a community sample and found the lifetime prevalence of DSM-III-R panic attacks to be 7.3%, and the prevalence in the preceding month to be 2.2% (Eaton *et al.*, 1994). With more inclusive criteria, in terms of severity and number of associated symptoms, the prevalence of a "fearful spell" was found to be more than twice higher: 15.6% over a lifetime and 5.8% during the last month (Eaton *et al.*, 1994). In other countries, the lifetime rates of panic attacks were more heterogeneous: 1.8% in Florence (Faravelli *et al.*, 1989), 2.4% in Japan (Aoki *et al.*, 1994), 1.7% in men and 4.8% in women in Paris (Lépine and Lellouch, 1994), 7.8% in New Zealand (Joyce *et al.*, 1989), 8.8% in Zurich (Angst and Dobler-Mikola, 1985) and 9.3% in Munich (Wittchen, 1986).

Thus, the best estimate of panic attack lifetime prevalence rates, according to diagnostic criteria, is between 7% and 9% in most countries.

The prevalence of panic disorder, assessed with diagnostic criteria and structured interviews, has been studied in 15 community epidemiologic surveys (Table 1.4). Eleven of these studies, conducted in 10 different countries with similar procedures and in a total of more than 40 000 subjects, have been presented together to examine the consistency of findings across various cultures (Weissman *et al.*, 1997). The lifetime prevalence rates for panic disorder ranged from 0.4% in Taiwan (Hwu *et al.*, 1989) to 3.5% in the NCS (Eaton *et al.*, 1994). Nevertheless, the majority of studies have found

Table 1.4. Prevalence rates per 100 of panic disorder in community-based surveys.

Sites	*N*	1-year	Lifetime Women	Men	Total	References
USA (ECA)	18 571	1.0	2.3	1.0	1.7	Eaton *et al.* (1991)
USA (NCS)	8 098	2.2	5.1	1.9	3.5	Eaton *et al.* (1994)
Canada (Edmonton)	3 258	0.9	1.9	0.9	1.4	Bland *et al.* (1988)
Puerto Rico	1 551	1.1	1.8	1.4	1.7	Canino *et al.* (1987)
France (Savigny)	1 746	0.9	3.0	1.3	2.2	Lépine *et al.* (1994)
Germany	481	1.7	3.8	1.4	2.6	Wittchen *et al.* (1992)
Italy (Florence)	1 100	1.3	3.9	1.2	2.9	Faravelli *et al.* (1989)
Lebanon (Beirut)	234	2.1	3.1	1.1	2.1	Karam (1992)
Taiwan	11 004	0.2	0.6	0.2	0.4	Hwu *et al.* (1989)
Korea (Seoul)	5 100	1.5	2.9	0.5	1.5	Lee *et al.* (1990)
New Zealand (Christchurch)	1 498	1.3	3.3	0.7	2.1	Wells *et al.* (1989)
Iceland	862				2.1	Lindal and Stefansson (1993)
Japan (Ichikawa)	207				1.0	Aoki *et al.* (1994)
USA (San Antonio)	1 306				3.4	Katerndahl and Realini (1993)

lifetime rates between 1.5 and 2.5%. As for major depression, prevalence rates were lower in Asia, and higher in the NCS in the USA. The age range of the population included in the NCS was 15–54 years of age, but convergent data have shown that panic disorder is relatively rare in the elderly (Flint, 1994).

The annual prevalence for panic disorder is generally about 1%, ranging from 0.2% in Taiwan to 3.1% in Zurich. There was also a high agreement in the ECA programme from one centre to another for 1-month prevalence of the disorder, ranging from 0.6 in New Haven to 1.0 in Baltimore (Weissman et al., 1988b).

Prevalence of panic in clinical settings

A recent world-wide survey conducted by the World Health Organization has explored the frequency and the nature of psychological problems in primary care or general health settings, with a modified version of the CIDI according to the International Classification of Disease (ICD-10) (Sartorius et al., 1993). The mean current prevalence of panic disorder was 1.1%, and the lifetime prevalence was 3.4% (Lecrubier, 1997; Üstün and Sartorius, 1995). The current prevalences of panic attacks and panic disorder in different countries are presented in Table 1.5. It can be noticed that, despite a great discrepancy in the prevalence rates of panic attacks, there is a better agreement (about 1%) for the prevalence of panic disorder. Low prevalence rates have been also reported in Asiatic sites (Nagasaki, Shanghai).

If prevalence rates of panic disorder in primary care patients seem to be close to those observed in the general population, this is not the case for patients referred to

Table 1.5. Current prevalence rates per 100 of panic attacks and panic disorder in primary care.

Sites	Panic attacks	Panic disorder
Rio de Janeiro	1.4	0.0
Bangalore	2.0	1.0
Athens	3.0	0.7
Nagasaki	3.3	0.2
Verona	3.3	1.5
Ankara	3.4	0.2
Shanghai	3.8	0.2
Ibadan	4.9	0.7
Santiago	5.5	0.6
Groningen	8.8	1.5
Berlin	10.0	0.9
Mainz	11.2	1.7
Paris	11.3	1.7
Seattle	11.5	1.9
Manchester	16.5	3.5

Data from Üstün and Sartorius (1995); Lecrubier (1997).

specialized consultations. Indeed, 15% of patients attending a clinic for vestibular disorders can be found to be suffering from panic disorder, as well as 16% of cardiac outpatients (Chignon *et al.*, 1993) and up to 35% of general hospital patients with hyperventilation symptoms.

Risk factors

The 1-month prevalence of panic attacks is consistently higher in women as compared with men in the NCS, with a prevalence more than twice as great among women at each level of severity (Eaton *et al.*, 1994). The same figures have been obtained in the ECA study (Von Korff *et al.*, 1985). The lifetime prevalence rates of panic disorder are also higher in women as compared with men, in all the countries (Table 1.4).

The age at onset of panic disorder is in general in the early to middle 20s in the NCS. By using life table survival methods, Burke *et al.* (1990) found the highest hazard rates in the ECA study to be between 25 and 34 years of age for women and between 30 and 44 years of age for men.

The prevalence of panic attacks and panic disorder is usually higher in young subjects, particularly between 15 and 45 years of age (Lépine and Lellouch, 1994). The age pattern in the NCS has suggested a bimodality, with an early mode in the range 15–24 years, and a later one in the range 45–54 years (Eaton *et al.*, 1994). In the ECA study, people of 65 years of age or more had very low prevalence rates, about 0.1% (Regier *et al.*, 1988), and panic disorder seems generally to be rare in the elderly (Flint, 1994).

Marital status is another significant risk factor for panic disorder: the highest life-time prevalence rates are found in widowed, separated or divorced subjects (Lépine and Lellouch, 1994).

Educational level is also associated with strong risk differences for panic disorder in the NCS (Eaton *et al.*, 1994). People with fewer than 12 years of education were more than ten times as likely to suffer from this disorder as the comparison sample with 16 or more years of education. However, no association was found between level of income and prevalence of panic disorder.

Another sociodemographic risk factor found to correlate with panic disorder is the fact of living in a city vs. a rural habitation (Hwu *et al.*, 1989). Regarding cultural impact, similar prevalence rates were found in Japan, in the USA and Canada, for example (Table 1.4); the only exception is Taiwan, where very low prevalence rates have been observed (Hwu *et al.*, 1989).

Lastly, several studies have suggested that life events such as major loss or separation before 15 years of age (Battaglia *et al.*, 1995; Servant and Parquet, 1995), early separation anxiety (Silove *et al.*, 1996) or other childhood trauma (Aoki *et al.*, 1994; Dumas *et al.*, 1995; David *et al.*, 1995) and more specifically parental indifference, physical or sexual abuse (Brown *et al.*, 1993; Stein *et al.*, 1996) may enhance the risk of panic attacks and panic disorder in adulthood.

Comorbidity

Evidence came from ECA data analysis that almost 50% of all subjects with a life-time anxiety disorder had at least one other anxiety disorder (Weissman *et al.*, 1986). At every cross-national site, panic disorder has been found to be significantly associated with an increased risk of agoraphobia (Table 1.6), with odds ratios ranging from 7.5 in the ECA survey to 21.4 in Puerto Rico (Weissman *et al.*, 1997). A comorbidity pattern with agoraphobia is observed in 29.5–58.2% of subjects with panic disorder. In the NCS, where 50% of subjects with panic disorder reported no symptoms of agoraphobia (Eaton *et al.*, 1994), the lifetime prevalence for panic disorder with agoraphobia was 1.5% and the 1-month prevalence of this association was 0.7%.

Social phobia is another condition frequently associated with panic disorder: 19.2–73.9% of subjects with social phobia have reported lifetime symptoms of panic disorder in the cross-national studies. Goisman *et al.* (1994) have suggested rates of 20% for generalized anxiety disorder, 14% for obsessive-compulsive disorder, and 6% for post-traumatic stress disorder in patients with panic disorder.

Based on the cross-national sites data (Table 1.7), the lifetime odds ratios for an association between panic disorder and major depression ranged from 3.8 in Savigny to 20.1 in Edmonton (Weissman *et al.*, 1994). In the French study (Lépine and Lellouch, 1994), the odds ratio for lifetime major depressive episodes in subjects with agoraphobia were the same for men (4.33; 95% CI 1.06–17.7) as for women (4.11; 2.10–8.03). In the WHO-ADAMHA CIDI Field Trial study, Lépine *et al.* (1993a) reported that, when studying retrospectively the time sequence of panic disorder and affective disorders in 55 comorbid subjects, both occurred in the same year in 50.9%, 25.5% experienced onset of an affective disorder before panic and 23.6% had the reverse pattern.

In the ECA study, 20.8% of subjects with panic disorder had a comorbid bipolar disorder (Chen and Dilsaver, 1995).

Table 1.6. Comorbidity between panic disorder and agoraphobia, with odds ratio adjusted by age and gender within each site.

	In subjects with panic disorder (%)	In subjects without panic disorder (%)	Odds ratio (95% CI)
USA (ECA)	33.3	5.5	7.5 (5.6–10.1)
USA (NCS)	38.8	5.1	10.6 (7.3–15.5)
Canada (Edmonton)	31.8	2.7	15.1 (7.6–29.9)
Puerto Rico	58.2	6.0	21.4 (9.2–50.2)
France (Savigny)	48.9	6.5	12.7 (8.0–24.0)
Taiwan	22.5	1.4	17.2 (10.6–27.8)
Korea (Seoul)	34.7	2.1	17.2 (4.2–21.2)
New Zealand (Christchurch)	29.5	3.4	10.6 (7.3–15.5)

From Weissman *et al.* (1997), with permission. Copyright 1997 American Medical Association.

Table 1.7. Comorbidity of panic disorder with major depression, with odds ratio adjusted by age and gender within each site.

	In subjects with panic disorder (%)	In subjects without panic disorder (%)	Odds ratio (95% CI)	
USA (ECA)	32.8	4.7	8.7	(6.4–11.7)
USA (NCS)	54.5	16.0	5.7	(4.0–8.1)
Canada (Edmonton)	68.2	9.2	20.1	(10.4–38.8)
Puerto Rico	38.2	3.7	15.3	(6.4–36.6)
France (Savigny)	48.9	17.3	3.8	(2.1–7.1)
Taiwan	22.5	1.3	19.6	(9.1–42.1)
Korea (Seoul)	28.4	2.5	13.2	(8.0–21.6)
New Zealand (Christchurch)	40.8	11.2	4.6	(2.2–9.4)

From Weissman *et al.* (1997), with permission. Copyright 1997 American Medical Association.

Lastly, Regier *et al.* (1990) have reported that 36% of subjects with panic disorder had a substance or alcohol abuse in the ECA survey. Evidence for this comorbidity pattern also appeared in clinical studies, where alcoholism is observed in 13–43% of patients with panic disorder (Wittchen and Essau, 1993).

Suicidality

A significant association between panic disorder and suicide attempt in the general population was originally reported by Weissman *et al.* (1989) and Johnson *et al.* (1990). In these findings, the majority of panic disorder subjects had other life-time psychiatric disorders, but non-comorbid cases were also associated with an increased risk of suicide attempts (7% vs. 1% in subjects without psychiatric disorders). In cross-national sites, significant odds ratios for history of suicide attempts in subjects with panic disorder vs. those without panic disorder were found, ranging from 11.4 in Christchurch to 78.4 in Edmonton.

Table 1.8. Rate of suicide attempts (%) in patients with panic disorder according to lifetime diagnoses of major depression (MD), alcoholism, and other substance abuse.

	Men (*N* = 37)	Women (*N* = 63)	Total (*N* = 100)
MD with alcoholism and/or substance abuse	57.1	81.8	72.2
MD without alcoholism and/or substance abuse	28.6	55.6	50.0
Alcoholism and/or other substance abuse without MD	42.9	50.0	46.2
No alcoholism, other substance abuse, or MD	12.5	21.1	17.1

From Lépine *et al.* (1993b), with permission. Copyright 1993 American Medical Association.

Further clinical studies have been conducted to address this issue, and Lépine et al. (1993b) have shown that 42% (30% in men and 49% in women) of outpatients with panic disorder had a history of suicide attempt, this rate being 17.1% in patients without lifetime comorbid disorder (Table 1.8). Regarding time sequencing of disorders, the majority (73.8%) of suicide attempts occurred after the first panic attack.

AGORAPHOBIA

As mentioned above, agoraphobia is frequently investigated in relation to panic disorder. In the ECA study, the lifetime prevalence of agoraphobia was 5.6% for four sites, with 6-month rates ranging from 2.7% in St Louis to 5.8% in Baltimore (Horwath and Weissman, 1995). Referring to DSM-III diagnostic criteria, other community surveys reported lifetime prevalence of 2.1% in Seoul (Lee et al., 1990), 2.9% in Edmonton (Bland et al., 1988), 5.7% in Munich (Wittchen et al., 1992), 6.9% in Puerto Rico (Canino et al., 1987), and 8.1% in Christchurch (Wells et al., 1989). In a French study, lifetime prevalence for DSM-III-R agoraphobia was 3.7% in males and 9.9% in females (Lépine and Lellouch, 1995).

Two community studies have explored specifically the prevalence of agoraphobia without panic disorder: the NCS, in which the lifetime prevalence was found to be 5.3% and the 12-month prevalence 2.8% (Kessler et al., 1994), and a survey in Basel where lifetime prevalence for agoraphobia without panic disorder was 10.8%, while the rate for agoraphobia with panic disorder was 2.1% (Wacker et al., 1992).

In all community studies, lifetime rates of agoraphobia were significantly higher for women than for men. Rates are also higher in young adults, i.e. between 18 and 29

Table 1.9. Lifetime comorbidity for subjects with agoraphobia in the NCS.

	Prevalence (%)	Odds ratio	95% CI
Major depression	45.9	4.81	3.65–6.35
Dysthymia	16.0	3.14	2.2–4.40
Mania	8.6	7.89	5.44–11.45
Any affective disorder	50.9	7.03	3.90–6.50
Generalized anxiety disorder	19.8	5.80	4.39–7.66
Simple phobia	45.6	8.67	6.77–11.11
Social phobia	46.5	7.07	5.65–8.83
Panic disorder	21.6	11.88	8.04–17.55
Panic attacks	35.8	10.01	7.55–13.28
PTSD	22.6	4.08	2.73–6.08
Any anxiety disorder	74.1	8.79	6.13–12.61
Any substance abuse or dependence	36.3	1.63	1.23–2.15
Any other disorder	87.6	6.80	4.87–11.37

From Magee et al. (1996), with permission. Copyright 1996 American Medical Association.

years, and higher in widowed, separated or divorced subjects than in married or never-married subjects (Lépine and Lellouch, 1995). The mean age at onset is about 20 years.

High comorbidity rates are obtained between agoraphobia and other anxiety disorders, and between agoraphobia and affective disorders. In Table 1.9 the life-time comorbidity rates for agoraphobia in the NCS are reported. In the French survey (Lépine and Lellouch, 1995), the highest odds ratios for agoraphobia life-time comorbidity were found with panic disorder (8.23) and social phobia (5.14), and then with major depressive episodes (3.30) and generalized anxiety disorder (3.15).

SOCIAL PHOBIA/SOCIAL ANXIETY DISORDER

Two comprehensive reviews on the epidemiology of social phobia have been published recently (Lépine and Pélissolo, 1999; Lecrubier *et al.*, 2000). They underlined the fact that several epidemiologic studies conducted in the community and in clinical samples have shown that social phobia is a frequent and disabling disorder, probably unrecognized and undertreated (Davidson *et al.*, 1993; Weiller *et al.*, 1996). Table 1.10 shows the lifetime prevalence rates of social phobia in various community studies using DSM-III or DSM-III-R diagnostic criteria. Some conceptual and methodological problems related to uncertainties about diagnostic thresholds may

Table 1.10. Lifetime prevalence of social phobia.

	Males	Females	Total	Reference
ECA (total USA)	2.5	2.9	2.7	Eaton *et al.* (1991)
ECA				
4 sites	2.0	3.1	2.4	
Saint-Louis			1.9	
Baltimore			3.1	Schneier *et al.* (1992)
Los Angeles			1.8	
Durham			3.2	
Duke			3.8	Davidson *et al.* (1993)
NCS	11.1	15.5	13.3	Kessler *et al.* (1993)
Puerto Rico	1.5	1.6	1.6	Canino *et al.* (1987)
Edmonton	1.4	2.0	1.7	Bland *et al.* (1988)
Paris	2.1	5.4	4.1	Lépine and Lellouch (1995)
Zurich	3.1	4.4	3.8	Degonda and Angst (1993)
Basel			16.0	Wacker *et al.* (1992)
Munich			2.5	Wittchen *et al.* (1992)
Florence			1.0	Faravelli *et al.* (1989)
Christchurch	4.3	3.0	3.5	Wells *et al.* (1989)
Seoul	0.0	1.0	0.5	Lee *et al.* (1990)
Taiwan	0.2	1.0	0.6	Hwu *et al.* (1989)

From Lépine and Lellouch (1995), reproduced by permission of Lippincott-Raven Publishers.

explain some of the variation in the rates which were reported. Indeed, the lifetime prevalence rates of social phobia in the general population was found to range from 2% to 4% in the earliest studies using the DIS for DSM-III (Schneier et al., 1992; Davidson et al., 1993). Subsequent studies, based on DSM-III-R criteria and diagnostic interviews which explored more abundant and diversified social situations, suggested more elevated lifetime prevalence rates for social phobia, between 4.1% and 16% (Wacker et al., 1992; Kessler et al., 1994; Lépine and Lellouch, 1995).

More recently, very similar lifetime prevalence rates for DSM-IV social anxiety disorder were found in four large community studies carried out in Germany, 7.3% (Wittchen et al., 1999), in France, 7.3% (Pélissolo et al., 2000), in Italy, 6.6% (Faravelli et al., 2000), and in the United States, 7.2% (Stein et al., 2000). It is also noteworthy that data from the United States suggest an increased prevalence of social phobia in recent cohorts, especially in generalized forms and in white, educated and married individuals (Heimberg et al., 2000).

In epidemiologic studies, subjects with social phobia are most frequently female (sex ratio about 1.5 : 1), are more likely to be younger, of lower socioeconomic status, less educated, and less likely to be married than subjects without social phobia (Schneier et al., 1992; Lépine and Lellouch, 1995). Most subjects had an onset of social phobia before the age of 25 years, with a peak in early childhood and another at 16–20 years (Schneier et al., 1992; Lépine and Lellouch, 1995).

Although social phobia by itself seems to be associated with a significant impairment, being a disorder with a very long-term unremitting course (Reich et al., 1994), its public health impact is also largely related to its comorbidity with other psychiatric disorders, which has been emphasized by many investigators (Liebowitz et al., 1985). Only 29% of subjects with social phobia had no other lifetime disorder in the ECA study reported by Schneier et al. (1992), and the proportion of pure social phobia in the NCS was 19% (Magee et al., 1996).

Comorbid disorders most frequently found in epidemiologic studies are other anxiety disorders, affective disorders and substance use disorders (Lépine and Pélissolo, 1996). In the NCS (Magee et al., 1996; Kessler et al., 1999), 56.9% of subjects with social phobia had at least one other anxiety disorder during the lifetime (odds ratio 5.80), most frequently simple phobia (37.6%) and agoraphobia (23.3%). Affective disorders were associated as lifetime comorbid conditions in 41.4% of subjects (odds ratio 3.74), with major depression found in 37.2% and dysthymia in 14.6%. Lastly, alcohol or drug abuse or dependence was observed in 39.6% of social phobia subjects (odds ratio 2.01). Importantly, in comorbid subjects, on the basis of a retrospective assessment, in most of the cases, social phobia predates the comorbid disorder.

SPECIFIC PHOBIA

According to NCS data, the lifetime prevalence for simple phobia was 11.3% (6.7% in males and 15.7% in females), and the 12-month prevalence was 8.8% (Kessler et al.,

1994). High comorbidity rates were found between simple phobia and all other anxiety disorders (odds ratios ranging from 3.68 for PTSD to 8.67 for agoraphobia), major depression (odds ratio 4.55), and drug dependence (odds ratio 2.47).

In the French study, the lifetime prevalence of simple phobia was 10.5% in males and 23.2% in females, with a significant comorbidity with anxiety disorders and major depression (Lépine and Lellouch, 1994).

GENERALIZED ANXIETY DISORDER

Although significant changes and revisions occurred in the diagnostic criteria for generalized anxiety disorder (GAD) between DSM-III and DSM-IV, community epidemiologic studies found consistent current prevalence rates between 1.2% and 2.8%, and lifetime prevalence rates between 4.0% and 6.6% (Table 1.11). Nevertheless, Wacker *et al.* (1992) have reported that the prevalence rates were markedly influenced by the diagnostic criteria applied. Prevalence rates are higher in primary care (8%) than reported in the general population (19%–5.1%).

GAD is twice as common among women as among men, with higher prevalence rates in subjects older than 24 years, and in separated, widowed, divorced or unemployed persons.

About 90% of subjects with GAD in the NCS had at least one other lifetime psychiatric disorder (Wittchen *et al.*, 1994). Dysthymia, panic disorder, mania and

Table 1.11. Prevalence rates for generalized anxiety disorder in community studies.

Sites	Diagnostic criteria	Current (%)	Lifetime (%)	12-month prevalence (%)	Reference
ECA	DSM-III				Robins and Regier (1991)
Durham		1.2	6.6		
St Louis		1.3	6.6		
Los Angeles		1.4	4.1		
Munich	DSM-III	2.4	4.0		Wittchen *et al.* (1992)
Florence	DSM-III	2.8	5.4		Faravelli *et al.* (1990)
Paris	DSM-III-R	M 3.7	M 6.6		Lépine Lellouch (1994)
		F 6.6	F 12.5		
Basel	DSM-III-R	—	1.9		Wacker *et al.* (1992)
	ICD-10	—	9.2		
NCS	DSM-III-R	1.6	5.1		Wittchen *et al.* (1994)
EDSP (Early developmental stages of psychopathology) study	DSM-IV			1.8	Wittchen *eta al.* (1998)
Australian				3.7	Andrews *et al.* (2000)
German National Survey (GHS)				1.5	Carter *et al.* (in press)

major depression were the most frequently associated disorders in the lifetime, with odds ratios between about 9 and 13. Other anxiety disorders and major depression were also found to be associated with GAD in the French study (Lépine and Lellouch, 1994).

Whether they were comorbid or not, the majority of subjects with GAD experienced significant impairment and reported a high level of seeking professional help and of drugs use in the NCS (Wittchen et al., 1994).

OBSESSIVE-COMPULSIVE DISORDER

Obsessive-compulsive disorder (OCD) was classically viewed as an uncommon disorder, but the ECA survey, referring to DSM-III criteria, revealed significant prevalence rates, with an overall lifetime rate as high as 2.6% (Robins and Regier, 1991). In this survey, the 6-month prevalences ranged between 0.7% in Los Angeles and 2.1% in North Carolina.

Other community studies have confirmed high lifetime prevalence rates for OCD, e.g. 2.1% in Seoul (Lee et al., 1990), 3.2% in Edmonton (Bland et al., 1988) and 3.2% in Puerto Rico (Canino et al., 1987). Nevertheless, Faravelli et al. (1990) in Florence and Hwu et al. (1989) in Taiwan reported lifetime prevalence rates lower than 1%.

In the ECA survey, OCD prevalence rates were found to be about the same magnitude in both sexes: 1.1% in male and 1.5% in female for 1-month prevalences (Regier et al. 1993). The higher prevalence rates were found in subjects aged 18–44 years, in separated or divorced subjects and in low socioeconomic groups.

POST-TRAUMATIC STRESS DISORDER

Until recently, little was known on the epidemiological characteristics of post-traumatic stress disorder (PTSD), despite a growing number of clinical works on this condition since the first codification of its diagnostic criteria in the DSM-III. Many publications describe selected samples of subjects as victims of traumas, showing high rates of PTSD even many years after the event. For example, in a group of 124 survivors of the Holocaust, Kuch and Cox (1992) reported that 57 subjects (46%) met the criteria for PTSD, and in two studies conducted on World War II prisoners, the prevalence of PTSD was still 20–29% 40 years after the traumatic events (Kluznik et al. 1986; Speed et al. 1989). Epidemiological data are nowadays available from community-based studies.

Two reports have been made from ECA data, from the sites of St Louis (Helzer et al., 1987) and the Piedmont region of North Carolina (Davidson et al., 1991). In the former study, in which 2500 subjects were analysed, the lifetime prevalence of PTSD was found to be 1.0% (0.5% in males and 1.3% in females). The prevalence of subthreshold PTSD, i.e. post-traumatic stress disorder not satisfying all DSM-III criteria, was 15% and even 45% for at least one symptom (Helzer *et al.*, 1987). The second ECA analyses included 2985 subjects and found that the lifetime and 6-month prevalence rates for PTSD were respectively 1.30% and 0.44%. The most frequently involved traumas were threat or close call, seeing someone hurt or killed, physical attack and accident. PTSD was associated with greater psychiatric comorbidity and suicide attempts, with increased somatic morbidity, and with impaired social support. Risk factors were job instability, family history of psychiatric illness, parental poverty, child abuse, and separation of parents before 10 years of age (Davidson *et al.*, 1991).

In a random sample of 1007 young adults in Detroit, Breslau *et al.* (1991) found the lifetime prevalence of DSM-III-R PTSD to be high: 9.2% in the total sample (11.3% in females and 6% in males). In a secondary analysis, Breslau *et al.* (1997) found that lifetime prevalence of exposure to traumatic events and number of traumatic events did not vary by sex, but that the vulnerability to PTSD in exposed females might be greater in childhood and increased by pre-existing anxiety disorders and major depressive disorders.

PTSD was also explored in the Part II subsample of 5877 subjects of the NCS, using DSM-III-R criteria (Kessler *et al.*, 1995). In the whole sample, 60.7% of men and 51.2% of women reported at least one traumatic event, and actually experienced generally several traumas. The estimated lifetime prevalence of PTSD in the total sample was 7.8% (5.0% in males and 10.4% in females). The traumas most frequently associated with PTSD were combat exposure and witnessing for men, rape and sexual abuse for women. PTSD was comorbid with a lifetime history of at least one other mental disorder in 88.3% of men and 79% of women, especially major depression (47.9% vs. 11.7% in subjects without history of PTSD), simple and social phobia, substance use disorder, and also conduct disorder in men. With respect to all other comorbid disorders, PTSD was primary between about 30% and 50% of the time among men, and between about 40% and 60% of the time among women. Sociodemographic risk factors for PTSD were female sex, and being separated, divorced or widowed for both men and women. Another important finding of this study is the fact that PTSD was found to be often persistent, with a median time to remission of 36 months among the subjects who ever sought professional help (58% of affected respondents), and 64 months among those who did not (Kessler *et al.*, 1995).

The prevalence rate of current DSM-IV PTSD in a survey carried out in Winnipeg (Canada) was 1.7% in males and 5% in females (Stein *et al.*, 1997). The most frequently traumatic events reported were the sudden death of a relative (34.7% in males and 33.5% in females), witnessing a death or a serious injury (18.8% in males and 38.9% in females), and physical attack (21% in males and 24.6% in females).

Two recent studies have been conducted in representative community samples in Munich (*n* = 3021, aged 14–24 years) and in Detroit (*n* = 2181, aged 18–45 years). In the German population, Perkonigg *et al.* (2000) found low rates of full PTSD (1% in males and 2.2% in females), although 26% of male subjects and 17.7% of female subjects reported at least one traumatic event. However, the rate of traumatic events obtained in the US population was higher, i.e. 89.6%, and the conditional probability for PTSD after experiencing traumas was 9.2%, with approximately a two-fold higher risk in women than in men (Breslau *et al.*, 1999).

CONCLUSION

Several epidemiologic studies have been conducted in the community during the past two decades in order to determine the prevalence and risk factors of affective and anxiety disorders. These studies have used the most recent methodological advances in the field for the definition of cases, namely reference to recent mental disorders classifications and, more importantly, the use of diagnostic criteria and structured diagnostic interviews. In such a framework, cross-cultural comparisons from one country to another can be allowed and have shown some consistencies as regards risk factors, but they have also underlined differences in prevalence rates, mostly for phobic disorders. Affective and anxiety disorders are frequent in the population; female sex, younger age and marital status have been consistently found to be risk factors for these disorders. A high lifetime comorbidity pattern has also been reported in these studies. Impairment associated with these disorders has a major impact in terms of public health.

New perspectives are offered in epidemiologic research. As previously mentioned, cross-cultural comparisons have stressed the consequences of methodological differences in the assessment procedures and study design. In terms of the need for treatment, more precise measurement of impairment and disability associated with specific disorders will play a crucial role (Regier *et al.*, 1998). Most of the studies reviewed in this chapter are cross-sectional and rely mainly on retrospective reports, although some prospective studies have been conducted or are ongoing. These studies are more suited to addressing some unresolved issues concerning, for example, the time sequence of disorders and the developmental risk factors. Finally, recent refinements in biological and genetic sampling will permit the testing of new hypotheses in epidemiologic studies in order to understand better the complex interactions between biological and psychosocial factors.

REFERENCES

Andrews G, Sanderson K, Slade T *et al.* (2000) Why does the burden of disease persist? Relating the burden of anxiety and depression to effectiveness of treatment. *Bull World Health Organ,* **78**, 446–454.

Angst J (1993) Comorbidity of anxiety, compulsions and depression. *Int Clin Psychopharmacol,* **8**, 21–25.

Angst J, Dobler-Mikola A (1984) The Zurich study: III. Diagnosis of depression. *Eur Arch Psychiatry Clin Neurosci,* **234**, 30–37.

Angst J, Dobler-Mikola A (1985) The Zurich study. V. Anxiety and phobia in young adults. *Eur Arch Psychiatry Clin Neurosci,* **235**, 171–178.

Angst J, Hochstrasser B (1994) Recurrent brief depression: the Zurich study. *J Clin Psychiatry*, **55** (4, suppl), 3–9.

Aoki Y, Fujihara S, Kitamura T (1994) Panic attacks and panic disorder in a Japanese non-patient population: epidemiology and psychosocial correlates. *J Affect Dis*, **32**, 51–59.

Battaglia M, Bertella S, Politi E, Bernardeschi L, Perna G, Gabriele A, Bellodi L (1995) Age at onset of panic disorder: influence of familial liability to the disease and of childhood. *Am J Psychiatry*, **152**, 1362–1364.

Bland RC, Orn H, Newman SC (1988) Lifetime prevalence of psychiatric disorders in Edmonton. *Acta Psychiatr Scand*, **77**(suppl 338), 24–32.

Breslau N, Davis GC, Andreski P, Peterson EL (1991) Traumatic events and posttraumatic stress disorder in an urban population of young adults. *Arch Gen Psychiat*, **48**, 216–222.

Breslau N, Davis GC, Andreski P, Peterson EL, Schultz LR (1997) Sex differences in post-traumatic stress disorder. *Arch Gen Psychiat*, **54**, 1044–1048.

Breslau N, Chilcoat HD, Kessler RC, Peterson EL, Lucia VC (1999) Vulnerability to assaultive violence: further specification of the sex difference in post-traumatic stress disorder. *Psychol Med*, **29**, 813–821.

Brown GW, Harris TO (1993) Aetiology of anxiety and depressive disorders in inner-city population. 1. Early adversity. *Psychol Med*, **213**, 143–154.

Burke KC, Burke JD, Regier DA, Rae DS (1990) Age at onset of selected mental disorders in five community populations. *Arch Gen Psychiat*, **47**, 511–518.

Canino GJ, Bird HR, Shrout PE, Rubio-Stipec M, Bravo M, Martinez R, Sesman M, Guevara LM (1987) The prevalence of specific psychiatric disorders in Puerto Rico. *Arch Gen Psychiat*, **44**, 727–735.

Carter RM, Wittchen H-U, Pfister H, Kessler RC (in press) One-year prevalence of subthreshold and threshold DSM-IV generalized anxiety disorder in a nationally representative sample. *Depression Anxiety*.

Chen YW, Dilsaver SC (1995) Comorbidity of panic disorder in bipolar illness: evidence from the epidemiologic catchment area survey. *Am J Psychiat*, **152**, 280–282.

Chignon JM, Lepine JP, Ades J (1993) Panic disorder in cardiac outpatients. *Am J Psychiat*, **150**, 780–785.

Cross-National Collaborative Group (1992) The changing rates of major depression. Cross-national comparisons. *JAMA*, **268**, 3098–3105.

David D, Giron A, Mellman JA (1995) Panic-phobic patients and developmental trauma. *J Clin Psychiat*, **56**, 113–117.

Davidson JRT, Hughes DL, Blazer DG, George LK (1991) Post-traumatic stress disorder in the community: an epidemiological study. *Psychol Med*, **21**, 713–721.

Davidson JRT, Hughes DL, George LK, Blazer DG (1993) The epidemiology of social phobia: findings from the Duke Epidemiologic Catchment Area Study. *Psychol Med*, **23**, 709–718.

Degonda M, Angst J (1993) The Zurich Study: XX. Social phobia and agoraphobia. *Eur Arch Psychiat Clin Neurosci*, **243**, 95–102.

Dumas CA, Katerndahl DA, Burge SK (1995) Familial patterns in patients with infrequent panic attacks. *Arch Fam Med*, **4**, 863–867.

Eaton WW, Drymon A, Weissman MM (1991) Panic and phobias. In: LN Robins, DA Regier (eds) *Psychiatric disorders in America: The Epidemiologic Catchment Area Study*. New York: Free Press, 155–179.

Eaton WW, Kessler RC, Wittchen HU, Magee WJ (1994) Panic and panic disorder in the United States. *Am J Psychiat*, **151**, 413–420.

Faravelli C, Degl'Innocenti BG, Aiazzi L, Incerpi G, Pallanti S (1989) Epidemiology of anxiety disorder in Florence. *J Affect Dis*, **19**, 1–5.

Faravelli C, Degl'Innocenti BG, Aiazzi L, Incerpi G, Pallanti S (1990) Epidemiology of mood disorders: a community survey in Florence. *J Affect Dis*, **20**, 135–141.

Faravelli C, Zucchi T, Viviani B, Salmoria R, Perone A, Paionni A, Scarpato A, Vigliaturo D, Rosi S, D'adamo D, Bartolozzi D, Cecchi C, Abrardi L (2000) Epidemiology of social phobia: a clinical approach. *Eur Psychiatry*, **15**, 17–24.

Flint AJ (1994) Epidemiology and comorbidity of anxiety disorders in the elderly. *Am J Psychiatry*, **151**, 640–649.

Goisman RM, Warshaw MG, Peterson LG, Rogers MP, Cuneo P, Hunt MF, Tomlin-Albanese JM, Kazim A, Golan JK, Epstein-Kaye T, Reich JH, Keller M (1994) Panic, agoraphobia and panic disorder with agoraphobia data from a multicenter anxiety disorders study. *J Nerv Ment Dis*, **182**, 72–79.

Goldberg DP, Lecrubier Y. (1995) Form and frequency of mental disorders across centres. In: Üstün TB, Sartorius N, eds, *Mental Illness in General Health Care: An International Study*. Chichester: John Wiley, 323–334.

Heimberg RG, Stein MB, Hiripi E, Kessler RC (2000) Trends in the prevalence of social phobia in the United States: a systematic cohort analysis of changes over four decades. *Eur Psychiatry*, **15**, 29–37.

Helzer JE, Robins LN, McEroy L (1987) Post-traumatic stress disorder in the general population. *N Engl J Med*, **317**, 1630–1634.

Horwath E Weissman MM (1995) Epidemiology of depression and anxiety disorders. In: MT Tsuang, M Tohen, GEP Zahner (eds) *Textbook of Psychiatric Epidemiology*. New York: Wiley-Liss, 317–344.

Hwu HG, Yeh EK, Chang LY (1989) Prevalence of psychiatric disorders in Taiwan defined by the Chinese Diagnostic Interview Schedule. *Acta Psychiat Scand*, **79**, 136–147.

Johnson J, Weissman MM, Klerman GL (1990) Panic disorder, comorbidity, and suicide attempts. *Arch Gen Psychiat*, **47**, 805–808.

Joyce PR, Bushnell JA, Oakley-Browne MA, Wells JE, Hornblow AR (1989) The epidemiology of panic symptomatology and agoraphobic avoidance. *Compr Psychiat*, **30**, 303–312.

Joyce PR, Oakley-Browne MA, Wells JE, Bushnell JA, Hornblow AR (1990) Birth cohort trends in major depression: increasing rates and earlier onset in New Zealand. *J Affect Dis*, **18**, 83–90.

Karam E (1992) Dépression et guerres du Liban: méthodologie d'une recherche. *Ann Psychol Sci Educ*, Univ St Joseph (Beyrouth), 99–106.

Kaaterndahl DA, Realini JP (1993) Lifetime prevalence of panic states. *Am J Psychiat*, **150**, 246–249.

Kessler RC, McGonagle KA, Swartz M, Blazer DG, Nelson CB (1993) Sex and depression in the National Comorbidity Survey. I: lifetime prevalence, chronicity and recurrence. *J Affect Dis*, **29**, 85–96.

Kessler RC, McGonagle KA, Zhao S, Nelson CB, Hughes M, Eshleman S, Wittchen HU, Kendler KS (1994) Lifetime and 12-month prevalence of DSM-III-R psychiatric disorders in the United States. Results from the National Comorbidity Survey. *Arch Gen Psychiat*, **51**, 8–19.

Kessler RC, Sonnega A, Bromet E, Hughes M, Nelson CB (1995) Posttraumatic stress disorder in the National Comorbidity Survey. *Arch Gen Psychiat*, **52**, 1048–1060.

Kessler RC, Nelson CB, McGonagle KA, Liu J, Swartz M, Blazer DG (1996) Comorbidity of DSM-III-R major depressive disorder in the general population: results from the US National Comorbidity Survey. *Br J Psychiat*, **168**(suppl 30), 17–30.

Kessler RC, Stang P, Wittchen HU, Stein M, Walters EE (1999) Lifetime co-morbidities between social phobia and mood disorders in the US National Comorbidity Survey. *Psychol Med*, **29**, 555–567.

Klerman GL, Weissman MM (1989) Increasing rates of depression. *JAMA*, **261**, 2229–2235.

Kluznik JC, Speed N, Van Valkenburg C, Magraw R (1986) Forty-year follow-up of United States prisoners of war. *Am J Psychiat*, **143**, 1443–1446.

✱Knauper B, Wittchen HU (1994) Diagnosing major depression in the elderly: evidence for response bias in standardized diagnostic interviews. *J Psychiat Res*, **28**, 147–164.

Kuch K, Cox BJ (1992) Symptoms of PTSD in 124 survivors of the Holocaust. *Am J Psychiat*, **149**, 337–340.

Lecrubier Y (1997) A worldwide primary care perspective. Paper presented at the 6th World Congress of Biological Psychiatry, Nice, France, June 22–27.

Lecrubier Y, Wittchen HU, Faravelli C, Bobes J, Patel A, Knapp M (2000) A European perspective on social anxiety disorder. *Eur Psychiatry*, **15**, 5–16.

Lee CK, Kwak YS, Yamamoto J, Rhee H, Kim YS, Han JH, Choi JO, Lee YH (1990) Psychiatric epidemiology in Korea. Part I: Gender and age differences in Seoul. *J Nerv Ment Dis*, **178**, 242–246.

Lépine, JP, Lellouch J (1994) Classification and epidemiology of anxiety disorders. In: G Darcourt, J Mendlewicz, G Racagni, N Brunello (eds) *Current therapeutic approaches to panic and other anxiety disorders. Int Acad Biomed Drug Res*, **8**, 1–14. Basel: Karger.

Lépine JP, Lellouch J (1995) Diagnosis and epidemiology of agoraphobia and social phobia. *Clin Neuropharmacol*, **18**(suppl 2), S15–S26.

Lépine JP, Pelissolo A (1996) Comorbidity of social phobia: clinical and epidemiological issues. *Int Clin Psychopharmacol*, **11**(suppl 3), 35–41.

Lépine JP, Pélissolo A (1999) Epidemiology and comorbidity of social anxiety disorder. In: *Social anxiety disorders*. In: Westenberg HGM, den Boer JA (eds) Syn-Thesis, Amsterdam, 29–45.

Lépine JP, Wittchen HU, Essau CA (1993a) Lifetime and current comorbidity of anxiety and affective disorders: results from the international WHO/ADAMHA CIDI field trials. *Int J Methods Psychiat Res*, **3**, 67–77.

✱ Lépine JP, Chignon JM, Teherani M (1993b) Suicide attempts in patients with panic disorder. *Arch Gen Psychiat*, **50**, 144–149.

Lépine JP, Lellouch J, Lovell A, Teherani M, Pariente P (1993c) L'épidémiologie des troubles anxieux et dépressifs dans une population générale française. *Confront Psychiat*, **35**, 139–161.

Lépine JP, Gastpar M, Mendlewicz J, Tylee A, on behalf of the DEPRES Steering Committee (1997) Depression in the community: the first pan-European study, DEPRES (Depression Research in European Society). *Int Clin Psychopharmacol*, **12**, 19–29.

Liebowitz MR, Gorman JM, Fyer AJ, Klein DF (1985) Social phobia. Review of a neglected anxiety disorder. *Arch Gen Psychiat*, **42**, 729–736.

Lindal E, Stefansson JG (1993) The lifetime prevalence of anxiety disorders in Iceland as estimated by the US National Institute of Mental Health Diagnostic Interview Schedule. *Acta Psychiat Scand*, **88**, 29–34.

Maier W, Gaensicke M, Freyberger HJ, Linz M, Heun R, Lecrubier Y. (2000) Generalized anxiety disorder (ICD-10) in primary care from a cross-cultural perspective: a valid diagnostic entity? *Acta Psychiatr Scand*, **101**, 29–36.

Magee WJ, Eaton WW, Wittchen HU, McGonagle KA, Kessler RC (1996) Agoraphobia, simple phobia, and social phobia in the National Comorbidity Survey. *Arch Gen Psychiat*, **53**, 159–168.

✱ Montgomery SA, Montgomery D, Baldwin D, Green M (1990) The duration, nature, and recurrence rate of brief depressions. *Prog Neuropsychopharmacol Biol Psychiat*, **14**, 729–735.

Pélissolo A, André C, Moutard-Martin F, Wittchen HU, Lépine JP (2000) Social phobia in the community: relationship between diagnostic threshold and prevalence. *Eur Psychiat*, **15**, 25–28.

Perkonigg A, Kessler RC, Storz S, Wittchen HU (2000) Traumatic events and post-traumatic stress disorder in the community: prevalence, risk factors and comorbidity. *Acta Psychiatr Scand*, **101**, 46–59.

Regier DA, Boyd JH, Burk JD Jr, Rae DS, Myers JK, Kramer M, Robins LN, George LK, Karno M, Locke BZ (1988) One-month prevalence of mental disorders in the United States: based on five Epidemiological Catchment Area sites. *Arch Gen Psychiat*, **45**, 977–986.

✳Regier DA, Farmer ME, Rae DS, Locke BZ, Keith SJ, Judd LL, Goodwin FK (1990) Comorbidity of mental disorders with alcohol and other drug abuse: results from the Epidemiologic Catchment Area (ECA) study. *JAMA*, **264**, 2511–2518.

Regier DA, Farmer ME, Rae DS, Myers JK, Kramer M, Robins LN, George LK, Kamo M, Locke BZ (1993) One-month prevalence of mental disorders in the United States and socio-demographic characteristics: the Epidemiological Catchment Area study. *Acta Psychiat Scand*, **88**, 35–47.

✳Regier DA, Kaelber CT, Rae DS, Farmer ME, Knauper B, Kessler RC, Norquist GS (1998) Limitations of diagnostic criteria and assessment instruments for mental disorders. *Arch Gen Psychiat*, **55**, 109–115.

Reich J, Goldenberg I, Vasile R, Goisman R, Keller M (1994) A prospective, follow-along study of the course of social phobia. *Psychiatry Res*, **54**, 249–258.

Robins LN, Regier DA (eds) (1981) *Psychiatric disorders in America: the Epidemiologic Catchment Area study*. New York: Free Press.

Sartorius N, Üstün B, Costa e Silva JA, Goldberg D, Lecrubier Y, Ormel J, Von Korff M, Wittchen HU (1993) An international study of psychological problems in primary care. *Arch Gen Psychiat*, **50**, 819–824.

Schneier FR, Johnson J, Hornig CD, Liebowitz MR, Weissman MM (1992) Social phobia. Comorbidity and morbidity in an epidemiological sample. *Arch Gen Psychiat*, **49**, 282–288.

Servant D, Parquet PJ (1995) Early life events and panic disorder: course of illness and comorbidity. *Prog Neuropsychopharmacol Biol Psychiat*, **18**, 373–379.

Silove D, Manicavasagar V, Curtis J, Blaszczynski A (1996) Is early separation anxiety a risk factor for adult panic disorder? a critical review. *Compr Psychiat*, **37**, 167–179.

✳Simpson HB, Nee JC, Endicott J (1997) First-episode major depression. Few sex differences in course. *Arch Gen Psychiat*, **54**, 633–639.

✳Stein MB, Walker JR, Anderson G, Hazen AL, Ross CA, Elridge G, Forde DR (1996) Childhood physical and sexual abuse in patients with anxiety disorders and in a community sample. *Am J Psychiat*, **153**, 275–277.

Stein MB, Torgrud LJ, Walker JR (2000) Social phobia symptoms, subtypes, and severity: findings from a community survey. *Arch Gen Psychiatry*, **57**, 1046–1052.

Stein MB, Walker JR, Hazen AL, Forde DR (1997) Full and partial Posttraumatic Stress Disorder: finding from a community survey. *Am J Psychiatry*, **154**, 1114–1119.

Speed N, Engdahl B, Schwartz J, Eberly R (1989) Posttraumatic stress disorder as a consequence of the POW experience. *J Nervs Ment Dis*, **177**, 147–153.

Tylee A, Gastpar M, Lepine JP, Mendlewicz J (1999a) DEPRES II (Depression Research in European Society II): a patient survey of the symptoms, disability and current management of depression in the community. DEPRES Steering Committee. *Int Clin Psychopharmacol*, **14**, 139–151.

Tylee A, Gastpar M, Lepine JP, Mendlewicz J (1999b) Identification of depressed patient types in the community and their treatment needs: findings from the DEPRES II (Depression Research in European Society II) survey. DEPRES Steering Committee. *Int Clin Psychopharmacol*, **14**, 153–165.

Üstün TB, Sartorius N (1995) *Mental Illness in General Health Care: An International Study*. Chichester: Wiley.

Von Korff MR, Eaton WW, Keyl PM (1985) The epidemiology of panic attacks and panic disorder: results of three community surveys. *Am J Epidemiol*, **122**, 970–981.

Wacker HR, Mullejans R, Klein KH, Battegay R (1992) Identification of cases of anxiety disorders and affective disorders in the community according to ICD-10 and DSM-III-R by using the Composite International Diagnostic Interview (CIDI). *Int J Methods Psychiat Res*, **2**, 91–100.

Weiller E, Boyer P, Lepine JP, Lecrubier Y (1994) Prevalence of recurrent brief depression in primary care. *Eur Arch Psychiat Clin Neurosci*, **244**, 174–181.

Weiller E, Bisserbe JC, Boyer P, Lepine JP, Lecrubier Y (1996) Social phobia in general health care: an unrecognised undertreated disabling disorder. *Br J Psychiat*, **168**, 169–174.

Weissman MM, Klerman GL (1985) Gender and depression. *Trends Neurosci*, **8**, 416–420.

Weissman MM, Leaf P, Blazer DG, Boyd JH, Florio L (1986) Panic disorder: clinical characteristics, epidemiology, and treatment. *Psychopharmacol Bull*, **22**, 787–791.

Weissman MM, Leaf PJ, Bruce ML, Florio L (1988a) The epidemiology of dysthymia in five communities: rates, risks, comorbidity and treatment. *Am J Psychiat*, **145**, 815–819.

Weissman MM, Leaf P, Tischler GL, Blazer DG, Karno M, Livingston Bruce M, Florio L (1988b) Affective disorders in five United States communities. *Psychol Med*, **18**, 141–153.

Weissman MM, Klerman GL, Markowitz JS, Ouelette R (1989) Suicidal ideation and suicide attempts in panic disorder and attacks. *N Engl J Med*, **321**, 1209–1241.

Weismann MM (1994) Panic disorder: epidemiology and genetics. In: BE Wolfe, JD Maser (eds) *Treatment of Panic Disorder. A Consensus Development Conference*. Washington, DC: American Psychiatric Press, 31–39.

Weissman MM, Bland RC, Canino G], Faravelli C, Greenwald S, Hwu HG, Joyce PR, Karam EG, Lee CK, Lellouch J, Lepine JP, Newman SC, Rubio-Stipec M, Wells JE, Wickramaratne PJ, Wittchen HU, Yeh EK (1996) Cross-national epidemiology of major depression and bipolar disorder. *JAMA*, **276**, 293–299.

Weissman MM, Bland RC, Canino GJ, Faravelli C, Greenwald S, Hwu HG, Joyce PR, Karam EG, Lee CK, Lellouch J, Lepine JP, Newman SC, Oakley-Brown MA, Rubio-Stipec M, Wells JE, Wickramaratne PJ, Wittchen HU, Yeh EK (1997) The cross-national epidemiology of panic disorder. *Arch Gen Psychiat*, **54**, 305–309.

Wells JE, Bushnell JA, Hornblow AR, Joyce PR, Oakley-Browne MA (1989) Christchurch psychiatric epidemiology study. I: Methodology and lifetime prevalence for specific psychiatric disorders. *Aust NZ J Psychiat*, **23**, 315–326.

Wittchen HU (1986) Natural course and spontaneous remissions of untreated anxiety disorders: results of the Munich Follow-up Study (MFS). *Panics and Phobias*, vol 2. Berlin: Springer-Verlag.

Wittchen HU, Essau CA (1993) Epidemiology of panic disorders: progress and unresolved issues. *J Psychiat Res*, **27**(suppl.1), 47–68.

Wittchen HU, Essau CA, von Zerssen D, Krieg JC, Zaudig M (1992) Lifetime and six-month prevalence of mental disorders in the Munich follow-up study. *Eur Arch Psychiat Clin Neurosci*, **241**, 247–258.

Wittchen HU, Zhao S, Kessler RC, Eaton WW (1994) DSM-III-R generalized anxiety disorder in the National Comorbidity Survey. *Arch Gen Psychiat*, **51**, 355–364.

Wittchen HU, Stein M, Kessler RC (1999) Social fears and social phobia in a community sample of adolescents and young adults: prevalence, risk factors and co-morbidity. *Psychol Med*, **29**, 309–323.

Wittchen HU, Nelson CB, Lachner G (1998) Prevalence of mental disorders and psychosocial impairments in adolescents and young adults. *Psychol Ed*, **28**, 109–126.

2

Biological aspects of anxiety disorders and depression

J.A. den Boer, B.R. Slaap and F.J. Bosker

INTRODUCTION

The degree to which the underlying brain mechanisms in anxiety and depression differ or overlap remains unknown. Anxiety and depression are complex emotions involving subjective, affective, physiological and neuroendocrine responses, as well as cognitive evaluations. The variety of response systems indicates that multiple brain mechanisms are involved. During the past 10 years our knowledge of the brain has expanded enormously. Different research strategies have been employed in an attempt to elucidate underlying pathogenetic mechanisms, including pharmacological challenge studies, studies of monoamine-metabolite concentrations in cerebrospinal fluid (CSF) as well as neuroimaging studies using a variety of techniques. Interestingly both pharmacological challenge studies and neuroimaging studies suggest that certain neurotransmitter systems and receptor subtypes as well as brain regions may be intimately involved in both anxiety disorders and depression. The fact, however, that to some extent the same neurotransmitter systems are involved in anxiety and depression does not mean that the mechanisms underlying these disorders are identical. The effects of neurotransmitter systems may vary according to their location in the brain and do not act in isolation. A multitude of influences maintain (and may threaten) the integrity and proper functioning of neurotransmitter systems; to mention a few, neuroendocrine and immunological factors all

SSRIs in Depression and Anxiety, Second Edition. Edited by S.A. Montgomery and J.A. den Boer.
© 2001 John Wiley & Sons Ltd.

influence the function of these systems in concert with a variety of environmental influences.

MONOAMINE FUNCTION IN DEPRESSION AND ANXIETY

Monoamine hypothesis

During the past 30 years the monoamine hypothesis of depression has taken on several forms. Since early studies indicated that depletion of the monoamines noradrenaline (NA) and serotonin (5-HT) by reserpine led to depression, the theory was advanced that reduced availability of monoamine neurotransmitters could play a role in the pathogenesis of depression (Schildkraut et al., 1977). In addition, based upon increasing knowledge of the working mechanism of antidepressants, the hypothesis was put forward that alterations in NA receptor functioning were involved. It has been suggested that enhanced sensitivity of presynaptic α_2- and postsynaptic β-adrenoceptors, and reduced sensitivity of postsynaptic α_2-adrenoceptors are possibly related to the pathophysiology of depression (Garcia-Sevilla et al., 1966; Mann et al., 1986). Preclinical research also indicated that 5-HT$_2$ binding sites can be down-regulated by several antidepressant treatments. These findings have led to the hypothesis that the action of antidepressant treatment depends on the down-regulation of β-adrenoceptors or 5-HT$_2$ receptors, and that enhanced sensitivity of these receptors is involved in the pathogenesis of depression.

More recently the role of monoamines in depression was further studied by using 5-HT and NA depletion paradigms. It was found that tryptophan depletion does not lead to depressive symptoms in healthy controls, but patients who experience remission on 5-HT reuptake inhibitors show a relapse of depressive symptoms after tryptophan depletion (Delgado et al., 1994). These findings indicate that 5-HT is somehow necessary for the maintenance of the antidepressant response.

Noradrenergic function in depression

A comprehensive review of all studies on NA function in depression is beyond the scope of this chapter; appropriate reviews have recently been published (e.g. Charney et al., 1994). Here we will review some recent work performed with α-methyl-p-tyrosine (αMPT) in depressed patients. αMPT is an inhibitor of tyrosine hydroxylase, the rate-limiting enzyme in the synthesis of dopamine (DA) and NA, thus leading to decreased levels of both DA and NA. Administration to healthy volunteers has been shown to lead to increased drowsiness, increases in negative mood and mild anxiety (McCann et al., 1995).

In depressed patients treated with antidepressants such as desipramine, αMPT administration led to rapid increases in depression scores, whereas αMPT administration was ineffective in patients treated with selective serotonin reuptake inhibitors (SSRIs) (Delgado *et al.*, 1993). Miller *et al.* (1996) administered αMPT to drug-free depressed patients in a double-blind cross-over design. Similar to other studies, αMPT reduced plasma homovanillic acid (HVA) by 70% and 3-methoxy-4-hydroxy-phenylethyleneglycol (MHPG) by 50%. In this study, no effects on mood were observed, indicating that catecholamine deficiency is not a sufficient explanation for the underlying neurobiological mechanisms in the pathogenesis of depression (Duman *et al.*, 1997).

Noradrenergic function in panic disorder

Challenge studies in panic disorder: α-adrenoceptors

Pharmacological challenge studies have attempted to shed light on adrenoceptor functioning in panic disorder (PD). Several studies have evaluated central α_2-adrenoceptor functioning in PD with the α_2-adrenoceptor antagonist yohimbine. A subgroup of PD patients (63%) experienced increased anxiety and panic symptoms in response to oral (Charney and Heninger, 1985; Charney *et al.*, 1987a) or intravenous (Charney *et al.*, 1992) administration of yohimbine, together with elevated plasma MHPG and cortisol levels, increased blood pressure and heart rate.

Another pharmacological probe of NA function in PD is the α_2-adrenoceptor agonist clonidine. Clonidine administration caused greater hypotension, greater decreases in plasma MHPG levels, and less sedation in panic patients than in controls (Charney and Heninger, 1986). These findings have also been consistently replicated (Nutt, 1989; Coplan *et al.*, 1992; Charney *et al.*, 1992).

The experiments with yohimbine and clonidine suggest that presynaptic α_2-adrenoceptor sensitivity is increased in PD. In addition, the growth hormone (GH) response to clonidine has been found to be blunted in PD patients, as compared to controls (Uhde *et al.*, 1986; Charney and Heninger, 1986; Nutt, 1989), suggesting subsensitivity of central postsynaptic α_2-adrenoceptors in PD. The GH finding is not specific for PD and has also been reported in depression and generalized anxiety disorder (Abelson *et al.*, 1991). On the other hand, it is also possible that processes beyond the α_2-adrenoceptor are dysregulated, such as intracellular second and third messenger systems linked to this receptor. Alternatively, there could be a dysregulation of non-NA neurotransmitter systems with significant input to the locus coeruleus (Redmond, 1987).

In conclusion, panic patients consistently show abnormal responses to α_2-adrenoceptor agonists and antagonists.

Challenge studies in panic disorder: β-adrenoceptors

Infusion of isoproterenol, a peripherally acting selective β-adrenoceptor agonist, has been reported to trigger anxiety responses in panic patients compared to controls

(Rainey et al., 1984; Pohl et al., 1985, 1988). Successful treatment with tricyclic antidepressants blunted isoproterenol-induced anxiety and systolic blood pressure responses (Pohl et al., 1990). These studies are consistent with the hypothesis of increased β_1-adrenoceptor sensitivity in PD, which is normalized by effective pharmacotherapy. However, Nesse et al. (1984) observed no differences between drug-free panic patients and controls in behavioural responses to intravenous isoproterenol. The mechanism of isoproterenol-induced panic remains to be clarified by future research.

Platelet studies in panic disorder: α-adrenoceptors

Clinical studies comparing PD patients to healthy control subjects have reported abnormalities in the α_2-adrenoceptor in PD patients. For example, Cameron et al. (1984, 1990) have observed a reduction in the density (B_{max}) of platelet α_2-adrenoceptors in PD patients. However, these changes have not been replicated in other studies (Nutt and Fraser, 1987; Norman et al., 1987; Charney et al., 1989a), indicating that peripheral indices of NA function are not consistently abnormal in PD.

Critique of the noradrenaline hypothesis of panic disorder

Several clinical findings are not in accordance with the NA hypothesis of PD. For example, sodium lactate did not alter plasma MHPG levels, a putative measure for central noradrenergic activity (Carr et al., 1986; den Boer et al., 1989) and clonidine was not able to block lactate-induced panic (Coplan et al., 1992). Moreover, at variance with the NA hypothesis, phobic exposure of panic patients did not significantly alter plasma MHPG (Woods et al., 1987). On the other hand, it should be emphasized that plasma MHPG may not be an accurate and sensitive measure of central noradrenergic activity. In addition, about one-third of the PD patients appeared insensitive to the yohimbine test. Yohimbine-induced panic, however, is relatively specific for PD (Charney et al., 1984; Glazer et al., 1987; Heninger et al., 1988; Rasmussen et al., 1987; Charney et al., 1989b), although a recent study has demonstrated that patients with post-traumatic stress disorder may also experience yohimbine-induced panic attacks (Southwick et al., 1993).

Chronic treatment with the antipanic agent imipramine, which significantly decreases noradrenergic function, was unable to block yohimbine-induced panic in 11 patients (Charney and Heninger, 1985). Finally, the clinical response of PD to a variety of pharmacotherapeutic agents, including benzodiazepines (Ballenger et al., 1988), tricyclics (Zitrin et al., 1983), monoamine oxidase inhibitors (Tyrer et al., 1973), SSRIs (Beaumont, 1977; den Boer et al., 1987; den Boer and Westenberg, 1990a,b; Evans et al., 1986), and cognitive-behavioural treatments (Barlow, 1988), suggests the involvement of other neurotransmitter systems in PD.

Noradrenergic function in obsessive-compulsive disorder

Challenge studies in obsessive-compulsive disorder: α-adrenoceptors

In other anxiety disorders such as PD, there is circumstantial evidence for an involvement of the noradrenergic system. To a large extent this is based on experiments with the α_2-adrenoceptor antagonist yohimbine, which enhances noradrenergic function by increasing the availability of noradrenaline in the synaptic cleft (for a review, see Charney *et al.*, 1994).

Challenging obsessive-compulsive disorder (OCD) patients with yohimbine led to increases in anxiety similar to those in healthy volunteers, yet no increases in obsessions or compulsive behaviours were reported in the OCD patients (Rasmussen *et al.*, 1987; Table 2.1).

Experiments with the α_2-adrenoceptor agonist clonidine, which decreases noradrenergic functioning, yielded equivocal results. One study reported a blunted growth hormone (GH) response to a clonidine challenge (Siever *et al.*, 1983), but another study failed to replicate these findings (Hollander *et al.*, 1991a). GH is used as a neuroendocrine marker since stimulation of α_2-adrenoceptors increases GH secretion from the pituitary.

The α_2-adrenoceptor agonist clonidine was without behavioural effects when administered to OCD patients. The effects of clonidine on plasma MHPG levels were similar in OCD patients and control subjects, indicating that the noradrenergic neuronal system is not abnormal in OCD (Lee *et al.*, 1990; Hollander *et al.*, 1991b).

In a study in which the GH response to the specific NA reuptake inhibitor desipramine was examined in OCD patients and control subjects, no differences were found in GH secretion between the two groups, suggesting that α_2-noradrenergic responsivity is normal in OCD (Lucey *et al.*, 1992a).

In sum, most studies do not support abnormalities in noradrenergic function in OCD.

Noradrenergic and dopaminergic function in social phobia

Challenge studies in social phobia: α-adrenoceptors and D2-dopamine receptors

Fear response with social phobia provokes symptoms which may be adrenergically mediated (e.g. sweating, palpitations, tremor). The function of the noradrenergic and dopaminergic nervous systems can be assessed in social phobics with specific pharmacological probes: clonidine for the former, and levodopa for the latter system. The response to clonidine is measured by its effect on GH release, and that to levodopa by its effect on plasma prolactin levels and eyeblink rate. Patients with social phobia, as well as those with panic disorder, appeared to have a blunted GH response to clonidine, indicating a disturbance of noradrenergic function; however,

Table 2.1. Noradrenergic challenge in obsessive-compulsive disorder.

Author	Substance	Patients N (Dep: N)	Design	Behavioural response		Compared to controls	
				OC symptoms	Other	Cortisol	Prolactin
Rasmussen et al., 1987	Yohimbine orally 20 mg	12(5)	Single-blind	=	—	↑(>C)	MHPG ↑ (= C)
Lee et al., 1990	Clonidine i.v. 2 μg/kg	10(0)	Single-blind placebo	=	sedation	—	GH ↑ (= C)MHPG =
Hollander et al., 1991a	Clonidine i.v. 2 μg/kg	18(0)	Double-blind	↓	sedation	=	GH ↑ (= C)MHPG =
Lucey et al., 1992a	Desipramine orally 1 mg/kg	10(0)	Open	—	—	—	GH ↑ (= C)

C = healthy controls; Dep = major depression; MHPG = 3-methoxy-4-hydroxyphenylethylenglycol; GH = growth hormone.

the results require replication (Schneier *et al.*, 1993). The prolactin/eyeblink rate response to levodopa was unchanged in social phobics compared to normal subjects, suggesting that there is no dopaminergic abnormality in social phobia (Schneier *et al.*, 1993).

Serotonin function in depression and anxiety

Several paradigms have been used to study serotonin (dys-)function in depression and anxiety. The use of serotoninomimetics in combination with the so-called neuroendocrine strategy seems most promising, but blood-platelet and CSF studies may also have their merit. The different paradigms will be outlined and discussed in the following sections. In addition, the involvement of serotonin receptor subtypes in the pathophysiology and treatment of depression and anxiety disorders will be discussed. Special attention will be paid to augmentation strategies with pindolol and its relation with Blier's desensitization hypothesis (Blier *et al.*, 1987).

A general remark on challenge studies

To elucidate the role of 5-HT, several investigators have used behavioural and neuroendocrine probes to evaluate 5-HT functions *in vivo*. This paradigm involves the administration of direct or indirect acting 5-HT agonists and the measurement of a function allegedly under 5-HT-ergic control. The pituitary–adrenal (e.g. the release of cortisol, prolactin and β-endorphin) response to 5-HT agonists is commonly used as a marker to assess the functional state of the 5-HT system in humans. This strategy promises to become increasingly useful as more selective drugs become available for clinical use. Other responses, besides the hormonal response, include body temperature and behaviour. Measurement of the hormonal, physiological or behavioural effects following administration of 5-HT-selective drugs permits an assessment of the responsivity of the central 5-HT system involved in the effects under investigation. There is extensive pharmacological and neuroanatomical evidence that 5-HT-containing neurones regulate the hypothalamo–pituitary–adrenal (HPA) axis in rats (Fuller, 1990).

5-HT-containing nerve terminals make synaptic contacts with the corticotrophin-releasing hormone (CRH)-containing cells in the hypothalamus, and direct and indirect 5-HT agonists all increase adrenocorticotrophic hormone (ACTH), β-endorphin and cortisol release. Another pituitary hormone that is regulated, in part, through 5-HT neurones is prolactin. There is circumstantial evidence that drugs that increase 5-HT function increase prolactin secretion as well.

Probes of 5-HT function are usually divided in those that increase brain 5-HT function (e.g. fenfluramine and 5-HT precursors like tryptophan and 5-hydroxy-tryptophan) and those that act directly on 5-HT receptors (e.g. *m*-chlorophenylpiper-azine, 5-HT_{1A} agonists).

Serotonin precursors in depression

Several studies have shown a blunted prolactin and GH response to intravenous administration of tryptophan in depression (Power and Cowen, 1992). Since the prolactin and GH responses to tryptophan can be attenuated by the 5-HT$_{1A}$ antagonist pindolol, it was hypothesized that the prolactin and GH responses to tryptophan are mediated through the postsynaptic 5-HT$_{1A}$ receptor. Thus, the endocrine abnormalities observed after tryptophan administration in depression could be indicative of a dysfunction at the level of this receptor subtype. Findings using 5-hydroxytryptophan (5-HTP) as a challenge in depressed patients are inconsistent, but in two studies increased plasma cortisol levels have been reported (for review, see Power and Cowen, 1992). In view of the fact that cortisol release is probably mediated by 5-HT$_2$ receptors, these findings may indicate the upregulation of postsynaptic 5-HT$_2$ receptors in depression (Meltzer and Maes, 1994).

Preliminary evidence suggests that 5-HTP-induced cortisol and prolactin responses in patients with either depression or OCD are not different during treatment with fluoxetine (Meltzer *et al.*, 1997).

Fenfluramine in depression

Fenfluramine has both 5-HT releasing and reuptake inhibiting properties. The 5-HT$_2$ receptor antagonist ritanserin (but not pindolol) has been shown to block the prolactin response to *d*-fenfluramine, indicating that the fenfluramine-induced prolactin release is mediated through 5-HT$_2$ receptors (Goodall *et al.*, 1993; Park and Cowen, 1995). Fenfluramine studies in depression have yielded inconsistent results, viz. only a limited number of studies have reported a blunted prolactin response to fenfluramine (for review, see Park *et al.*, 1996). This may relate to the fact that a particular subgroup of depressed patients, who are inpatients with melancholic symptoms, show this blunted prolactin response. Another subgroup consists of patients with impulsive traits and a history of suicide attempts (Coccaro *et al.*, 1989; Lichtenberg *et al.*, 1992a).

Fenfluramine and serotonin precursors in panic disorder

A summary of serotonergic challenge studies in panic disorder is depicted in Table 2.2. Targum and Marshall (1989), using an oral dose of 60 mg fenfluramine, found significantly greater prolactin and cortisol responses in PD patients than in either depressed patients or healthy controls. PD patients also revealed a significantly greater anxiogenic response to fenfluramine administration than either depressed patients or healthy controls. Alterations in mood after administration of fenfluramine are unlikely to occur (Lichtenberg *et al.*, 1992b). A more recent study reported an increased prolactin response to a single oral dose of 60 mg fenfluramine in PD patients compared to controls (Apostolopoulos *et al.*, 1993). These data offer circumstantial evidence for the idea that an impaired 5-HT system is an important element in the

Table 2.2. Serotonergic challenges in panic disorder.

Authors	Challenge	Route	Dose	Effects	Hormonal response	Remarks
den Boer and Westenberg, 1990b	L-5-HTP, Placebo	i.v., 20 PD, 20 C	60 mg		↑ Cortisol, β-endorphin	↑ Similar in PD and C, Severe GI side-effects
van Vliet, Slaap, den Boer and Westenberg, 1996	L-5-HTP, Placebo	i.v., 7 PD, 7 C	10, 20, 40 mg		↑ Cort PD = C, ↑ Cort PD = C, ↑ Cort PD > C	All underwent four infusions (placebo, 10, 20, 40 mg 5-HTP). Mild GI side effects only in the 40 mg group
Charney and Heninger, 1986	Tryptophan Placebo	i.v., 23 PD, 21 C	7 g		Prolactin	↑ Similar in PD vs. C
Targum and Marshall, 1989	Fenfluramine Placebo	Oral, 9 PD, 9 MDD, 9 C	60 mg	PD ↑, MDD =, C =	Prol/Cort ↑, PD > MDD = C	Suggests hyper-responsivity in PD
Apostolopoulos et al., 1993	Fenfluramine Placebo	Oral, 11 PD, 12 C	60 mg	ND	Prol PD ↑↑, C ↑	Indicative of ↑ 5-HT function
Kahn et al., 1988a	mCPP	Oral, 11 C, 10 PD, 10 MDD	0.25 mg/kg	PD ↑, C =, MDD =	ND	↑ Depression, anxiety and hostility in PD. No criteria given for panic attacks
Kahn et al., 1988b	mCPP Placebo	Oral, 13 PD, 17 MDD, 15 C	0.25 mg/kg	ND	Cort ↑ PD	Augmented Cort response in PD vs. other groups
Charney et al., 1987b	mCPP Placebo	i.v., 23 PD, 19 C	0.1 mg/kg	PD =, C =	GH, Cort, Prol: PD = C	i.v. dose possibly too high
Klein et al., 1991	mCPP Caffeine Placebo	Oral, 10 PD	0.5 mg/kg, 480 mg	anx Caf > mCPP	mCPP: Cort ↑, Prol ↑ Caf: Cort = Prol ↑	mCPP: panic 70%, Caf: 70%
Lesch et al., 1992	Ipsapirone Placebo	Oral, 14 PD, 14 C	0.3 mg/kg		PD: Cort ↓, PD: ACTH ↓, C: both =	Slight increase in nervousness in C

i.v. = intravenous; C = healthy controls; MDD = major depressive disorder; PD = panic disorder; Prol = prolactin; Cort = cortisol; ND = not done; mCPP = m-chlorphenylpiperazine; UDP = unipolar depression; OCD = obsessive-compulsive disorder; ACTH = adrenocorticotrophic hormone; GI = gastrointestinal; Caf = caffeine-treated group; anx Caf = anxiety in the caffeine-treated group is greater than in the MNCP-treated group.

pathophysiology of PD and are consistent with the hypothesis of an increased 5-HT receptor function in panic disorder. The question is, which 5-HT receptor subtype is involved in the increased prolactin release following the fenfluramine challenge? Animal experiments have implicated both 5-HT_{2C} and 5-HT_{2A} receptors in prolactin release. In human volunteers ritanserin appears to be able to abolish the fenfluramine anorectic effects, as well as the fenfluramine-induced increases in oral temperature and plasma prolactin, thus supporting the idea that 5-HT_{2A} or 5-HT_{2C} receptors mediate the effects of fenfluramine (Goodall *et al.*, 1993). Other investigators, however, have debated the idea that the 5-HT/HPA interaction is abnormal in PD patients. Charney *et al.* (1987b) using 0.1 mg/kg *m*CPP (see below) intravenously, found similar cortisol and prolactin responses in PD patients and healthy controls. They also reported a similar anxiogenic effect of *m*CPP in PD patients and controls. Differences in design (dosage and route of administration) may account for these discrepancies (Murphy *et al.*, 1989). Using prolactin as hormonal probe of 5-HT activity, Charney and Heninger (1986) also reported similar increases in both patients and controls after loading with tryptophan. The validity of the latter test has been questioned by van Praag *et al.* (1987), who contended that prolactin release after high doses of tryptophan can affect catecholamine as well as 5-HT neurones. The argument is that tryptophan competes with tyrosine at the same carrier in the blood–brain barrier, thereby reducing the tyrosine influx into the brain, which in turn could lead to decreased catecholamine levels.

Den Boer and Westenberg (1990b) evaluated the responsivity of the 5-HT system in PD patients and healthy controls by measuring the neuroendocrine and behavioural concomitants of 5-HTP administration. Cortisol and β-endorphin plasma levels were used as hormonal probes of the 5-HT responsivity. Following an intravenous dose of 60 mg 5-HTP in combination with 150 mg of carbidopa, a peripheral decarboxylase inhibitor, significant but similar increases of both hormones were found in patients and controls. Administration of 5-HTP appeared to decrease rather than to increase levels of anxiety in PD patients. Despite severe gastrointestinal side effects, most patients became less anxious by the end of the test. In contrast, controls did not consider 5-HTP administration as a relief; they developed a dysphoric mood with organic brain syndrome-like symptoms instead. The relatively high dose of 5-HTP and the side effects may have obscured differences in hormonal response, which prompted us to conduct a double-blind placebo-controlled 5-HTP dose–response study (van Vliet *et al.*, 1996). In this study we administered 5-HTP intravenously in doses ranging from 10 to 40 mg in PD patients and healthy controls. We found that 10 and 20 mg 5-HTP elicited dose-dependent, albeit comparable, increases in cortisol in patients with PD and controls. At dosages below 40 mg no side effects were reported, supporting the idea that the hormonal response was the result of 5-HTP-induced rather than stress-induced HPA activity.

In the 40 mg dose, however, an augmented cortisol response was found in PD compared to controls, thus supporting the idea of increased 5-HT receptor sensitivity in PD (van Vliet *et al.*, 1996).

m-*Chlorophenylpiperazine challenge in panic disorder*

Most challenge studies to date have been performed with *m*-chlorophenylpiperazine (*m*CPP). Originally this compound was thought to bind with high selectivity to 5-HT_{1B} receptors, but more recent studies have pointed out that it also binds to some degree to 5-HT_{1A}, 5-HT_{1D}, α_1-, α_2-, and β-adrenergic and dopamine receptors (Hamik and Peroutka, 1989). Nowadays *m*CPP is considered to be a non-selective 5-$HT_{2A/2C}$ receptor agonist, and it is commonly used to assess possible dysfunctions related to these receptor subtypes. Needless to say, claims for specificity cannot be made, but at present better ligands for the 5-HT_2 receptor are not available for challenge studies.

Using the neuroendocrine strategy, Kahn *et al.* (1988a) studied the responsivity of 5-HT receptors in PD patients by measuring the cortisol release after administration of *m*CPP, the metabolite of the antidepressant trazodone. When given orally (0.25 mg/kg), *m*CPP induced an augmented cortisol release in PD patients as compared to normal controls and depressed patients. These authors also found *m*CPP to increase anxiety in PD patients but not in healthy controls (Kahn *et al.*, 1988b). Based on these findings the authors postulated that 5-HT receptors in PD patients might be supersensitive and that drugs that reduce 5-HT function should be useful therapeutic agents in PD. Anxiogenic effects of *m*CPP in PD patients were also reported by Klein *et al.* (1991). In view of *m*CPP's lack of specificity, it is not clear which receptor subtype would be functioning abnormally in PD. A recent study in normal controls revealed that pretreatment with ritanserin was able to diminish the *m*CPP-induced increases in anxiety and prolactin, and to abolish the *m*CPP-induced cortisol increase, suggesting that the neuroendocrine and behavioural responses to *m*CPP might be mediated through 5-HT_{2C} receptors (Seibyl *et al.*, 1991).

m-*Chlorophenylpiperazine challenge in obsessive-compulsive disorder*

In several studies in which *m*CPP was administered orally, a transient increase in obsessive-compulsive symptoms has been reported (Zohar *et al.*, 1987, 1988; Hollander *et al.*, 1988, 1992; Pigott *et al.*, 1991; see Table 2.3). In addition, OCD patients became more anxious, depressed or dysphoric after *m*CPP administration. Interestingly, intravenous administration failed to induce the same increases in obsessions or compulsions (Charney *et al.*, 1988; Pigott *et al.*, 1993a), while in a recent study no evidence was found for increases in obsessions or compulsive behaviours after either oral or intravenous administration of *m*CPP (Goodman *et al.*, 1995). The reason for these inconsistencies is unclear. In volunteers, changing the route of *m*CPP administration also elicited a different response: intravenous administration induced more anxiety and physical symptoms than oral administration (Murphy *et al.*, 1989). Another reason for the contradictory results could be the time elapsing before *m*CPP reaches the receptor. In addition, the reliability of psychometric assessments determines to a large extent the interpretation of results. The most widely used scale for the

Table 2.3. Challenge studies with serotonergic compounds in OCD.

Author	Substance	Patients (N) (Dep: N)	Design	Behavioural response	OC symptoms Other	Compared to controls Cortisol	Prolactin
Zohar et al., 1987	mCPP orally, 0.5 mg/kg	12 (0)	Double-blind placebo	↑↑	Anxiety ↑, depression ↑, dysphoria ↑	= (<C)	↑(= C)
	Metergoline orally, 4 mg	8		→	—		
Charney et al., 1988	mCPP, i.v., 0.1 mg/kg	21 (10)	Double-blind placebo	=	Anxiety ↑, sedation	↑(= C)	↑(= ♂C, <♀C)
	Tryptophan i.v., 7 g	21 (11)		=	Sedation	↑(= C)	↑(= C)
Zohar et al., 1988	mCPP orally, 0.5 mg/kg	9 (?)	Double-blind placebo: Before treatment	↑↑	—	=	↑
			After 3 months' treatment with clomipramine	↑	—	=	↑(At baseline already raised)
Pigott et al., 1990	mCPP orally, 0.5 mg/kg	13 (?)	Double-blind placebo After clomipramine (N = 6)	=	—	=	↑
			After fluoxetine (N = 11)	=	—	↑	
Hollander et al., 1991b	mCPP orally, 0.5 mg/kg	6 (?)	Double-blind placebo Before treatment	↑↑	—	↑(<C)	↑(<C)
			After 3 months' treatment with fluoxetine	=	—	↑ (After correction for mCPP-plasma level: =)	↑
Pigott et al., 1991	mCPP orally, 0.5 mg/kg Metergoline orally, 4 mg	12 (0)	Double-blind placebo mCPP (N = 6)	↑↑	Anxiety ↑		
			Metergoline (N = 12)	=	—	=	→
			Metergoline + mCPP (N = 6)	=	—	=	=

Study	Drug, dose	N (Dep)	Design					
Hollander et al., 1992	mCPP orally, 0.5 mg/kg	20 (0)	Double-blind placebo	—	↑↑	—	↑(= C)	↑(< C)
	Fenfluramine orally, 60 mg	14 (0)		—	=	—	↑(= C)	↑(= C)
Pigott et al., 1993a,b	mCPP orally, 0.5 mg/kg	17 (0)	Double-blind placebo	—	=	—		
	mCPP i.v. 0.1 mg/kg	10 (0)	Double-blind	Anxiety ↑, depression ↑, dysphoria ↑	=	—		
	Metergoline orally (dose?)	12 (0)	MTG + plac (N = 10), Plac + mCPP (N = 5)	—	↑↑	—		
	mCPP i.v. 0.1 mg/kg		MTG + mCPP (N = 5)	—	↑↑	—		
Goodman et al., 1995	mCPP orally 0.5 mg/kg		All three tests: double-blind/placebo	Anxiety ↑	=	—	↑(no C)	↑
	mCPP i.v. 0.1 mg/kg			Anxiety ↑	=	—	↑(no C)	↑
	Placebo			—	=	—		
McBride et al., 1992	Fenfluramine orally, 60 mg	21 (0)	Single-blind placebo	—	=	—		↑(= C)
Lucey et al., 1992a	Fenfluramine orally 30 mg	10 (0)	Open	—	=	—	↑(< C)	↑(< C)
Hewlett et al., 1993	Fenfluramine orally 60 mg	26 (0)	Open	—	—	—		↑(< C; ♀ < C, ♂ = C)
Bastani et al., 1990	MK-212 orally, 20 mg	17 (0)	Double-blind placebo	Anxiety ↑, depression ↑, derealization ↑	=	—	↑(< C)	↑(< C)
Lesch et al., 1991a	Ipsapirone orally, 0.3 mg/kg	12 (0)	Double-blind placebo	Sedation ↑, anxiety ↑	=	—	↑(= C)	↑(= C)
Lesch et al., 1991b	Ipsapirone orally, 0.3 mg/kg	10 (0)	Double-blind placebo after treatment with fluoxetine	—	=	—	↑(< before treatment)	
Lucey et al., 1992c	Buspirone, orally 30 mg	10 (0)	Open	—	=	—		
de Leeuw et al., 1997	5-HTP i.v., 40 mg	7 (0)	Double-blind placebo	—	=	—	↑(= C)	↑(= C)

C = controls; Dep = major depression; Dep: N = number of patients who were depressed.

assessment of changes in frequency and/or severity of obsessions or compulsive behaviours during provocation studies is the challenge version of the Yale–Brown Obsessive-Compulsive Scale (Y-BOCS) (Goodman *et al.*, 1989, 1991). It is conceivable that discrete changes in obsessions or compulsions are simply not detected by the present psychometric instruments.

Based on the fact that the release of several hormones like prolactin, cortisol and corticotrophin is under serotonergic control, these hormones have been studied during serotonergic challenges. In healthy volunteers, *m*CPP induces increases in plasma concentrations of prolactin, cortisol and adrenocorticotrophic hormone (ACTH). Similar to the behavioural findings, the effects of *m*CPP on neuroendocrine parameters in patients suffering from OCD are equivocal. Two studies reported a blunted prolactin response to *m*CPP challenge in OCD patients (Charney *et al.*, 1988; Hollander *et al.*, 1992). Other studies failed to confirm these findings and reported normal increases of prolactin after *m*CPP challenge (Zohar *et al.*, 1987). In one study, patients were rechallenged with *m*CPP after 4 months' treatment with clomipramine. After this treatment period, the plasma prolactin response (increase) to *m*CPP remained unchanged (Zohar *et al.*, 1988). On the other hand, the blunted prolactin response reported by Hollander and coworkers (1992) was found to normalize during rechallenge with *m*CPP after chronic fluoxetine treatment (Hollander *et al.*, 1991a). Likewise, the non-specific $5-HT_2$ receptor antagonist metergoline has been shown to attenuate the *m*CPP-induced increase in plasma prolactin levels in OCD (Pigott *et al.*, 1991).

Cortisol response was found to be blunted in OCD patients compared to healthy controls (Zohar *et al.*, 1987; Hollander *et al.*, 1991b). Treatment with antidepressants like clomipramine or fluoxetine (which normalized the blunted prolactin response to *m*CPP) was without effect on the blunted cortisol response. A more recent study failed to replicate these findings (Hollander *et al.*, 1992).

In a recent preliminary study, *m*CPP was administered to patients with trichotillomania, a disorder which shares many phenomenological features with OCD. It was found that cortisol and prolactin responses to *m*CPP did not differ from those in controls. There was, however, a somewhat more robust prolactin response to *m*CPP in OCD, which was positively correlated with the urge to pull hair (Stein *et al.*, 1995).

In summary, the effects of *m*CPP on behavioural ratings of obsessions and compulsive behaviours, as well as the neuroendocrine responses to *m*CPP, are subject to debate. If anything, there is circumstantial evidence for an increased behavioural response and a blunted neuroendocrine response to the *m*CPP challenge in OCD patients. Despite *m*CPP's lack of selectivity, the challenge studies may hint at a dysfunction of $5-HT_{2A/2C}$ receptors in OCD patients, or a subgroup.

Serotonin precursors in obsessive-compulsive disorder

Stimulation of the serotonergic system by 5-HTP, the precursor of 5-HT, failed to increase obsessions or compulsions, nor were there any differences in cortisol response between patients and controls (de Leeuw *et al.*, 1997). Two studies have been published in which OCD patients were challenged with the 5-HT precursor tryptophan. Charney and co-workers (1988) found that administration of tryptophan led to a significant enhancement of tryptophan-induced prolactin release, and a non-significant increase in growth hormone (GH) release. In a recent study, Fineberg and co-workers (1994) reported a significantly greater GH release in 16 OCD patients compared to healthy controls after intravenous administration of tryptophan. These findings suggest that OCD patients have modest increases in neuroendocrine responses to tryptophan. It is unlikely that studies with tryptophan and 5-HTP will shed more light on the 5-HT subtypes involved, since both compounds lack selectivity with respect to 5-HT receptor subtypes.

Tryptophan depletion in OCD patients, who demonstrated symptom reduction with SSRIs, failed to influence mean ratings of obsessions or compulsions (Barr *et al.*, 1994). This indicates that the maintenance of the anti-OCD effects of SSRIs does not depend on the availability of 5-HT.

These findings indicate that the relationship between 5-HT and OCD cannot be explained in terms of 5-HT availability, but it is still possible that the sensitivity of one or more receptor subtypes is altered, and that challenging with tryptophan, 5-HTP or tryptophan depletion is not able to detect these changes.

Fenfluramine and other serotoninomimetics in obsessive-compulsive disorder

Fenfluramine possesses 5-HT-releasing and reuptake inhibiting properties and therefore acts as a 5-HT agonist at all the pre- and postsynaptic receptors. Challenge studies with fenfluramine in OCD are scarce, but available evidence indicates that OCD patients and healthy controls show similar cortisol responses to fenfluramine (Hollander *et al.*, 1992; Hewlett and Martin, 1993). Controversial results have been reported for the prolactin response to fenfluramine, which was found to be identical in OCD patients and controls (Hollander *et al.*, 1992; Price *et al.*, 1989). A blunted plasma prolactin response to a challenge with fenfluramine, which was only present in females and could be reversed by treatment with clonazepam, was reported by Hewlett and Martin (1993). In drug-free patients a blunted prolactin response was reported to the challenge with fenfluramine in OCD (Lucey *et al.*, 1992b; Monteleone *et al.*, 1997a). Prolactin response to fenfluramine challenge was normalized following treatment with the SSRI fluvoxamine (Monteleone *et al.*, 1997a).

The abnormal cortisol and prolactin responses are not confined to OCD: in depressed patients similar blunted responses to fenfluramine challenge have been reported (Lucey *et al.*, 1992b). Considering the fact that the prolactin response to fenfluramine is mediated through $5-HT_{2A/2C}$ receptors, it is conceivable that these receptor subtypes are involved in the pathogenesis of OCD. Similar to the gender differences observed with respect to the prolactin response to fenfluramine challenge, Monteleone *et al.* (1997b) reported that the cortisol response to fenfluramine challenge was significantly reduced in female patients but not in males. The notion of altered receptor sensitivity is, however, not easily explained in terms of super- or subsensitivity. An exaggerated behavioural response to mCPP could indicate supersensitivity of the 5-HT_2 receptor subtype(s). On the other hand, in studies in which a blunted prolactin response to a challenge with, for example, fenfluramine was found, this finding was interpreted as evidence for subsensitivity of the same receptor subtype. A reason for the lack of consistency in the behavioural and neuroendocrine results of challenge studies in OCD may be that the dysfunction is possibly confined to a subgroup of OCD patients (e.g. "checkers" or "cleaners"), whereas virtually all studies have been on "OCD", irrespective of subtype.

Since 5-HT precursors and fenfluramine do not discriminate between the 5-HT receptor subtypes, research has focused recently on challenge studies with compounds that are more selective, such as the $5\text{-}HT_{1A}$ agonists buspirone and ipsapirone. The latter has been shown to produce increased cortisol levels in controls. In a study in which ipsapirone was administered to OCD patients, Lesch and co-workers have shown that ipsapirone does not lead to increased severity or frequency of obsessions or compulsive behaviours (Lesch *et al.*, 1991a). They also found no differences between OCD and controls in corticotrophin-releasing hormone (CRH) and plasma cortisol responses to ipsapirone challenge. CRH is synthesized in the hypothalamus and regulates the release of ACTH in the pituitary. Since there were no differences in behavioural or neuroendocrine responses to ipsapirone, the hypothesis that the $5\text{-}HT_{1A}$ receptor is critically involved in the pathogenesis of OCD should be rejected. In a subsequent study of the same group it was found that long-term treatment with fluoxetine decreased the ipsapirone-induced neuroendocrine responses after a rechallenge with fenfluramine (Lesch *et al.*, 1991b).

Lucey and co-workers (1992c) challenged 10 OCD patients with buspirone and found similar prolactin responses in OCD patients and controls, which strengthens the idea that there is no dysfunction at the level of the $5\text{-}HT_{1A}$ receptor in OCD.

Another serotonergic agent which has been investigated in OCD is the experimental drug MK-212, a $5\text{-}HT_{2A/2C}$ agonist, which increased, like mCPP, plasma levels of cortisol and prolactin in controls (Lowy and Meltzer, 1988). In OCD, the neuroendocrine responses to MK-212 were revealed in a blunting of the plasma cortisol and prolactin levels, whilst at the behavioural level obsessions or compulsive symptoms were not induced (Bastani *et al.*, 1990).

Is there evidence for a dysfunctional $5\text{-}HT_{1D}$ receptor in obsessive-compulsive disorder?

$5\text{-}HT_{1D}$ receptors have a high density in the basal ganglia and frontal cortex. These brain areas have consistently been implicated in the pathophysiology of OCD (see below).

Preliminary evidence suggests that challenging OCD patients with sumatriptan, a selective $5\text{-}HT_{1D}$ receptor agonist used for the treatment of migraine, results in an exacerbation of obsessive compulsive symptoms (Zohar, 1996). We have recently investigated the effects of a challenge with sumatriptan in a double-blind, placebo-controlled cross-over study (Ho Pian *et al.*, 1998a). Although sumatriptan was found to induce a significant rise in plasma concentration of GH, no changes in obsessions or compulsive behaviours were reported. In view of the fact that sumatriptan does not cross the blood–brain barrier, we recently performed a study using zolmitriptan, because this compound does cross the blood–brain barrier (Boshuisen and den Boer, 2000). In this placebo-controlled double-blind cross-over study we were unable to detect any changes in obsessions or compulsive behaviors during challenge with zolmitriptan.

In summary, challenge studies with mCPP, fenfluramine and MK-212, despite inconsistent results, do provide circumstantial evidence for a subsensitivity of 5-$HT_{2A/2C}$ receptors in OCD. Interestingly, this would imply a biological difference between PD and OCD. Challenge studies with mCPP, though likewise equivocal, have led to the hypothesis of a supersensitivity of 5-$HT_{2A/2C}$ receptors in panic disorder (for a review, see den Boer and Westenberg, 1996). This conclusion should of course be taken as tentative, since mCPP is a non-specific agent which also shows affinity for α_2-adrenoceptors, among others. Therefore, some of the effects of mCPP could be attributed to interactions with the noradrenergic system through α_2-adrenoceptors. The role of other receptor subtypes in OCD is unclear. Challenge with buspirone and ipsapirone could not supply evidence for the existence of a dysfunction of 5-HT_{1A} receptors. The functional state of the 5-HT_3 receptor is presently unknown. A preliminary study reported anxiolytic and anti-obsessive-compulsive effects of 5-HT_3 receptor antagonist ondansetron (Pigott et al., 1993b). Two double-blind studies showed that the 5-HT_{1D} receptor agonists sumatriptan and zolmitriptan did not lead to an exacerbation of OCD symptoms.

Further challenge and treatment studies are necessary to expand our insight into the pathogenetic mechanisms involved in OCD.

Fenfluramine in social phobia

Fenfluramine has been used as a pharmacological probe to assess serotonergic function in patients with social phobia; the response to fenfluramine is measured by its effect on two biological markers, cortisol and prolactin. In social phobics, fenfluramine produced a significantly greater rise in cortisol compared with control subjects but had no effect on prolactin. These findings have been interpreted as evidence of supersensitivity of postsynaptic serotonin receptors but require replication and confirmation (Sheehan et al., 1993; Schneier et al., 1993).

Additional support for a serotonergic mechanism in social phobia can be derived from the efficacy of serotoninomimetics and clonazepam in social phobia (den Boer, 1997). For instance, the 5-HT_{1A} receptor agonist buspirone and ondansetron, a 5-HT_3 receptor antagonist normally used as an anti-emetic, have been shown to improve the symptoms of social phobics (Davidson et al., 1993; Pratt et al., 1979). The benzodiazepine clonazepam also has demonstrable efficacy in social phobia (Rosenbaum et al., 1991), an effect possibly mediated through a change in serotonin utilization in the brain (Gabbard, 1992).

Discussion of serotonergic challenge studies

A general problem of the neuroendocrine paradigm is the lack of selectivity of the challenge agents used so far and the complexity of the mechanisms controlling the hormones allegedly under 5-HT control. There is considerable pharmacological evidence that activation of either 5-HT_{1A} or $5\text{-HT}_{2A}/5\text{-HT}_{2C}$ receptors leads to a stimulation of the HPA axis (Fuller, 1990). In man, elevated plasma cortisol levels have also been observed after acute administration of selective 5-HT_{1A} ligands such as ipsapirone and gepirone (Lesch *et al.*, 1990; Rausch *et al.*, 1990). In contrast to *m*CPP, these selective 5-HT_{1A} ligands induce a blunted response in depressed patients (Lesch *et al.*, 1990), suggesting that these effects may occur through separate pathways. 5-HTP affects HPA activity through stimulation of the 5-HT release, which may interact with all 5-HT receptor subsets, both pre- and postsynaptically. It has been suggested, though, that the neuroendocrine effects of 5-HTP are mediated through $5\text{-HT}_{2A}/5\text{-HT}_{2C}$ receptors, since ritanserin, a $5\text{-HT}_{2A}/5\text{-HT}_{2C}$ antagonist, was able to inhibit the 5-HTP-induced cortisol secretion (Lee *et al.*, 1991). The failure of 5-HTP to increase plasma MHPG levels suggests that central noradrenergic activity was not affected by 5-HTP administration (den Boer and Westenberg, 1990b).

In summary, the *m*CPP and fenfluramine findings are intriguing and putatively indicative of an impaired 5-HT function in PD patients. They suggest that an increase in 5-HT activity is positively correlated to anxiety. However, the data cited above do not permit any definite conclusion, because the effects are not unequivocal and were elicited by rather non-selective agents. The data beg for further clinical investigations with more selective 5-HT agonists and antagonists.

Blood platelet and CSF studies in depression and anxiety

Inferences about 5-HT functions in the brain may also be based on measurements in readily accessible biological fluids, such as blood, urine and cerebrospinal fluid (CSF).

Blood platelets Blood platelets are considered as peripheral markers for some functions of the 5-HT neurones. They share with 5-HT neurones the ability to store and release 5-HT. In contrast to neurones, 5-HT is not synthesized in platelets, but derived from blood. It is taken up into the platelets by a 5-HT-specific transporter which resembles the transporter in the brain. Platelets also contain other constituents that are found in the brain. Thus, specific high-affinity binding sites for [³H]-imipramine or [³H]-paroxetine have been found in brain and platelet membranes (Paul *et al.*, 1980). There is circumstantial evidence that these sites are associated with, but not identical to, the 5-HT uptake mechanism in both platelets and neurones (Langer *et al.*, 1980). It has been suggested, therefore, that [³H]-imipramine binding labels a physiological relevant site that modulates 5-HT reuptake. A reduction in the maximum concentration or density of platelet [³H]-imipramine binding sites has been reported in depressed patients by many investigators (Paul *et al.*, 1981; Raisman *et al.*, 1981; Roy *et al.*, 1987; Innis *et al.*, 1987).

Studies conducted so far in patients with PD do not reveal abnormal [^{3}H]-imipramine binding characteristics (Norman *et al.*, 1986; Innis *et al.*, 1987; Nutt and Fraser, 1987; Schneider *et al.*, 1987; Uhde *et al.*, 1987; Norman *et al.*, 1989). In spite of the fact that the number of subjects was relatively small in most studies, it can be concluded that [^{3}H]-imipramine binding in PD patients is normal, thus pointing to a different pathogenesis of PD as opposed to depression (for review of pathogenetic differences and similarities between depression and anxiety disorders, see den Boer and Sitsen, 1994). Platelet 5-HT uptake is also considered to share several properties with the presynaptic terminal of 5-HT-containing fibres and is therefore used as a peripheral marker of presynaptic 5-HT function in the brain (Stahl *et al.*, 1982). Platelet 5-HT uptake has been reported to be lowered among depressed patients (Tuomisto and Tukiainen, 1976; Meltzer *et al.*, 1984). In two studies an augmented maximal uptake rate (V_{max}) and a similar affinity for uptake (K_m) was found in patients with PD relative to healthy controls (Norman *et al.*, 1986, 1989). In contrast, Pecknold *et al.* (1988) found a reduced V_{max} in patients with PD, whereas den Boer and Westenberg (1990a) found no difference in the platelet kinetics between patients with PD and healthy controls. Another similarity between platelets and the 5-HT system is that they contain 5-HT$_{2A}$ binding sites. Studying peripheral markers of 5-HT activity in PD patients, Butler *et al.* (1992) found that the density of 5-HT$_{2A}$ binding sites on platelets is elevated and that it remained increased after successful treatment, suggesting that it is a trait marker rather than a state marker in PD. In contrast, a decrease in [^{3}H]-LSD binding, which among others labels the 5-HT$_{2A}$ sites, on platelets of PD patients was found by Norman *et al.* (1990).

CSF studies in depression   In the 1970s and 1980s several studies have shown a reduced CSF 5-hydroxyindole-acetic acid (5-HIAA) concentration in some depressed patients, although this was not a consistent finding. More recent studies point towards a relation between lowered CSF 5-HIAA and a subtype of depression in which violent suicide or aggression towards others may play a pivotal role (Brown *et al.*, 1992). Interestingly, this relationship appeared not to be confined to depressed patients, as violent suicide attempts in patients with personality disorders and schizophrenia were also characterized by lowered CSF 5-HIAA (for review, see Smith and Cowen, 1997). Since it was established that a lowered CSF 5-HIAA correlated with a cluster of symptoms which cuts across the boundaries of different axis I and axis II diagnoses, it has been hypothesized that a subgroup of depression exists which does justice to this dimensional approach. This concept, coined by van Praag, was named "stressor-precipitated cortisol-induced 5-HT-related anxiety/aggression-driven depression" (van Praag, 1997).

CSF studies in panic disorder   Measurement of 5-HIAA, the major metabolite of 5-HT, in CSF has also been used to evaluate brain 5-HT turnover. A number of studies have used lumbar CSF 5-HIAA as marker for 5-HT turnover. Studies in depression have revealed a decrease in CSF 5-HIAA levels in a subgroup of patients (Westenberg and Verhoeven, 1988). There is only one report on CSF 5-HIAA concentrations in PD patients (Eriksson *et al.*, 1991). In this study PD patients did not differ significantly from age- and sex-matched normal controls. Taking these data together, one may tentatively conclude that these peripheral indices of 5-HT function do not consistently disclose a 5-HT abnormality in PD. They might point, however, to a neurobiological difference between PD and depression.

CSF studies in obsessive-compulsive disorder   Only a small number of studies have investigated CSF levels of 5-HIAA in patients with OCD. A trend towards an increase was reported by Thoren *et al.* (1980), whereas a significant increase was found by Insel *et al.* (1985) in a small number of patients (8).

A complete discussion of all methodological problems in CSF research is beyond the scope of this chapter. Suffice it to say that CSF data should be interpreted with caution. Moreover, there is considerable evidence that CSF 5-HIAA relates to other clinical characteristics such as impulsivity and aggression, and not specifically with an axis I diagnosis.

Involvement of serotonin receptor subtypes in depression and anxiety

Serotonin receptor subtypes   At present four major classes of 5-HT receptors have been identified in the brain; they have been classified into 5-HT_1, 5-HT_2, 5-HT_3 and 5-HT_4 receptors. With the exception of the 5-HT_3 receptor, they all belong to the superfamily of G protein-linked receptors. These receptors transduce signals by activating G proteins, producing relatively slow responses through second messengers. The 5-HT_3 receptor is unique among the 5-HT receptors in that it is a ligand-gated ion channel, producing rapid depolarizing responses when stimulated. The 5-HT_1 family can be subdivided into at least five different subtypes, all of which appear to be seven-transmembrane-domain receptors. They are denoted as 5-HT_{1A}, 5-HT_{1B}, 5-HT_{1C}, 5-HT_{1D} and 5-HT_{1E}. In this chapter we use the accepted new terminology of 5-HT receptor subtypes: 5-HT_2 receptors are now designated as 5-HT_{2A}, and 5-HT_{1C} receptors are named 5-HT_{2C} receptors (Humphrey *et al.*, 1993).

The 5-HT_1 receptors were originally identified by their high affinity for $[^3\text{H}]5\text{-HT}$. Although the relatively high affinity of the 5-HT_{2C} receptor for 5-HT resulted in its classification as a 5-HT_1-like receptor, subsequent studies have called this classification into question. Unlike the 5-HT_1 receptors, the 5-HT_{2C} receptor is not coupled to adenylate cyclase. Similar to 5-HT_{2A} receptor, stimulation of the 5-HT_{2C} receptor promotes the hydrolysis of phosphoinositide. Apart from the analogy in signal transduction, these receptor subtypes share a high degree of amino acid sequence homology. The 5-HT_{1A}, 5-HT_{1B} and 5-HT_{1D} receptors are all negatively linked to adenylate cyclase activity. The 5-HT_{1B} receptor is found only in some rodents and has been suggested to represent the species equivalent of the 5-HT$_{1D}$ receptor in higher species, where the 5-HT$_{1B}$ receptors are absent (Hoyer and Middlemiss, 1989). This is supported by recent cloning work which has led to a further differentiation of this receptor subtype into a human 5-HT$_{1D\alpha}$ and 5-HT$_{1D\beta}$ site; a closely related rat 5-HT$_{1D\beta}$ clone is identical to the rat 5-HT$_{1B}$ receptor (Hartig, 1992). The 5-HT$_{1E}$ is a novel 5-HT receptor subtype, also linked to adenylate cyclase, but whose exact localization and function in the brain is as yet unknown. Preliminary studies using in situ hybridization techniques have revealed that this receptor subtype is present in cortical areas, caudate, putamen and amygdala (Bruinvels, 1993). The existence of the 5-HT$_4$ receptor is based on pharmacological studies, which indicate that it is closely related to the 5-HT$_1$ receptor family, but differs in that it is positively coupled to adenylate cyclase (Bockaert *et al.*, 1987). As yet its molecular structure is unknown.

Several new 5-HT receptor subtypes have been cloned, e.g. the 5-HT$_{5A}$, 5-HT$_{5B}$, 5-HT$_6$ and 5-HT$_7$ receptors (Erlander *et al.*, 1993; Matthes *et al.*, 1993; Plassat *et al.*, 1992; Monsma *et al.*, 1993). In view of the lack of information on the pharmacological properties and physiological functions of these receptor subtypes, they will not be discussed here.

5-HT$_{1A}$ receptors in depression and anxiety Selective serotonin reuptake inhibitors (SSRIs) are effective in the treatment of depression (Delgado *et al.*, 1990; Briley and Moret, 1993), panic (den Boer and Westenberg, 1988) and obsessive-compulsive disorder (Kahn *et al.*, 1984; Turner *et al.*, 1985; Perse *et al.*, 1987). Azapirones, 5-HT$_{1A}$ receptor partial agonists, are well established anxiolytics and may possess antidepressant properties as well (Schweizer *et al.*, 1986; Robinson *et al.*, 1989). Chronic lithium therapy in mania could involve a 5-HT$_{1A}$ receptor-mediated mechanism (Newman *et al.*, 1992; Uchitomi and Yamawaki, 1993). Moreover, the addition of lithium or buspirone to ongoing serotonin reuptake inhibitor (SRI) therapy has been reported effective in treatment-resistant obsessive-compulsive disorder (see Goodman *et al.*, 1993). Thus, evidence is accumulating for a critical involvement of the serotonergic system, in particular 5-HT$_{1A}$ receptors, in the treatment of both depression and anxiety disorders.

An additional argument for the involvement of serotonergic pathways in the treatment of depression comes from 5-HT depletion studies. Inhibition of 5-HT synthesis by *p*-chlorophenylalanine (Shopsin *et al.*, 1975, 1976) or L-tryptophan depletion (Delgado *et al.*, 1990) caused a relapse of symptoms in depressed patients, successfully treated with SRIs or bright light (Lam *et al.*, 1996). Tryptophan depletion also produced a transient exacerbation of depressive symptoms in obsessive-compulsive disorder patients responding to serotonin reuptake inhibitors (Barr *et al.*, 1994).

As regards the involvement of 5-HT in the pathophysiology of depression and anxiety disorders, 5-HT depletion studies have produced mixed results. Tryptophan depletion was able to lower the mood of healthy volunteers (Young *et al.*, 1985; see also Young, 1994), especially in those persons with high normal depression rate scores or with a genetic risk (Benkelfat *et al.*, 1994). Combined with a yohimbine challenge,

Goddard *et al.* (1995) reported a significant increase in nervousness in healthy volunteers. In patients with OCD, however, tryptophan depletion did not worsen the obsessive and compulsive symptoms (Smeraldi *et al.*, 1996). Moreover, it did not induce anxiogenic or panicogenic effects in unmedicated PD patients (Goddard *et al.*, 1994), and it also failed to modify the panicogenic effects of CCK-4 in healthy volunteers (Koszycki *et al.*, 1996). It is of note that Bel and Artigas (1996) have reported a decrease of cortical 5-HT levels following tryptophan depletion in rats chronically treated with fluvoxamine, an SSRI, but not in control animals. Thus, depletion studies reinforce the idea that 5-HT is critically involved in the treatment of depression in particular, but they may be less indicative for a role of 5-HT in the pathogenesis of depression and anxiety.

In this respect the neuroendocrine strategy seems more promising. Neuroendocrine markers for central serotonergic activity have shown a blunted response following administration of serotoninomimetics in untreated depressed patients (Charney *et al.*, 1981; Siever *et al.*, 1984; Upadhyaya *et al.*, 1991; Ansseau *et al.*, 1997). This may indicate the desensitization of particular 5-HT receptor subtypes or their signal transduction systems in depression.

Pindolol augmentation strategies in depression   The desensitization hypothesis by Blier *et al.* (1987a) proposes that SSRIs increase the 5-HT synaptic efficacy through a gradual desensitization of 5-HT_{1A} autoreceptors. This would compensate for a reduced responsiveness of postsynaptic 5-HT receptors in depression. The idea was prompted by the delay in therapeutic effect of SRIs and is supported by electrophysiological studies in rats chronically treated with SRIs. However, animal studies do not unequivocally support the desensitization of 5-HT autoreceptors following repeated administration of SRIs. Using different experimental procedures, investigators have reported decreased (Chaput *et al.*, 1986; Schechter *et al.*, 1990; Kreiss and Lucki, 1993; Rutter *et al.*, 1994), normal (Schechter *et al.*, 1990; Hjorth and Auerbach, 1994; Bosker *et al.*, 1995) and increased (O'Connor and Kruk, 1994) sensitivity of 5-HT_{1A} autoreceptors after chronic treatment with SRIs. The varying outcome may partly be attributed to lack of attention to the pharmacokinetic aspects of SSRI administration in animals. Plasma half lives of SSRIs are much shorter in rodents compared to humans. A practicable way to obtain steady-state conditions in rodents is to use osmotic minipumps. In combination with a highly soluble SSRI, such as citalopram, plasma levels comparable to those in humans can be attained. Using this approach desensitization of 5-HT_{1A} receptors was demonstrated recently by Cremers *et al.* (2000). Similarly, desensitization of the release controlling $5\text{-HT}_{1B/1D}$ receptors has been advanced to explain the latency in therapeutic effects of SRIs in psychiatric disorders (Blier *et al.*, 1987a), but contradictory findings have also been reported for the effect of SRIs on the sensitivity of these receptors (Sleight *et al.*, 1989; Moret and Briley, 1990; Chaput *et al.*, 1991; O'Connor and Kruk, 1994; Bosker *et al.*, 1995). Interestingly, using the minipump approach, Cremers *et al.* (2000) could not demonstrate desensitization of $5\text{-HT}_{1B/D}$ receptors.

A key point in Blier's hypothesis is that the secondary effects of SRIs on the release-controlling autoreceptors limit the effect of uptake inhibition on the 5-HT release in terminal areas. This is supported by microdialysis experiments in rats, showing that the increase in extracellular 5-HT elicited by a single dose of an SRI is augmented by co-administration of a 5-HT_{1A} autoreceptor antagonist (Invernizzi *et al.*, 1992; Hjorth, 1993). This approach may also have clinical relevance, as pointed out by Artigas (1993). A preliminary study with previously untreated depressed patients indeed suggests an improvement in both latency and efficacy by combined treatment with paroxetine, an SSRI, and pindolol, a mixed $\beta/5\text{-HT}_{1A}$ receptor antagonist (Artigas *et al.*, 1994). These initial clinical findings were replicated by Blier and Bergeron (1995). Importantly, measurement of pulse rate and arterial pressure indicated only minimal activation of β-adrenoceptors at the pindolol dose used. A double-blind placebo-controlled study with fluoxetine and pindolol (Berman *et al.*, 1997), however, did not confirm the findings of the previous open studies. Part of this discrepancy may be due to differences in patient groups with regard to drug history or severity of the illness. It has also been suggested that non-response to pindolol augmentation may relate to 5-HT_{1A} receptor genetic polymorphism (Isaac, 1997), allelic variants of the 5-HT transporter (Artigas, 1997) or temperament factors (Tome *et al.*, 1997a). For all that, the increasing number of reports (Kraus, 1996; Maes *et al.*, 1996; Bakish *et al.*, 1997; Erfurth *et al.*, 1997; Perez *et al.*, 1997; Tome *et al.*, 1997b; Thomas *et al.*, 1997; Zanardi *et al.*, 1997; Bordet *et al.*, 1998; Perez *et al.*, 1999) and letters (Anderson, 1996; Bordet *et al.*, 1997; Isaac and Tome, 1997; Terao, 1997; Bell *et al.*, 1998; McAllister-Williams and Young, 1998) indicates that augmentation with pindolol is still a matter of debate. Recently McAskill *et al.* (1998) have compared six open label studies and six controlled studies with pindolol. The open label studies strongly suggest that pindolol may accelerate and augment the antidepressant response; however, controlled studies do not fully support these findings. The authors plead for larger, well-designed, controlled studies.

Lately several PET scan studies have been published on pindolol binding in the human brain (Andree *et al.*, 1999; Rabiner *et al.*, 2000a; Martinez *et al.*, 2000a). The studies agree that pindolol binds to somatodendritic 5-HT_{1A} autoreceptors at the doses used in clinical studies; however, receptor occupancy is moderate and highly variable. The latter may partly explain the varying outcomes of pindolol augmentation studies (Martinez *et al.*, 2000b; Rabiner *et al.*, 2000b).

In addition to major depression, the merit of pindolol augmentation has been investigated in psychotic depression (Kraus, 1997), obsessive-compulsive disorder (Blier and Bergeron, 1996; Koran *et al.*, 1996), treatment-resistant obsessive-compulsive disorder (Dannon *et al.*, 2000) and panic disorder (Dannon *et al.*, 1997).

In animal research the pindolol augmentation strategy has also gained attention. Data from electrophysiological (Arborelius *et al.*, 1995; Davidson and Stamford, 1995; Romero *et al.*, 1996) and microdialysis studies (Arborelius *et al.*, 1996; Gardier *et al.*, 1996; Romero *et al.*, 1996) in rats indicate a potentiation of the chronic effects of SSRIs on 5-HT neurotransmission by 5-HT_{1A} receptor antagonists, which is broadly compatible with the hypothesis raised by Artigas (1993). Recently, a microdialysis study in guinea pigs raised questions whether the pindolol doses used in the clinical studies were sufficient to augment 5-HT concentrations in the brain. In that particular study pindolol plasma levels 10–100 times higher than those reported in clinical studies were needed to augment the effect of paroxetine on extracellular 5-HT. On the other hand pindolol completely blocked central β-adrenoceptor function at plasma levels comparable with those measured in humans (Cremers et al., 2001).

The situation on the 5-HT$_{1A}$ receptor front has been becoming more and more complex since it was found that postsynaptic 5-HT$_{1A}$ receptors may also have a role in the regulation of 5-HT release. The idea was first hypothesized by Blier et al., 1987b and Blier & de Montigny, 1987. Since then several studies on this topic have been published (Ceci et al., 1994; Romero et al., 1994; Bosker et al., 1997; Casanovas et al., 1999). Interestingly, chronic treatment with citalopram via osmotic minipumps reduced postsynaptic 5-HT$_{1A}$ receptor-mediated feedback in the amygdala. Moreover, local infusion of WAY 100635, a 5-HT$_{1A}$ receptor antagonist, into the amygdala augmented the effect of citalopram, but the effect of WAY 100635 disappeared after chronic citalopram treatment (Bosker et al., 2001).

The notion that both pre-and postsynaptic 5-HT$_{1A}$ receptors may desensitize following chronic SSRI treatment makes augmentation strategies based on blockade of this receptor subtype even more interesting. It is to be hoped that registration of a potent and selective 5-HT$_{1A}$ receptor antagonist will not take too long.

Involvement of postsynaptic 5-HT$_{1A}$ and other 5-HT receptor subtypes in depression and anxiety An interesting but puzzling aspect of the pindolol augmentation strategy is the concomitant blockade of postsynaptic 5-HT$_{1A}$ receptors not involved in long feedback loops. Since pindolol is devoid of antidepressant properties and does at least not compromise SRI treatment, it can be argued that these postsynaptic 5-HT$_{1A}$ receptor-mediated processes are not crucial in the treatment of depression. This would also imply that the antidepressant effect of 5-HT$_{1A}$ (partial) receptor agonists (and SSRIs) is mediated through non-5-HT$_{1A}$ postsynaptic receptors.

Similar arguments can be raised against the involvement of 5-HT$_{2A}$ and 5-HT$_3$ receptors in the treatment of depression. The "5-HT and NA specific" antidepressant mirtazapine increases 5-HT in terminal areas through blockade of α_2-adrenoceptors (de Boer et al., 1995). It is also an antagonist at 5-HT$_{2A}$ and 5-HT$_3$ receptors (de Boer et al., 1995), and selective antagonists for the latter receptor subtypes seem devoid of antidepressant properties. Interestingly, the effect of the SSRI fluvoxamine on forced-swimming-induced immobility in mice, a model for depression, has been reported not to involve the 5-HT$_{1A}$ and 5-HT$_2$ receptor subtypes (Egawa et al., 1995). Similarly de Vry et al. (1997) hypothesized that 5-HT$_{1B/1D}$, 5-HT$_{2C}$, 5-HT$_3$ and 5-HT$_4$ receptors may not be critically involved in the therapeutic effects of SSRIs.

In contrast, postsynaptic 5-HT$_{1A}$, 5-HT$_2$ and 5-HT$_3$ receptors are likely to play a role in the treatment of certain dimensions of anxiety, as witnessed by the anxiolytic activity of compounds selective for these subtypes.

Summarizing, treatment of depression and anxiety may benefit from the same adaptive processes at the presynaptic level. Yet it is likely that therapeutic effects are brought about through divergent postsynaptic 5-HT receptors.

CHOLECYSTOKININ INVOLVEMENT IN ANXIETY

Cholecystokinin (CCK) is recognized as the most widely distributed neuropeptide in the brain. CCK-like immunoreactivity has been demonstrated in the cerebral cortex, olfactory bulb, hypothalamus, amygdala, hippocampus, striatum and spinal cord (Emson, 1982).

The functional role of CCK in the central nervous system has been an area of intensive investigation over the past 20 years. As a result of these investigations, a role for neuronal CCK has been proposed in feeding and satiety (for review, see Morley, 1990), pain perception (for review, see Wang *et al.*, 1990) and psychiatric diseases like schizophrenia and anxiety disorders (for review, see van Megen *et al.*, 1994a).

Evidence has been found for interactions between CCK and dopamine, γ-aminobutyric acid, serotonin, noradrenaline, excitatory amino acids and opioid peptides. In addition, CCK was found to be co-localized with several of these neurotransmitters (Yaksh *et al.*, 1987; Boden *et al.*, 1991; Harro *et al.*, 1992).

Distribution of cholecystokinin and cholecystokinin receptors in the human brain

CCK is distributed in many different brain areas (Rehfeld, 1978). The highest levels of CCK immunoreactivity are found in the (temporal and frontal) cortex, caudate nucleus, putamen, and in the hippocampus and subiculum; intermediate levels are found in the nucleus accumbens, septum, ventromedial thalamus, periaqueductal grey and substantia nigra, and pars compacta and low amounts are found in the globus pallidus, lateral thalamic nuclei and other mesoencephalic and metencephalic nuclei (Emson, 1982; Cross *et al.*, 1988).

CCK binding sites have been classified into CCK_A (alimentary) receptors, mainly found in the periphery, and CCK_B (brain) receptors, exclusively found in the brain, although more recent studies suggest that the CCK_B receptor may be homologous with the gastrin receptor. In humans, CCK_A receptors are found in the alimentary tract and discrete areas of the brain like the area postrema and nucleus solitarius, dorsal horn of the spinal cord, vagus nerve complex, hypothalamus, interpeduncular nucleus and substantia nigra (primates). CCK_B receptors are more widely distributed in the CNS and have been found in the cortex, olfactory bulb, nucleus accumbens, amygdala, hippocampus, caudate nucleus, cerebellum and hypothalamus.

Cholecystokinin challenge as a human panic model

According to the DSM-IV criteria, panic attacks are defined by a crescendo of extreme fear or apprehension concomitant with at least four out of 12 somatic symptoms

(American Psychiatric Association, 1994). Panic attacks do not exclusively occur in the course of PD, but are also found in other anxiety disorders (e.g. simple phobia, social phobia and obsessive-compulsive disorder according to DSM-IV). Panic attacks can also be provoked by a number of challenge agents such as mCPP, yohimbine, CO_2 inhalation and sodium lactate infusion (Liebowitz *et al.*, 1984, 1985, 1986; van den Hout and Griez, 1984; Griez *et al.*, 1987; den Boer *et al.*, 1989; Kahn and Wetzler, 1991; Zandbergen *et al.*, 1991; Klein *et al.*, 1991; Charney *et al.*, 1992; Albus *et al.*, 1992).

In an open label study, de Montigny (1989) found that the CCK_B receptor agonist CCK_4, in doses ranging from 20 to 150 mg, elicited panic-like symptoms in seven out of 10 healthy volunteers. Administration of the mixed $CCK_{A/B}$ receptor agonist CCK_8 to two subjects induced only gastrointestinal complaints, but no anxiety, suggesting that CCK_B receptors mediate the CCK induced anxiety (see Table 2.4).

To further elucidate the putative panicogenic effect of CCK_4, others have investigated the effect of CCK_4 in PD patients. In a double-blind study, 11 PD patients were challenged with 50 mg CCK_4 and saline on two separate occasions (Bradwejn *et al.*, 1990). All patients panicked with CCK_4 while none of the subjects panicked on saline. Patients judged CCK_4-induced symptomatology as identical to their naturally occurring panic attacks, but more abrupt in onset and more condensed in time. These findings have been confirmed in a single-blind placebo-controlled study using an unbalanced incomplete block design in PD patients (van Megen *et al.*, 1992). In this study, the panic rate with 50 mg CCK_4 was 71%, while 25 mg CCK_4 induced a panic rate of 44%. Again, none of the patients panicked on placebo. Bradwejn *et al.* (1992) conducted a dose-finding study in 29 PD patients with i.v. bolus injections of 0 mg, 10 mg, 15 mg, 20 mg and 25 mg CCK_4. He reported panic rates of 0%, 17%, 64%, 75% and 75%, respectively, suggesting a plateau in panic rate at dosages ranging from 20 mg and higher.

In a subsequent study, an enhanced sensitivity of PD patients to CCK_4 was found (Bradwejn *et al.*, 1991a). In this study, 10 out of 11 patients (91%) reported a panic attack following a 25 mg bolus injection of CCK_4, whereas only two out of 12 healthy controls (17%) experienced panic-like symptoms. The panic rate with 50 mg of CCK_4 was 100% for patients and 47% for controls.

Studies with the CCK_B receptor agonist pentagastrin, a synthetic analogue of CCK_4, have confirmed these observations (Abelson and Nesse, 1990, 1994; van Megen *et al.*, 1994b).

Effects of antidepressants and CCK_B receptor antagonists on CCK_4-induced panic

Bradwejn and Koszycki (1994a) reported that PD patients successfully treated with 100–300 mg imipramine showed a reduced sensitivity to the panicogenic effects of CCK_4. Only 18% had an panic attack after a 20 mg CCK_4 challenge. Imipramine has consistently been found clinically effective in the treatment of PD (for review, see Liebowitz *et al.*, 1985). Bradwejn and Koszycki's findings (1994a) suggest that a well established antipanic agent such as imipramine is able to abolish the panicogenic effects of CCK_4. These findings have been confirmed by van Megen *et al.* (1997a), who investigated the treatment effect of 150 mg fluvoxamine on CCK_4-induced panic attacks in PD patients. The reason for selecting fluvoxamine was that this drug has been found to be clinically effective in reducing both panic attacks and avoidance behaviour (den Boer *et al.*, 1987, 1989; den Boer and Westenberg, 1988; Hoehn Saric *et al.*, 1993; Black *et al.*, 1993). Before and after an 8-week double-blind placebo-controlled treatment phase, 26 PD patients were challenged with 50 mg CCK_4. In contrast to the patients treated with placebo, patients receiving fluvoxamine showed a statistically significant decrease of the CCK_4-induced panic after treatment (the panic rate dropped from 76% before treatment to 29% after 8 weeks of treatment). This effect was even more robust when comparing patients who responded to treatment versus those who did not. In the responder group the panic rate declined from 75% to 13%.

Bradwejn *et al.* (1994b) studied the effect of the GABA antagonist flumazenil (2 mg) on CCK_4 panic in 30 healthy volunteers. Flumazenil did not change the panic elicited by CCK_4, indicating that the anxiogenic effects of CCK_4 are not mediated through GABA receptors.

In a collaborative study Bradwejn *et al.* (1994c) investigated the effect of a selective CCK_B receptor antagonist L-365,260 on CCK_4-induced panic attacks in PD patients. In this double-blind placebo-controlled study, 24 PD patients were treated with two different dosages of L-365,260 (10, 50 mg) on two separate occasions and were subsequently challenged with 20 mg CCK_4. Both L-365,260 dosages significantly reduced the likelihood of PD patients to respond to CCK_4 with a panic attack. Moreover, 50 mg L-365,260 was able to block the CCK_4-elicited panic attacks completely. Similarly, L-365,260 significantly reduced the number of somatic anxiety symptoms induced by CCK_4. These results are in line with the findings of Lines *et al.* (1995), who investigated the effect of L-365,260 (10 mg and 50 mg) or placebo on an i.v. bolus injection of pentagastrin (0.3 mg/kg) in 15 healthy volunteers. In accordance with the effect of L-365,260 in Bradwejn *et al.*'s study (1994c), 10 mg partially reversed the pentagastrin-induced symptoms, while 50 mg blocked the effects completely. In contrast to these findings, we found that the CCK_B receptor antagonist CI-988 was unable to block CCK_4-induced panic in patients with PD (van Megen *et al.*, 1997b).

This raises the question whether the effect of CCK_B receptor antagonists on CCK_4-induced panic can be generalized to panic induced by other panicogenic agents and, ultimately, to naturally occurring panic attacks.

In a double-blind placebo-controlled study in which PD patients were pretreated with 50 mg L-365,260, significantly less anxiety was reported following lactate infusion compared to patients pretreated with placebo (van Megen *et al.*, 1994c). L-365,260 treatment resulted in a 50% reduction of the panic rate; however, this reduction was not statistically significant. In contrast to the effect on fear and apprehension, L-365,260 was unable to block the physical symptoms elicited by lactate

Table 2.4. Cholecystokinin challenge in humans.

Author/year	Design/compound	N/diagnosis	Dose (Panic rate, %)				
de Montigny, 1989	Open, CCK4	10 Volunteers	20–100 µg (70)				
Bradwejn et al., 1990	Double-blind, CCK4	11 PD	0 (0)		50 µg (100)		
Abelson and Nesse, 1990	Open, pentagastrin		0.6 µg				
		4 PD	(60–80)				
		4 Controls	(0–25)				
Bradwejn et al., 1991	Double-blind, CCK4	12 PD	0 (9)	25 µg (91)	50 µg (100)		
		15 controls	0 (0)	25 µg (17)	50 µg (47)		
Bradwejn et al., 1992	Double-blind CCK4	29 PD	0 (0)	10 µg (17)	15 µg (64)	20 µg (75)	
van Megen et al., 1992	Single-blind, CCK4	12 PD	0 (0)	25 µg (44)	50 µg (71)	25 µg (75)	
van Megen et al., 1994b	Double-blind, pentagastrin	15 PD	0 (0)	0.1 µg (50)	0.3 µg (67)	0.6 µg/kg (50)	
		15 Controls	0 (0)	0.1 µg (0)	0.3 µg (0)	(13)	
van Megen et al., 1994c	Double-blind, L-365, 260-placebo 0.5 M/min/kg lactate infusion	24 PD	0 (50)		50 µg (25)		
van Megen et al., 1997a	Double-blind, treatment fluvoxamine-placebo, CCK4 challenge	26 PD	Pretreatment Placebo (67)	150 mg (76)	Post-treatment Placebo (56)	150 mg (29)	
Bradwejn et al., 1994c	Double-blind, L-365,260 20 µg CCK4	24 PD	Placebo (87)	10 mg (33)	50 mg L-365,260 (0)		

Study	Design	Subjects			
Bradwejn et al, 1994b	Double-blind cross-over, flumazenil 20 µg CCK$_4$	30 Volunteers	0 (47)	20 mg (43)	
Bradwejn et al, 1994d	Double-blind, placebo-saline placebo-50 µg CCK$_4$, 100 mg CI-988 50 µg CCK$_4$	30 Volunteers	Placebo + saline (0)	Placebo + CCK$_4$ (53)	CI-988 + CCK$_4$ (27)
Bradwejn et al, 1994a	Treatment with 100–300 mg of imipramine, challenge with 20 µg CCK$_4$	11 PD patients	18% on treatment		
Abelson and Nesse, 1994	Single-blind, pentagastrin	10 PD 9 Controls	Saline (0)(0)	0.6 µg (70)(11)	
Lines et al, 1995	Double-blind five-period cross-over design; a. placebo–saline b. placebo–pentagastrin 0.3 µg/kg c. L-365,260 10 mg–pentagastrin 0.3 µg/kg d. L-365,260 50 mg–pentagastrin 0.3 µg/kg e. L-365,260 0.3 µg/kg 50 mg–saline	15 Volunteers			

Group	a	b	c	d	e
VAS score	16	123	39	16	14
PSS score	1.1	19.3	7.0	3.0	0.6

PD = panic disorder. Adapted from van Megen *et al.* (1996), with permission.

infusion. These data suggest that L-365,260 may possess anxiolytic but not antipanic properties.

In a 6-week multi-centre placebo-controlled trial, the effect of L-365,260 (30 mg q.i.d.) on PD was investigated in 88 patients (Kramer et al., 1995). This study revealed no clinically significant differences between L-365,260 and placebo in global improvement ratings, Hamilton anxiety ratings, panic attack frequency and intensity or disability measurements. These results suggest that L-365,260, at the dose tested, is not effective in the treatment of PD. Although these preliminary findings with repeated dosing of L-365,260 are not encouraging, it is possible that the bioavailability of L-365,260 is too low. Interestingly, in one study, (Cutler et al., 1994), an anxiolytic effect was reported in PD, as measured by the inter-panic Hamilton Rating Scale of anxiety.

In summary, in PD several studies have shown that CCK_B receptor agonists like CCK_4 and pentagastrin are able to induce panic attacks in PD. Pretreatment with the CCK_B receptor antagonist L-365,260 dose-dependently blocks the ability of CCK_4 to induce panic attacks, which could not be corroborated with the CCK_B receptor antagonist CI-988. In addition, treatment with the SSRI fluvoxamine protects against the panic-inducing properties of CCK_4. The outcome of treatment studies with CCK_B receptor antagonists is disappointing in that no clinically relevant anxiolytic effect was found.

Cholecystokin in obsessive-compulsive disorder and social phobia

In a recent study we hypothesized that pentagastrin would increase anxiety in OCD without a concomitant increase in obsessions or compulsive behaviours. Seven female patients and seven matched healthy controls entered the study. Subjects were tested on two separate occasions, one week apart, in a double-blind, placebo-controlled design. Included were patients who fulfilled DSM-III-R criteria for OCD and whose Hamilton Depression Rating Scale (HAMD) scores did not exceed 15. The dosage of pentagastrin was 0.6 mg/kg.

In this study none of the patients showed increases in the severity of obsessions or compulsive complaints. In five out of seven patients a panic attack occurred shortly after the bolus injection of pentagastrin. In the control group only one volunteer showed a panic-like response on pentagastrin. Placebo was without effect in all subjects (de Leeuw et al., 1996).

In patients with social phobia, too, provocation with pentagastrin resulted in panic-like reactions in five out of seven social phobic patients (71%) and two out of seven controls (29%; van Vliet et al., 1997).

These results indicate an enhanced sensitivity for pentagastrin in PD, OCD and social phobic patients compared to controls. The results with pentagastrin obtained so far, indicate that patients with anxiety disorders, irrespective of nosological background, are more sensitive to the panic-inducing properties of this agent than are healthy controls.

Based upon these findings it may be hypothesized that the propensity to react with anxiety symptoms may be detected with pentagastrin challenge in different psychiatric syndromes. If this hypothesis is true, then patients with anxious depression should also exhibit panic attacks after pentagastrin challenge, whereas patients with major depression without anxiety symptoms should not. To date, no studies with CCK_4 or pentagastrin have been performed in depression.

BRAIN REGIONS INVOLVED IN DEPRESSION AND ANXIETY: NEUROIMAGING STUDIES

This section reviews the literature on neuroimaging research in panic disorder (PD), obsessive-compulsive disorder (OCD) and major depressive disorder (MDD). Other anxiety disorders will not be mentioned here, because neuroimaging studies are very scarce in those fields. In this section neuroimaging techniques are restricted to structural imaging techniques like computed tomography (CT) and magnetic resonance imaging (MRI) and functional imaging techniques such as positron emission tomography (PET), single photon emission computerised tomography (SPECT) and functional MRI.

Neuroimaging in depression

Neuroimaging research in mood disorders has focused on both primary and secondary mood disorders. In primary depression structural imaging studies have shown demonstrable results only in studies where large groups of patients were compared with healthy controls (Jeste *et al.*, 1988; Nasrallah *et al.*, 1989). Subtle reductions in size of the hippocampus (Krishnan *et al.*, 1991; Mervaala *et al.*, 2000), basal ganglia (Husain *et al.*, 1991), frontal lobes (Dolan *et al.*, 1990; Coffey *et al.*, 1993; Kumar *et al.*, 1997) and temporal lobes (Hauser *et al.*, 1989) were reported. A finding of some consistency, at least in older depressed patients, is so-called subcortical hyperintensities which have been found in subcortical white matter, basal ganglia and frontal lobes (Hickie *et al.*, 1995; Greenwald *et al.*, 1996). Recently, a "vascular depression" hypothesis was raised to account for these findings (Alexopoulos *et al.*, 1997; Krishnan *et al.*, 1997). Briefly, this hypothesis stated that depression (mainly late-onset depression) can be caused by cerebrovascular disease (in the form of white matter hyperintensities) affecting white matter pathways and subcortical structures involved in mood regulation. Evidence has been found for this hypothesis, but it is possible that the higher rates of white matter hyperintensities in older depressed patients are in part a reflection of a greater prevalence of cerebrovascular risk factors in this group. The data of Lenze and co-workers (1999), who tried to untangle the effects of depression and cerebrovascular risk factors, seem to point in that direction.

Increased ventricular size has also been reported by several researchers (Shima *et al.*, 1984; Kellner *et al.*, 1986; Schlegel *et al.*, 1989a). Two recent MRI studies investigated differences in ventricular size and brain tissue volume between MDD patients and healthy controls, but were unable to replicate previously reported findings (Greenwald et al., 1997; Pillay et al., 1997). Meta-analyses have shown that ventricular enlargement is apparent in older depressed patients, and that patients with mood disorders have less ventricular enlargement than patients with schizophrenia (Elkis et al., 1995). Apart from the fact that the aetiology and significance of this non-specific finding is still unclear, it is also a matter of debate why equivocal results have been reported. Currently it is impossible to make a positive diagnosis of depression in individual patients on the basis of CT or MRI findings (George et al., 1993; Drevets, 1998).

PET and SPECT studies have implicated several brain regions in primary depression (see Table 2.5). The dorsolateral prefrontal area, the anterior cingulate cortex, the basal ganglia and the temporal lobes have all been shown to be implicated in primary depression (Ebert and Ebmeier, 1996; Videbech, 2000). In a classic PET study Baxter and co-workers (1989) have shown that hypometabolism in the left anterolateral prefrontal cortex was characteristic of patients with unipolar depression, bipolar depression or OCD with comorbid depression. OCD patients without comorbid depression or healthy control did not show this hypometabolism. The study of Martinot et al. (1990a) confirmed this finding.

Using PET, Bench and co-workers (1992) reported on regional cerebral blood flow (r-CBF) differences in patients with primary depression, as compared to healthy controls. They found patients were characterized by a decreased r-CBF in the left dorsolateral prefrontal cortex and the left anterior cingulate cortex.

Bench and co-workers (1995) reported on changes in r-CBF on recovery from depression. In this study patients were rescanned following clinical remission. An increased r-CBF was evident in the left dorsolateral prefrontal cortex and the medial prefrontal cortex, which includes the anterior cingulate. It appears that the relationship between brain perfusion and clinical symptoms is state-dependent, because the abnormal r-CBF findings dissolved together with the depressed symptoms. This normalization of brain perfusion has been reported in several studies using various treatment modalities (Wu et al., 1992; Goodwin et al., 1993; Buchsbaum et al., 1997; Smith GS et al., 1999).

Short-term tryptophan depletion in remitted depressed patients has been shown to result in depressive relapse (see above). Bremner and co-workers (1997) investigated this phenomenon with ^{18}F-fluorodeoxyglucose (^{18}F-DG) PET. Tryptophan depletion induced relapse in seven out of 21 patients. In these patients a decrease in brain metabolism was evident in the dorsolateral prefrontal cortex, thalamus and orbitofrontal cortex. Another study, using $H_2^{15}O$ PET, reported similar findings in a group of eight recovered depressed men (Smith KA et al., 1999).

Recently Mayberg and co-workers (1997) have further elucidated the relationship between depression and hypometabolism. They investigated the relationship between pretreatment cerebral glucose metabolism and antidepressant drug response. Metabolism in the rostral anterior cingulate uniquely differentiated responders and non-responders to antidepressant treatment at baseline. As a group the depressed

Table 2.5. Functional imaging studies in major depressive disorder.

Method	Control/MDD	Laterality	Findings
^{133}Xenon			
Sackeim *et al.*, 1990	40/41	None	Global ↓; frontal ↓; temporal ↓; parietal ↓
^{195m}Au			
Schlegel *et al.*, 1989b	21/21	None	Global ↓; temporal ↓
^{99m}Tc-exametazime			
Austin *et al.*, 1992	20/40	None	Interior frontal ↓; temporal ↓; parietal ↓
Yazici *et al.*, 1992	10/14	L > R	Temporal ↓
Goodwin *et al.*, 1993	—/28 (twice)	Yes	On remission: inferior anterior cingulate ↑; basal ganglia ↑; R thalamus ↑; R posterior cingulate ↑
Maes *et al.*, 1993	12/31	None	None
Mayberg *et al.*, 1994a	11/31	None	Inferior frontal ↓; cingulate ↓
^{18}F-DG PET			
Post *et al.*, 1987	18/13	R > L	Temporal ↓
Baxter *et al.*, 1989	12/14 OCD/ 10 OCD + MDD/ 10 bipolar/10	L > R	In MDD, bipolar and OCD + MDD: anterolateral prefrontal ↓
Martinot *et al.*, 1990a	10/10	L > R	Inferior and superior frontal ↓
Francois *et al.*, 1995	12/12	None	Frontal ↓
Bremner *et al.*, 1997	—/21 (twice)	None	After tryptophan depletion induced relapse: dorsolateral prefrontal ↓; thalamus ↓; orbitofrontal ↓
Mayberg *et al.*, 1997	15/18	None	Rostral anterior cingulate: ↓ in non-responders, ↑ in responders
^{15}O PET			
Bench *et al.*, 1992	23/33	L > R	Dorsolateral prefrontal ↓; anterior cingulate ↓
Dolan *et al.*, 1992	—/33	Yes	Cognitive impaired MD: L anterior medial prefrontal cortex ↓; cerebellar vermis ↑
Drevets and Raichle, 1992	33/13	L > R	Prefrontal ↑; amygdala ↑; medial caudate ↓
Bench *et al.*, 1995	—/25 (twice)	L > R	On remission: dorsolateral prefrontal cortex ↑; medial prefrontal cortex ↑

Control/MDD means number of controls and patients; laterality is given when the effect is evident more in one side; findings are shown in comparison to healthy controls, unless stated otherwise.

patients were characterized by hypometabolism in this brain area, as compared to controls, but further analyses revealed that non-responders were characterized by hypometabolism, whereas responders to treatment were hypermetabolic.

Other studies have also reported a decreased metabolism in the frontal lobes using PET (Dolan *et al.*, 1992; Francois *et al.*, 1995) or SPECT (Sackeim *et al.*, 1990; Austin *et al.*, 1992; Mayberg *et al.*, 1994a). Not all studies could replicate this finding: Maes and co-workers (1993) did not see any r-CBF abnormalities using SPECT. Drevets and Raichle (1992) reported on a PET study where they found an increased r-CBF in the left prefrontal cortex, amygdala and the medial thalamus and a decreased r-CBF in the medial caudate in patients with familial pure depressive disease, a subtype of unipolar depression (Winokur, 1982). Whether these findings can be explained by differences in methodology or patient group remains unclear.

Hypometabolism, or a reduced r-CBF, in the temporal lobes has been described by several researchers (Post *et al.*, 1987; Schlegel *et al.*, 1989b; Austin *et al.*, 1992; Yazici *et al.*, 1992). In most studies this was found together with abnormalities in the paralimbic region, or more specifically the inferior frontal and cingulate cortex. In the study of Mayberg and co-workers (1994a) the paralimbic region showed the most pronounced decrease.

Research in secondary depression has focused on the fact that injury to some brain areas is much more likely to produce depression than injury to other brain areas (Cummings, 1993). In several neurological diseases depression is common, particularly with diseases involving the basal ganglia (Mayberg, 1994b). Changes in both mood and cognitive performance are very common in Parkinson's disease, in Huntington's disease and following ischaemic lesions of the striatum (Mendez *et al.*, 1989; McHugh, 1990). In diseases with generalized or randomly distributed pathologies, such as multiple sclerosis or Alzheimer's disease, secondary depression is also quite common (Salloway *et al.*, 1988; Rabins *et al.*, 1991; Kumar *et al.*, 1993; Hirono *et al.*, 1998). Because the clinical presentation of depressive symptoms in neurological patients is similar to those seen in primary depression, it has been argued that neurological depressions are useful and appropriate models in the study of the pathophysiology of mood disorders in general (Mayberg, 1994b).

The affected regions thought to be responsible for secondary depression in neurological diseases are very similar to those regions which appear associated with primary depression. Studies using functional imaging techniques suggest that bilateral hypometabolism in the paralimbic regions (orbital-inferior prefrontal cortex and anterior temporal cortex) is associated with depression, independent of disease aetiology (Mayberg, 1994b). In her excellent review of frontal lobe dysfunction in secondary depression, Mayberg (1994b) proposed a depression model which attempts to explain this finding. The regional localization of the metabolic abnormalities matches two known pathways: the orbitofrontal–basal ganglia–thalamic circuit and the basotemporal limbic circuit that links the orbitofrontal cortex and the anterior temporal cortex. Neurologic disease-specific interruptions in these pathways could explain the characteristic paralimbic frontal and temporal metabolic defects that have been identified and could reconcile the presence of similar clinical symptomatology in the settings of different disease aetiologies.

Neuroimaging in panic disorder

Neuroimaging techniques have not been used as extensively in PD as in obsessive-compulsive disorder (OCD) or major depressive disorder (MDD). Panic disorder patients do not appear to be characterized by anatomical abnormalities that could be detected with CT (Uhde and Kellner, 1987; Lepola *et al.*, 1990; de Cristofaro *et al.*, 1993). Two studies using qualitative MRI reported an increased rate of focal atrophy or abnormal signal intensities in the temporal lobes, as compared to healthy controls (Ontiveros *et al.*, 1989; Fontaine *et al.*, 1990). Recently, a quantitative MRI study was carried out which reported that the mean volume of the temporal lobes in PD patients was smaller than in healthy subjects (Vythilingam *et al.*, 2000). These authors also measured hippocampal volumes, but no differences were found in that brain region. The authors speculate on the relation between PD symptoms and decreased temporal lobe volumes, but more evidence is needed to elucidate this link.

Several neuroimaging studies have focused on the panic-provoking properties of sodium lactate. An infusion with sodium lactate has consistently been shown to provoke panic-like attacks in PD patients, but not in healthy volunteers (Liebowitz *et al.*, 1985; Aronson *et al.*, 1989; den Boer *et al.*, 1989; Shear *et al.*, 1991; Goetz *et al.*, 1997).

Reiman and co-workers investigated differences in r-CBF using PET in PD patients with a positive response to sodium lactate, while at rest (Reiman, 1987; Reiman *et al.*, 1984, 1986) and during an infusion (Reiman *et al.*, 1989). In resting PD patients, sensitive to sodium lactate, they found an abnormal asymmetry (left less than right) in r-CBF in the region of the parahippocampal gyrus, which was absent in normal controls (Reiman *et al.*, 1984, 1986; see Table 2.6). They also reported an abnormally high whole-brain metabolism in this group (Reiman *et al.*, 1986; Reiman, 1987).

De Cristofaro and co-workers (1993) also reported a left (less than) right asymmetry in r-CBF in a similar patient sample. This asymmetry was found in the inferior frontal cortex by using SPECT with ^{99m}Tc-hexamethylpropylene amine oxime (HMPAO) as tracer. They also reported an increased r-CBF in the left occipital cortex and a bilateral decrease in the hippocampal region.

Nordahl *et al.* (1990) investigated regional glucose metabolic rates in PD patients during an auditory discrimination task using PET. Similar to Reiman *et al.* (1986, 1987) they also found an asymmetry in the hippocampal region, but did not find an increased whole-brain metabolism. Furthermore, a metabolic decrease was observed in the left inferior parietal lobule and in the anterior cingulate. An increase was seen in the metabolic rate of the medial orbital frontal cortex.

Bisaga *et al.* (1998), using ^{18}F-DG PET, also reported on the involvement of the hippocampal and parahippocampal areas in PD. They also reported a decrease in metabolic rate in the right inferior parietal and the right superior temporal areas.

Table 2.6. Functional imaging studies in panic disorder.

Method	Control/PD	Laterality	Findings
[133]Xenon			
Stewart et al., 1988	5/10	None	PD panickers during lactate: global ↑ or ↓
[99]Tc HMPAO			
de Cristofaro et al., 1993	5/7	Yes	L ↓/R asymmetry inferior frontal; L occipital ↑; hip-pocampal ↓
[123]I Iomazenil			
Schlegel et al., 1994	10/10	None	Compared to epileptic patients: frontal ↓; occipital ↓; temporal ↓
Kaschka et al., 1995	9/9	L > R	PD + MD compared to dysthymic patients: inferior temporal ↓; inferior frontal ↓
Kuikka et al., 1995	17/17	Yes	L/R ↑ asymmetry middle and inferior frontal
^{18}F-DG PET			
Nordahl et al., 1990	30/12	Yes	L ↓/R asymmetry PHG; L inferior parietal ↓; anterior cingulate ↓; medial orbitofrontal ↑
[15]O PET			
Reiman et al., 1984	6/10	Yes	L ↓/R asymmetry PHG
Reiman et al., 1986	25/16	Yes	L ↓/R asymmetry PHG; global ↑
Reiman et al., 1989	18/24	Yes	PD panickers during lactate: temporal ↑; insular ↑; claustrum ↑; sup. colliculis ↑; L anterior cerebellar vermis ↑

Control/PD means number of controls and patients; laterality is given when the effect is evident more in one side; findings are shown in comparison to healthy controls, unless stated otherwise; PHG = parahippocampal gyrus.

Stewart et al. (1988), using ^{133}Xe SPECT, and Reiman et al. (1989), using PET, reported on changes in r-CBF during sodium lactate infusion, but with conflicting results. Stewart and co-workers (1988) noted an increase in r-CBF in healthy volunteers and non-panicking PD patients. Patients who panicked either showed a minimal increase or a decrease in r-CBF. Reiman et al. (1989) reported an increased r-CBF in panicking PD patients in a several brain areas (temporal poles, insular cortex, claustrum, or lateral putamen, superior colliculus, left anterior cerebellar vermis). This increase in r-CBF was not seen in healthy volunteers or non-panicking PD patients.

Differences in study design might explain these inconsistent findings, but the fact remains that most studies implicate the hippocampal region in PD. Other regions, like the anterior cingulate or the inferior frontal/orbital frontal cortex, are less consistently reported to be implicated in PD.

Several studies have investigated the benzodiazepine receptor function in PD with SPECT (Schlegel et al., 1994; Kaschka et al., 1995; Kuikka et al., 1995, Bremner et *al.*, 2000) or PET (Malizia *et al.*, 1998) All the SPECT studies used ^{123}I-iomazenil as a ligand. In the PET study ^{11}C-flumazenil was used. Schlegel and co-workers (1994) found lower ^{123}I-iomazenil uptake rates in the frontal, occipital and temporal cortex, as compared to epileptic patients. Kaschka *et al.* (1995) compared PD patients with a comorbid depression with a group of dysthymic patients. They reported a decreased regional activity in the lateral and the medial inferior temporal lobes and in the interior frontal lobes. Apart from the decrease in the medial inferior temporal lobe, which was only evident on the left side of the brain, all effects were bilateral. Kuikka and co-workers (1995) compared PD patients to healthy controls. They found an increased right : left ratio of benzodiazepine uptake in a majority of the patients. Magnetic resonance imaging (MRI) indicated that the affected region was located in the right middle and inferior frontal gyri. Bremner and co-workers (2000) recently reported on decreased benzodiazepine receptor binding in the left hippocampus. A significant decrease was also evident in the precuneus. They also had the opportunity to compare the receptor binding of PD patients who had a panic attack at the time of the scan with PD patients who did not. The panickers showed a decrease in the prefrontal cortex.

In the only PET study to date, Malizia and co-workers (1998) reported a global decrease in benzodiazepine receptor binding, with the greatest magnitude in the right orbitofrontal cortex and insula.

All the imaging studies which investigated benzodiazepine receptor function in PD patients consistently report a reduced uptake/binding in the frontal cortex. Findings in other brain regions are less consistent. Methodological differences between the studies might explain the different findings.

Neuroimaging in obsessive-compulsive disorder

In anxiety disorders most research using neuroimaging techniques has focused on obsessive-compulsive disorder (OCD). Structural imaging studies using techniques like CT or MRI have gathered evidence for brain structural abnormalities in the frontostriatal circuits, such as significantly smaller striatal volumes (Robinson *et al.*, 1995; Rosenberg and Keshavan, 1998) and increased volume of the prefrontal cortex (Rosenberg and Keshavan, 1998). Whether OCD patients are also characterized by ventricular enlargement is still a matter of debate, as conflicting results have been reported. Two studies in early-onset OCD reported an increase in ventricle-to-brain ratio (VBR) (Behar *et al.*, 1984; Luxenberg *et al.*, 1988). Apart from this non-specific measure of generalized atrophy, both studies also reported a decrease in the volume of the caudate nucleus. Robinson and co-workers (1995), studying a more general OCD population, also reported a significantly smaller caudate nucleus volume, but they did not find differences in VBR. Four further studies of more general OCD populations were unable to find any differences in volumetric parameters (Insel *et al.*, 1983; Kellner *et al.*, 1991; Zitterl *et al.*, 1994; Aylward *et al.*, 1996). Jenike and co-workers (1996) recently reported lower white-matter volume in OCD patients as compared to healthy controls. These results suggest a widely distributed brain abnormality in OCD. Functional imaging studies should further explore the significance of this finding.

Research in OCD using functional imaging techniques has focused on differences between normal subjects and patients while at rest and during induction of psychopathology, and on changes due to treatment (see Tables 2.7 and 2.8).

Baxter and co-workers (1987, 1988) were among the first researchers to use PET in OCD. They reported an increased metabolic rate in resting OCD patients in the left orbital gyrus and bilaterally in the caudate nuclei. In further studies a more or less consistent pattern of hypermetabolism in several brain areas has been reported (Swedo *et al.*, 1989; Benkelfat *et al.*, 1990; Machlin *et al.*, 1991; Perani *et al.*, 1995).

This hypermetabolism, which differentiates OCD patients from normal controls, is evident in the orbitofrontal cortex, anterior cingulate, caudate nuclei and thalamus. Maliza and Nutt (1997) remark that these brain regions are in accordance with a postulated neural circuitry for a comparator system which results in willed action. The observed overactivity while at rest should account for the spontaneous generation of classical OCD psychopathology. (For a recent overview of the theory of the functional neuroanatomy of OCD, see Saxena and Rauch, 2000.)

A few studies reported hypometabolism in the same anatomical locations (Martinot *et al.*, 1990b; Edmonstone *et al.*, 1994). In both studies patients were receiving treatment, whereas in the other studies this was not the case. Lucey and co-workers (1997) reported reduced r-CBF in the caudate nucleus of OCD patients as compared to PD patients and normal controls. Even when the medicated patients (four in each group) were removed, the decreased r-CBF remained statistically significant. Apparently, medication status alone can not account for the different findings.

A recent voxel-based SPECT study with a large sample of unmedicated patients did not find any significant r-CBF differences in subcortical nuclei (Busatto *et al.*, 2000). The authors suggest that functional abnormalities in that brain region are not invariably present in OCD. This may be due to the fact that OCD patients are not a phenotypically homogeneous group. An often-used subdivision is made between patients with compulsive washing (washers) and patients with compulsive checking (checkers). In a functional MRI study Phillips and co-workers (2000) investigated whether washers and checkers show different neural responses to disgusting visual stimuli. Both groups, and normal controls, were shown pictures which were cued to elicit responses from washers. A differential neural response was observed in washers versus checkers, with, surprisingly, the latter group showing more activation of the frontostriatal brain regions, which are thought to be associated with the urge to ritualize (McGuire *et al.*, 1994; Rauch *et al.*, 1994; Breiter *et al.*, 1996). The authors suggest that washers directed their attention more to the emotive component of the pictures, at the expense of the urge to ritualize (Phillips *et al.*, 2000). This study highlights the need for further investigations in OCD subgroups to further clarify this issue, but it also demonstrates the complexity of visual information processing in pathological states.

Table 2.7. Functional imaging studies in obsessive-compulsive disorder: PET and f-MRI studies.

Method	Control/OCD	Laterality	Findings
^{18}F-DG PET			
Baxter *et al.*, 1987	14/14/14 MD	Yes	OCD compared to both groups: L orbital gyrus ↑; caudate nucleus ↑
Baxter *et al.*, 1988	10/10	None	Global ↑; head caudate nucleus ↑; orbital gyri ↑
Swedo *et al.*, 1989	18/18	Yes	L orbitofrontal ↑; R sensimotor ↑; prefrontal ↑; anterior cingulate ↑
Benkelfat *et al.*, 1990	—/8 (twice)	Yes	During treatment with clomipramine: L caudate ↓; orbitofrontal ↓; anterior putamen ↑
Martinot *et al.*, 1990b	8/16	None	Global ↓; prefrontal lateral ↓
Baxter *et al.*, 1992	—/18 (twice)	R > L	After treatment with either fluoxetine or behaviour therapy: head caudate nucleus ↓
Swedo *et al.*, 1992	—/13 (twice)	None	After 1 year of pharmacotherapy: orbitofrontal ↓
Perani *et al.*, 1995	15/11	None	Cingulate ↑; thalamus ↑; pallidum/putamen ↑ After SSRI treatment: cingulate ↓
Schwartz *et al.*, 1996	—/9 (twice)	None	After behavioural and cognitive treatment: caudate nucleus ↓
[15]O PET			
McGuire *et al.*, 1994	—/4	Yes	During *in vivo* exposure: R inferior frontal ↑; caudate nucleus ↑; striatum ↑; L hippocampus ↑; L posterior cingulate ↑
Rauch *et al.*, 1994	—/8	Yes	During *in vivo* exposure: R caudate nucleus ↑; L anterior cingulate ↑; orbitofrontal ↑
f-MRI			
Breiter *et al.*, 1996	5/10	None	During *in vivo* exposure: medial orbitofrontal ↑; lateral frontal ↑; anterior temporal ↑; anterior cingulate ↑; insular ↑; caudate ↑; lenticulate ↑; amygdala ↑

Control/OCD means number of controls and patients; laterality is given when the effect is evident more in one side; findings are shown in comparison to healthy controls, unless stated otherwise.

Table 2.8. Functional imaging studies in obsessive-compulsive disorder: SPECT studies.

Method	Control/OCD	Laterality	Findings
[133]Xenon			
Zohar *et al.*, 1989	—/10	None	During *in vivo* exposure: global ↓
Rubin *et al.*, 1992	10/10	None	None
Hollander *et al.*, 1995	—/14	None	In patients responding to *m*CPP: global ↑
Rubin *et al.*, 1995	—/8 (twice)	None	During treatment with clomipramine: none
[99m]Tc-exametazime			
Edmonstone *et al.*, 1994	12/12/12 MD	None	OCD compared to both groups: basal ganglia ↓
[99]Tc HMPAO			
Hoehn Saric *et al.*, 1991	—/6 (twice)	None	During treatment with fluoxetine: hyperfrontality ↓
Machlin *et al.*, 1991	8/10	None	Mediofrontal ↑
Rubin *et al.*, 1992	10/10	Yes	L posterofrontal ↑; high dorsal parietal ↑; orbitofrontal ↑
Rubin *et al.*, 1995	—/8 (twice)	None	During treatment with clomipramine: orbitofrontal ↓; posterofrontal ↓; high dorsal parietal ↓
Ho Pian *et al.*, 1997	8/7	None	After *m*-CPP: frontal ↓; parietal ↓; caudate nucleus ↓; thalamus ↓
Lucey *et al.*, 1997	15/15/15 PD	Yes	R caudate nucleus ↓

Control/OCD means number of controls and patients; laterality is given when the effect is evident more in one side; findings are shown in comparison to healthy controls, unless stated otherwise.

A few studies have investigated metabolic changes due to the induction of psychopathology using *m*CPP as a challenge (Hollander *et al.*, 1995; Ho Pian *et al.*, 1998b) or exposure to provocative stimuli (Zohar *et al.*, 1989; McGuire *et al.*, 1994; Rauch *et al.*, 1994; Breiter *et al.*, 1996).

The serotonin agonist *m*CPP has been reported to induce obsessive-compulsive symptoms in some patients (for a review, see den Boer and Westenberg, 1997). Hollander and co-workers (1995) reported an increase in global perfusion in patients who responded to *m*CPP with an exacerbation of obsessive-compulsive symptoms. The patients in the study of Ho Pian and co-workers (1998b) did not show an increase of obsessive-compulsive symptoms on *m*CPP, but it nevertheless produced changes in r-CBF. On placebo, patients showed an increased r-CBF in the frontal and parietal cortex, caudate nucleus and thalamus, as compared to controls. *m*CPP induced a significant reduction in r-CBF in these brain regions in patients, but not in controls. The effects of *m*CPP in OCD patients are a still a matter of debate, as different studies show different results (den Boer and Westenberg, 1997).

Zohar *et al.* (1989) reported on a ^{133}Xe SPECT study, where patients were scanned during *in vivo* exposure to provocative stimuli. They found a decrease in cortical blood flow during exposure. Two PET studies also reported changes in r-CBF during *in vivo* exposure (McGuire *et al.*, 1994; Rauch *et al.*, 1994). They found increased metabolic activity in the caudate nucleus, frontal cortex, anterior cingulate, thalamus, putamen and globus pallidus. Recently a study was performed with functional MRI (f-MRI), using the same challenge paradigm (Breiter *et al.*, 1996). In patients, but not in controls, statistical maps showed activation in the medial orbitofrontal, lateral frontal, anterior temporal, anterior cingulate and insular cortex, as well as caudate, lenticulate and amygdala. It appears that the f-MRI study and PET studies show similar results. A possible explanation why Zohar and co-workers (1989) found different results may be the use of ^{133}Xe SPECT. Rubin *et al.* (1992) carried out a SPECT study with both ^{133}Xe and ^{99m}Tc HMPAO. Metabolic changes, evident with ^{99m}Tc HMPAO, were not visible with ^{133}Xe. Apparently ^{133}Xe SPECT has less resolution, which may account for different findings.

Several studies have looked at response to treatment with selective serotonin reuptake inhibitors (SSRIs) (Hoehn Saric *et al.*, 1991; Baxter *et al.*, 1992; Swedo *et al.*, 1992; Perani *et al.*, 1995; Rubin *et al.*, 1995; Saxena *et al.*, 1999) or behavioural therapy (Baxter *et al.*, 1992; Schwartz *et al.*, 1996). Most studies reported a reduction of the typical "hyperfrontality" in OCD patients, or, more specifically, a decrease in metabolism in the caudate nucleus (particularly right) and in the orbitofrontal cortex. Interestingly this change occurred irrespective of treatment: pharmacotherapy and behavioural therapy produced comparable changes in cerebral functioning.

CONCLUDING REMARKS

Neuroimaging techniques have become an indispensable tool in modern-day psychiatric research. These techniques all allow us a view inside the living brain. Unfortunately the field is difficult to overview because of the equivocal results. There are quite a few factors, which vary between studies, that might account for these different findings. One of the main differences is in the patient groups that are studied. Not only do group size, medication status and age differ between studies, but also factors like comorbid diagnoses and comparison groups vary greatly. Another major difference between studies is the acquisition and analysis of the data. The scanning method, quantification method and statistical analysis all influence the results to a large extent. If incontestable results are wanted, comparable methods are essential. Until then neuroimaging research will possibly raise more questions than it can answer.

REFERENCES

Abelson JL, Glitz D, Cameron OG *et al.* (1991) Blunted growth hormone response to clonidine in patients with generalized anxiety disorder. *Arch Gen Psychiat,* **48**, 157–162.

Abelson JL, Nesse RM (1990) Cholecystokinin-4 and panic. *Arch Gen Psychiat,* **47**, 395.

Abelson JL, Nesse RM (1994) Pentagastrin infusion in patients with panic disorder. I. Symptoms and cardiovascular responses. *Biol Psychiat,* **36**, 73–83.

Albus M, Zahn TP, Breier A (1992) Anxiogenic properties of yohimbine. I. Behavioral, physiological and biochemical measures. *Eur Arch Psychiatry Clin Neurosci,* **241**, 337–344.

Alexopoulos GS, Meyers BS, Young RC, Campbell S, Silbersweig D, Charlson M (1997) "Vascular depression" hypothesis. *Arch Gen Psychiat,* **54**, 915–922.

American Psychiatric Association (1994) *Diagnostic and Statistical Manual of Mental Disorders (DSM-IV).* Washington, DC: American Psychiatric Association.

Anderson GM (1996) Comments on "Effectiveness of pindolol with selected antidepressant drugs in the treatment of major depression" (letter). *J Clin Psychopharmacol,* **16**, 256–257.

Andree B, Thorberg SO, Halldin C, Farde L (1999) Pindolol binding to 5-HT$_{1A}$ receptors in the human brain confirmed with positron emission tomography. *Psychopharmacol,* **144**, 303–305.

Ansseau M, Pitchot W, Hansenne M (1997) Neuroendocrine assessment of 5-HT$_{1A}$ receptors. *Eur Neuropsychopharmacol,* **7** (suppl 2), S126 S127.

Apostolopoulos M, Judd FK, Burrows GD, Norman TR (1993) Prolactin response to dl-fenfluramine in panic disorder. *Psychoneuroendocrinology,* **18**(5/6), 337–342.

Arborelius L, Nomikos GG, Grillner P, Hertel P, Hook BB, Hacksell U, Svensson TH (1995) 5-HT$_{1A}$ receptor antagonists increase the activity of serotonergic cells in the dorsal raphe nucleus in rats treated acutely or chronically with citalopram. *Naunyn-Schmiedeberg's Arch Pharmacol,* **352**, 157–165.

Arborelius L, Nomikos GG, Hertel P, Salmi P, Grillner P, Hook BB, Hacksell U, Svensson TH (1996) The 5-HT$_{1A}$ receptor antagonist (S)-UH-301 augments the increase in extracellular concentrations of 5-HT in the frontal cortex produced by both acute and chronic treatment with citalopram. *Naunyn-Schmiedeberg's Arch Pharmacol,* **353**, 630–640.

Aronson TA, Carasiti I, McBane D, Whitaker Azmitia P (1989) Biological correlates of lactate sensitivity in panic disorder. *Biol Psychiat,* **26**, 463–477.

Artigas F (1993) 5-HT and antidepressants; new views from microdialysis studies. *Trends Pharmacol Sci,* **14**, 262–263.

Artigas F (1997) Potential rapid onset: mechanisms of action. Abstract S.11.03. Vienna: ECNP.

Artigas F, Perez V, Alvarez E (1994) Pindolol induces a rapid improvement of depressed patients treated with serotonin reuptake inhibitors. *Arch Gen Psychiat,* **51**, 248–251.

Austin MP, Dougall N, Ross M, Murray C, O'Carroll RE, Moffoot A, Ebmeier KP, Goodwin GM (1992) Single photon emission tomography with ^{99m}Tc-exametazime in major depression and the pattern of brain activity underlying the psychotic/neurotic continuum. *J Affect Dis,* **26**, 31–43.

Aylward EH, Harris GJ, Hoehn Saric R, Barta PE, Machlin SR, Pearlson GD (1996) Normal caudate nucleus in obsessive-compulsive disorder assessed by quantitative neuroimaging. *Arch Gen Psychiat,* **53**, 577–584.

Bakish D, Hooper CL, Thornton MD, Wiens A, Miller CA, Thibaudeau CA (1997) Fast onset: an open study of the treatment of major depressive disorder with nefazodone and pindolol combination therapy. *Int Clin Psychopharmacol,* **12**, 91–97.

Ballenger JC, Burrows GD, DuPont RLJ et al. (1988) Alprazolam in panic disorder and agoraphobia: results from a multicenter trial. I. Efficacy in short-term treatment. *Arch Gen Psychiat,* **45**, 413–422.

Barlow DH (1988) *Anxiety and Its Disorders: The Nature and Treatment of Anxiety and Panic.* New York: Guilford.

Barr LC, Goodman WK, McDougle CJ (1994) Tryptophan depletion in obsessive-compulsive disorder patients responding to serotonin uptake inhibitors. *Arch Gen Psychiat,* **51**, 309–317.

Bastani B, Nash F, Meltzer H (1990) Prolactin and cortisol responses to MK-212, a serotonin agonist, in obsessive-compulsive disorder. *Arch Gen Psychiat,* **47**, 946–951.

Baxter LR Jr, Phelps ME, Mazziotta JC, Guze BH, Schwartz JM, Selin CE (1987) Local cerebral glucose metabolic rates in obsessive-compulsive disorder. A comparison with rates in unipolar depression and in normal controls (published erratum appears in *Arch Gen Psychiat* 1987, **44**, 800) (see comments). *Arch Gen Psychiat*, **44**, 211–218.

Baxter LR Jr, Schwartz JM, Mazziotta JC, Phelps ME, Pahl JJ, Guze BH, Fairbanks L (1988) Cerebral glucose metabolic rates in nondepressed patients with obsessive-compulsive disorder. *Am J Psychiat*, **145**, 1560–1563.

Baxter LR Jr, Schwartz JM, Phelps ME, Mazziotta JC, Guze BH, Selin CE, Gerner RH, Sumida RM (1989) Reduction of prefrontal cortex glucose metabolism common to three types of depression. *Arch Gen Psychiat*, **46**, 243–250.

Baxter LR Jr, Schwartz JM, Bergman KS, Szuba MP, Guze BH, Mazziotta JC, Alazraki A, Selin CE, Ferng HK, Munford P *et al.* (1992) Caudate glucose metabolic rate change with both drug and behavior therapy for obsessive-compulsive disorder. *Arch Gen Psychiat*, **49**, 681–689.

Beaumont G (1977) A large open multicenter trial of clomipramine (Anafranil) in the management of phobic disorder. *J Int Med Res*, **5**, 116–123.

Behar D, Rapoport JL, Berg CJ, Denckla MB, Mann L, Cox C, Fedio P, Zahn T, Wolfman MG (1984) Computerized tomography and neuropsychological test measures in adolescents with obsessive-compulsive disorder. *Am J Psychiat*, **141**, 363–369.

Bel N, Artigas F (1996) Reduction of serotonergic function in rat brain by tryptophan depletion: effects in control and fluvoxamine-treated rats. *J Neurochem*, **67**, 669–676.

Bell C, Wilson S, Nutt DJ (1998) Pindolol augmentation of sertraline in resistant depression and its effect on sleep. *J Psychopharmacol*, **12**, 105–107.

Bench CJ, Friston KJ, Brown RG, Scott LC, Frackowiak RS, Dolan RJ (1992) The anatomy of melancholia—focal abnormalities of cerebral blood flow in major depression. *Psychol Med*, **22**, 607–615.

Bench CJ, Frackowiak RS, Dolan RJ (1995) Changes in regional cerebral blood flow on recovery from depression. *Psychol Med*, **25**, 247–261.

Benkelfat C, Nordahl TE, Semple WE, King AC, Murphy DL, Cohen RM (1990) Local cerebral glucose metabolic rates in obsessive-compulsive disorder. Patients treated with clomipramine. *Arch Gen Psychiat*, **47**, 840–848.

Benkelfat C, Ellenbogen MA, Dean P, Palmour RM, Young SN (1994) Mood-lowering effect of tryptophan depletion: enhanced susceptibility in young men at genetic risk for major affective disorders. *Arch Gen Psychiat*, **51**, 687–697.

Berman RM, Darnell AM, Miller HL, Anand A, Charney DS (1997) Effect of pindolol in hastening response to fluoxetine in the treatment of major depression: a double-blind, placebo-controlled trial. *Am J Psychiat*, **154**, 37–43.

Bisaga A, Katz JL, Antonini A, Wright CE, Margouleff C, Gorman JM, *et al.* (1998) Cerebral glucose metabolism in women with panic disorder. *Am J Psychiat*, **155**, 1178–1183.

Black DW, Wesner R, Bowers W, Gabel J (1993) A comparison of fluvoxamine, cognitive therapy and placebo in the treatment of panic disorder. *Arch Gen Psych*, **50**, 44–50.

Blier P, Bergeron R (1995) Effectiveness of pindolol with selected antidepressant drugs in the treatment of major depression. *J Clin Psychopharmacol*, **15**, 217–222.

Blier P, Bergeron R (1996) Sequential administration of augmentation strategies in treatment-resistant obsessive-compulsive disorder: preliminary findings. *Int Clin Psychopharmacol*, **11**, 37–44.

Blier P, de Montigny C (1987) Modification of 5-HT neuron properties by sustained administration of the 5-HT1A agonist gepirone: electrophysiological studies in the rat brain. *Synapse*, **1**, 470–480.

Blier P, de Montigny C, Chaput Y (1987a) Modifications of the serotonin system by antidepressant treatments: implications for the therapeutic response in major depression. *J Clin Psychopharmacol*, **7** (suppl 6), 24S–35S.

Blier P, de Montigny C, Tardif D (1987b) Short-term lithium treatment enhances responsiveness of postsynaptic 5-HT$_{1A}$ receptors without altering 5-HT autoreceptor sensitivity: an electrophysiological study in the rat brain. *Synapse*, **1**, 225–232.

Bockaert J, Demuis A, Bouhelal R, Seblin M, Cory RN (1987) Piperazine derivatives including the putative anxiolytic drugs, buspirone and ipsapirone, are agonists at 5-HT$_{1A}$ receptors negatively coupled with adenylcyclase in hippocampal neurons. *Naunyn-Schmiedeberg's Arch Pharmacol*, **335**, 588–592.

Boden PR, Woodruff GN, Pinnock RD (1991) Pharmacology of a chlolecystokinin receptor on 5-hydroxytryptamine neurones in the dorsal raphe of the rat brain. *Br J Pharmacol*, **102**, 635–638.

Bordet R, Thomas P, Dupuis B (1997) Selective serotonin reuptake inhibitors plus pindolol (letter). *Lancet*, **350**, 289.

Bordet R, Thomas P, Dupuis B (1998) Effect of pindolol on onset of action of paroxetine in the treatment of major depression: intermediate analysis of a double-blind, placebo-controlled trial. Réseau de Recherche et d'Expérimentation Psychopharmacologique. *Am J Psychiat*, **155**, 1346–1351.

Boshuisen MI, den Boer JA (2000) Zolmitriptan (a 5-HT$_{1B}$ receptor agonist) with central action does not increase symptoms in obsessive compulsive disorder. *Psychopharmacology*, **152**, 74–79.

Bosker FJ, van Esseveldt KE, Klompmakers AA, Westenberg HGM (1995) Chronic treatment with fluvoxamine fails to induce functional changes in central 5-HT$_{1A}$ and 5-HT$_{1B}$ receptors, as measured by *in vivo* microdialysis in dorsal hippocampus of conscious rats. *Psychopharmacology*, **117**, 358–363.

Bosker FJ, Klompmakers AA, Westenberg HGM (1997) Postsynaptic 5-HT$_{1A}$ receptors mediate 5-hydroxytryptamine release in the amygdala through a feedback to the caudal linear raphe. *Eur J Pharmacol*, **333**, 147–157.

◁ Bosker FJ, Cremers TIFH, Jongsma ME, Westerink BHC, Wikström HV, den Boer JA (2001) Acute and chronic effects of citalopram on postsynaptic 5-hydroxytryptamine1A (5-HT$_{1A}$) receptor mediated feedback: a microdialysis study in the amygdala. *J Neurochem*, **76**, 1645–1653.

Bradwejn J, Koszycki D, Meterissian G (1990) Cholecystokinin tetrapeptide induces panic attacks in patients with panic disorder. *Can J Psychiat*, **35**, 83–85.

Bradwejn J, Koszycki D, Shriqui C (1991) Enhanced sensitivity to cholecystokinin tetrapeptide in panic disorder. *Arch Gen Psychiat*, **48**, 603–610.

Bradwejn J, Koszycki D, Annable L, Couetoux du tertre A, Reines S, Karkanias C (1992) A dose-ranging study of the behavioural and cardiovascular effects of CCK-tetrapeptide in panic disorder. *Biol Psychiat*, **32**, 903–912.

Bradwejn J, Koszycki D (1994a) Imipramine antagonism of the panicogenic effects of cholecystokinin tetrapeptide in panic disorder patients. *Am J Psychiat*, **151**, 261–263.

Bradwejn J, Koszycki D, Annable L, Couetoux du tertre A, Paradis M, Bourin M (1994b) Effects of flumazenil on cholecystokinin-tetrapeptide-induced panic symptoms in healthy volunteers. *Psychopharmacology*, **114**, 257–261.

Bradwejn J, Koszycki D, Couetoux du tertre A, van Megen HJGM, Westenberg HGM, den Boer JA, Karkanias C, Haigh J (1994c) The panicogenic effects of cholecystokinin tetrapeptide are antagonized by L-365,260, a central cholecystokinin receptor antagonist in patients with panic disorder. *Arch Gen Psychiat*, **51**, 486–493.

Bradwejn J, Paradis J, Kozycki D, Reece P, Sedman A (1994d) The effects of CI-988 on CCK-4 panic in healthy volunteers. *Neuropsychopharmacology*, **10**, 27–42.

Breiter HC, Rauch SL, Kwong KK, Baker JR, Weisskoff RM, Kennedy DN, Kendrick AD, Davis TL, Jiang A, Cohen MS, Stern CE, Belliveau JW, Baer L, O'Sullivan RL, Savage CR, Jenike MA, Rosen BR (1996) Functional magnetic resonance imaging of symptom provocation in obsessive-compulsive disorder. *Arch Gen Psychiat*, **53**, 595–606.

Bremner JD, Innis RB, Salomon RM, Staib LH, Ng CK, Miller HL, Bronen RA, Krystal JH, Duncan J, Rich D, Price LH, Malison R, Dey H, Soufer R, Charney DS (1997) Positron emission tomography measurement of cerebral metabolic correlates of tryptophan depletion-induced depressive relapse. *Arch Gen Psychiat*, **54**, 364–374.

Bremner JD, Innis RB, White T, Fujita M, Silbersweig D, Goddard AW, *et al.* (2000) SPECT [I-123]iomazenil measurement of the benzodiazepine receptor in panic disorder. *Biol Psychiat*, **47**, 96–106.

Briley M, Moret C (1993) Neurobiological mechanisms involved in antidepressant therapies. *Clin Neuropharmacol*, **16**, 387–400.

Brown SL, Botsis AJ, van Praag HM (1992) Suicide: CSF and neuroendocrine challenge studies. *Int Rev Psychiat*, **4**, 141–148.

Bruinvels AT (1993) 5-HT$_{1D}$ receptors reconsidered, radio-ligand binding assays, receptor autoradiography and *in situ* hybridisation histochemistry in the mammalian nervous system. Academic Thesis, University of Utrecht.

Buchsbaum MS, Wu J, Siegel BV, Hackett E, Trenary M, Abel L, *et al.* (1997) Effect of sertraline on regional metabolic rate in patients with affective disorder. *Biol Psychiat*, **41**, 15–22.

Busatto GF, Zamignani DR, Buchpiguel CA, Garrido GEJ, Glabus MF, Rocha ET, *et al.* (2000) A voxel-based investigation of regional cerebral blood flow abnormalities in obsessive-compulsive disorder using single photon emission computed tomography (SPECT). *Psychiat Res Neuroimaging*, **99**, 15–27.

Butler J, O'Halloran A, Leonard BE (1992) The Galway study of panic disorder II: changes in some peripheral markers of noradrenergic and serotonergic function in DSM-III-R panic disorder. *J Affect Dis*, **26**, 89–100.

Cameron OG, Smith CB, Hollingworth PF *et al.* (1984) Platelet α_2-adrenergic receptor binding and plasma catecholamines: before and during imipramine treatment in patients with panic anxiety. *Arch Gen Psychiat*, **41**, 1144–1148.

Cameron OG, Smith CB, Lee MA *et al.* (1990) Adrenergic status in anxiety disorders: platelet α_2-adrenergic receptor binding, blood pressure, pulse and plasma catecholamines in panic and generalized anxiety disorder patients and in normal subjects. *Biol Psychiat*, **28**, 3–20.

Carr DB, Sheenan DV, Surman OS *et al.* (1986) Neuroendocrine correlates of lactate-induced anxiety and their response to chronic alprazolam therapy. *Am J Psychiat*, **143**, 483–494.

Casanovas JM, Hervas I, Artigas F (1999) Postsynaptic 5-HT$_{1A}$ receptors control 5-HT release in the rat medial prefrontal cortex. *Neuroreport*, **10**, 1441–1445.

Ceci A, Baschirotto A, Borsini F (1994) The inhibitory effect of 8-OH-DPAT on the firing activity of dorsal raphe serotoninergic neurons in rats is attenuated by lesion of the frontal cortex. *Neuropharmacology*, **33**, 709–713.

Chaput Y, de Montigny C, Blier P (1986) Effects of a selective 5-HT reuptake blocker, citalopram, on the sensitivity of the 5-HT autoreceptors: electrophysiological studies in the rat. *Naunyn-Schmiedeberg's Arch Pharmacol*, **333**, 342–345.

Charney DS, Heninger GR (1985) Noradrenergic function and the mechanism of action of anti-anxiety treatment. II. The effect of long-term imipramine treatment. *Arch Gen Psychiat*, **42**, 473–481.

Charney DS, Heninger GR (1986) Abnormal regulation of noradrenergic function in panic disorders: effects of clonidine in healthy subjects and patients with agoraphobia and panic disorders. *Arch Gen Psychiat*, **43**, 1042–1054.

Charney DS, Menkes DB, Heninger GR (1981) Receptor sensitivity and the mechanism of action of antidepressant treatment: implications for the etiology and therapy of depression. *Arch Gen Psychiat*, **38**, 1160–1180.

Charney DS, Heninger GR, Breier A (1984) Noradrenergic function in panic anxiety: effects of yohimbine in healthy subjects and patients with agoraphobia and panic disorder. *Arch Gen Psychiat*, **41**, 751–763.

Charney DS, Woods SW, Goodman WK, Heninger GR (1987a) Neurobiological mechanisms of panic anxiety: biochemical and behavioral correlates of yohimbine-induced panic attacks. *Am J Psychiat*, **144**, 1030–1036.

Charney DS, Woods SW, Goodman WK, Heninger GR (1987b) Serotonin function in anxiety. II. Effects of the serotonin agonist *m*CPP in panic disorder patients and healthy subjects. *Psychopharmacology*, **92**, 14–24.

Charney DS, Goodman WK, Price LH, Woods SW, Rasmussen SA, Heninger GR (1988) Serotonin function in obsessive-compulsive disorder. *Arch Gen Psychiat*, **45**, 177–185.

Charney DS, Innis RB, Duman RS *et al.* (1989a) Platelet α_2-adrenergic receptor binding and adenylate cyclase activity in panic disorder. *Psychopharmacology*, **98**, 102–107.

Charney DS, Woods SW, Heninger GR (1989b) Noradrenergic function in generalized anxiety disorder: effects of yohimbine in healthy subjects and patients with generalized anxiety disorder. *Psychiatry Res*, **27**, 173–182.

Charney DS, Woods SW, Krystal JH *et al.* (1992) Noradrenergic neuronal dysregulation in panic disorder: the effects of intravenous yohimbine and clonidine in panic disorder patients. *Acta Psychiat Scand*, **86**, 273–282.

Charney DS, Krystal JH, Southwick SM, Delgado PL (1994) The role of noradrenergic functioning in human anxiety and depression. In: JA den Boer, JMA Sitsen (eds) *Handbook of depression and anxiety*. New York: Marcel Dekker, 573–597.

Coccaro EF, Siever LJ, Klar HM *et al.* (1989) Serotonergic studies in patients with affective and personality disorders. *Arch Gen Psychiat*, **46**, 587–599.

Coffey CE, Wilkinson WE, Weiner RD, Parashos IA, Djang WT, Webb MC, Figiel GS, Spritzer CE (1993) Quantitative cerebral anatomy in depression. A controlled magnetic resonance imaging study. *Arch Gen Psychiat*, **50**, 7–16.

Coplan JD, Liebowitz MR, Gorman JM *et al.* (1992) Noradrenergic function in panic disorder: effects of intravenous clonidine pretreatment on lactate induced panic. *Biol Psychiat*, **31**, 135–146.

Cremers TIFH, Spoelstra EN, de Boer P, Bosker FJ, Mork A, den Boer JA, Westerink BHC, Wikstrom HV (2000) Desensitization of 5-HT autoreceptors upon pharmacokinetically monitored chronic treatment with citalopram. *Eur J Pharmacol*, **397**, 351–357.

Cremers TIFH, Wiersma LJ, Bosker FJ, den Boer JA, Westerink BHC, Wikstrom HV (2001) Is the beneficial antidepressive effect of co-administration of pindolol really due to somatodendritic autoreceptor antagonism? *Biol Psychiat*, in press.

Cross AJ, Slater P, Skan W (1988) Characteristics of ^{125}I-Bolton-Hunter labelled cholecystokinin binding in human brain. *Neuropeptides*, **11**, 73–76.

Cummings JL (1993) The neuroanatomy of depression. *J Clin Psychiat*, **54** (suppl), 14–20.

Cutler NR, Sramek JJ, Kramer MS, Reines SA (1994) Pilot study of a CCK-B antagonist in panic disorder. NCDEU 34th annual meeting, Marco Island, FL.

Dannon PN, Hirschmann S, Kindler S, Iancu T, Dolberg OT, Grunhaus LJ (1997) Pindolol augmentation in the treatment of resistant panic disorder: A double-blind placebo-controlled trial. Abstract P.3.013. Vienna: ECNP.

Dannon PN, Sasson Y, Hirschmann S, Iancu I, Grunhaus LJ, Zohar J (2000) Pindolol augmentation in treatment-resistant obsessive compulsive disorder: a double-blind placebo controlled trial. *Eur Neuropsychopharmacol*, **10**, 165–169.

Davidson C, Stamford JA (1995) The effect of paroxetine on 5-HT efflux in the rat dorsal raphe nucleus is potentiated by both $5\text{-}HT_{1A}$ and $5\text{-}HT_{1B/D}$ receptor antagonists. *Neurosci Lett*, **188**, 41–44.

Davidson JRT, Potts N, Richichi E, Krishnan R, Ford SM, Smith R, Wilson WH (1993) Treatment of social phobia with clonazepam and placebo. *J Clin Psychopharmacol*, **13**, 423–28.

de Boer T, Ruigt GSF, Berendsen HHG (1995) The α_2-selective adrenoceptor antagonist Org 3770 (mirtazapine, Remeron) enhances noradrenergic and serotonergic transmission. *Hum Psychopharmacol*, **10**, S107–S118.

de Cristofaro MT, Sessarego A, Pupi A, Biondi F, Faravelli C (1993) Brain perfusion abnormalities in drug-naive, lactate-sensitive panic patients: a SPECT study. *Biol Psychiat*, **33**, 505–512.

de Leeuw AS, den Boer JA, Slaap BR, Westenberg HG (1996) Pentagastrin has panic-inducing properties in obsessive compulsive disorder. *Psychopharmacology*, **126**, 339–344.

de Leeuw AS, den Boer JA, Westenberg HGM (2000) Unaltered behavioral and neuroendocrine responsivity to 5-HTP challenge in obsessive compulsive disorder. A double blind placebo controlled study. Submitted.

Delgado PL, Charney DS, Price LH, Aghajanian GK, Landis H, Heninger GR (1990) Serotonin function and the mechanism of antidepressant action: reversal of antidepressant induced remission by rapid depletion of plasma tryptophan. *Arch Gen Psychiat*, **47**, 411–418.

Delgado PL, Miller HL, Salomon RM, Licinio J, Heninger GR, Gelenberg AJ, Charney DS (1993) Monoamines and the mechanism of antidepressant action: effects of catecholamine depletion on mood of patients treated with antidepressants. *Psychopharmacol Bull*, **29**, 389–396.

Delgado PL, Price LH, Miller HL *et al.* (1994) Serotonin and the neurobiology of depression: effects of tryptophan depletion in drug-free depressed patients. *Arch Gen Psychiat*, **51**, 865–874.

de Montigny C (1989) Cholecystokinin tetrapeptide induces panic like attacks in healthy volunteers. *Arch Gen Psychiat*, **46**, 511–517.

den Boer JA (1997) Social phobia: epidemiology, recognition and treatment. *Br Med J*, **315**, 796–800.

den Boer JA, Sitsen JMA (eds) (1994) *Handbook of Depression and Anxiety: A Biological Approach.* New York: Marcel Dekker.

den Boer JA, Westenberg HGM (1988) Effect of a serotonin and noradrenaline uptake inhibitor in panic disorder; a double-blind comparative study with fluvoxamine and maprotiline. *Int Clin Psychopharmacol*, **3**, 59–74.

den Boer JA, Westenberg HGM (1990a) Serotonin function in panic disorder: a double-blind placebo controlled study with fluvoxamine and ritanserin. *Psychopharmacology*, **102**, 85–94.

den Boer JA, Westenberg HGM (1990b) Behavioral, neuroendocrine, and biochemical effects of 5-hydroxytryptophan administration in panic disorder. *Psychiat Res*, **31**, 367–378.

den Boer JA, Westenberg HGM (1995) Serotonin receptor sensitivity in panic disorder: a critical appraisal of the evidence. In HGM Westenberg, JA den Boer, DS Murphy (eds), *Advances in the Neurobiology of Anxiety Disorders.* Chichester: Wiley.

den Boer JA, Westenberg HGM (1997) Challenge studies in obsessive-compulsive disorder. In: JA den Boer, HGM Westenberg (eds) *Obsessive Compulsive Spectrum Disorders.* Amsterdam: Syn-thesis Publishers, 123–134.

den Boer JA, Westenberg HGM, Kamerbeek WDJ (1987) Effect of serotonin uptake inhibitors in anxiety disorders: a double-blind comparison of clomipramine and fluvoxamine. *Int Clin Psychopharmacol*, **2**, 21–32.

den Boer JA, Westenberg HGM, Klompmakers AA, and van Lint LE (1989) Behavioral biochemical and neuroendocrine concomitants of lactate-induced panic anxiety. *Biol Psychiat*, **26**, 612–622.

de Vry J, Melon C, Jentzsch KR, Schreiber R (1997) Identification of 5-HT receptor subtypes responsible for the therapeutic effects of selective 5-HT reuptake inhibitors (SSRIs) Abstract 24–8, *Biol Psych.*

Dolan RJ, Poynton AM, Bridges PK, Trimble MR (1990) Altered magnetic resonance white-matter T1 values in patients with affective disorder. *Br J Psychiat*, **157**, 107–110.

Dolan RJ, Bench CJ, Brown RG, Scott LC, Friston KJ, Frackowiak RS (1992) Regional cerebral blood flow abnormalities in depressed patients with cognitive impairment. *J Neurol Neurosurg Psychiat*, **55**, 768–773.

72   J.A. den Boer, B.R. Slaap and F.J. Bosker

Dolberg OT, Sasson Y, Cohen R, Zohar J (1995) The relevance of behavioural probes in obsessive-compulsive disorder. *Eur Neuropsychopharmacol*, **5**, S161.

Drevets WC (1998) Functional neuroimaging studies of depression: the anatomy of melancholia. *Annu Rev Med*, **49**, 341–361.

Drevets, WC Raichle ME (1992) Neuroanatomical circuits in depression: implications for treatment mechanisms. *Psychopharmacol Bull*, **28**, 261–274.

Duman RS, Heninger GR, Nestler EJ (1997) A molecular and cellular theory of depression. *Arch Gen Psychiat*, **54**, 597–606.

Ebert D, Ebmeier KP (1996) The role of the cingulate gyrus in depression: from functional anatomy to neurochemistry. *Biol Psychiat*, **39**, 1044–1050.

Edmonstone Y, Austin MP, Prentice N, Dougall N, Freeman CP, Ebmeier KP, Goodwin GM (1994) Uptake of ^{99m}Tc-exametazime shown by single photon emission computerized tomography in obsessive-compulsive disorder compared with major depression and normal controls. *Acta Psychiat Scand*, **90**, 298–303.

Egawa T, Ichimaru Y, Imanishi T, Sawa A (1995) Neither the 5-HT$_{1A}$ nor the 5-HT$_2$ receptor subtype mediates the effect of fluvoxamine, a selective serotonin reuptake inhibitor, on forced-swimming-induced immobility in mice. *Jap J Pharmacol*, **68**, 71–75.

Elkis H, Friedman L, Wise A, Meltzer HY (1995) Meta-analyses of studies of ventricular enlargement and cortical sulcal prominence in mood disorders. Comparisons with controls or patients with schizophrenia. *Arch Gen Psychiat*, **52**, 735–746.

Emson PC, Rehfeld JF, Rossor MN (1982) Distribution of cholecystokinin in the human brain. *J Neurochem*, **38**, 1177–1179.

Erfurth A, Kammerer C, Ackenheil M, Moller HJ (1997) Effect of pindolol in hastening response to serotoninergic antidepressants: an open study in severely depressed female inpatients. Abstract P.1.041. Vienna: ECNP.

Eriksson E, Westberg P, Alling C, Thursson K, Modigh K (1991) Cerebrospinal fluid levels of monoamine metabolites in panic disorder. *Psychiat Res*, **36**, 243–251.

Erlander MG, Lovenberg TW, Baron BM, de Lecca L, Danielson PE, Racke M, Slone AL, Siegel BW, Foye PE, Burns JE, Sutcliffe JG (1993) Two members of a distinct subfamily of 5-hydroxytryptamine receptors differentially expressed in rat brain. *Proc Natl Acad Sci USA*, **90**, 3452–3456.

Evans L, Kenardy J, Schneider P, Hoey H (1986) Effect of a selective serotonin uptake inhibitor in agoraphobia with panic attacks. *Acta Psychiat Scand*, **73**, 49–53.

Fineberg NA, Cowen PJ, Kirk JW, Montgomery SA (1994) Neuroendocrine responses to intravenous L-tryptophan in obsessive-compulsive disorder. *J Affect Dis*, **32**, 97–104.

Fontaine R, Breton G, Dery R, Fontaine S, Elie R (1990) Temporal lobe abnormalities in panic disorder: an MRI study. *Biol Psychiat*, **27**, 304–310.

Francois A, Biver F, Goldman S, Luxen A, Mendlewicz J, Lotstra F (1995) Decrease in the frontal-superobasal metabolic ratio in unipolar depression. Reduction du rapport metabolique frontal supero-basal dans la depression unipolaire. *Acta Psychiat Belg*, **95**, 234–245.

Fuller W (1990) Serotonin receptors and neuroendocrine responses. *Neuropsychopharmacology*, **3**, 495–502.

Gabbard GO (1992) Psychodynamics of panic disorder and social phobia. *Bull Menninger Clin*, **56** (2, suppl A), A3–A13.

Garcia-Sevilla JA, Guimon P, Garcia-Vallejo P, Fuster MJ (1966) Biochemical and functional evidence of supersensitive platelet α_2-adrenoreceptors in major affective disorder: effect of long-term lithium carbonate treatment. *Arch Gen Psychiat*, **43**, 51–57.

Gardier AM, Malagie I, Trillat AC, Jacquot C, Artigas F (1996) Role of 5-HT$_{1A}$ autoreceptors in the mechanism of action of serotoninergic antidepressant drugs: Recent findings from *in vivo* microdialysis studies. *Fund Clin Pharmacol*, **10**, 16–27.

George MS, Ketter TA, Post RM (1993) SPECT and PET imaging in mood disorders. *J Clin Psychiat*, **54** (suppl), 6–13.

Glazer WM, Charney DS, Heninger GR (1987) Noradrenergic function in schizophrenia. *Arch Gen Psychiat*, **44**, 898–904.

Goddard AW, Sholomskas DE, Walton KE, Augeri FM, Charney DS, Heninger GR, Goodman WK, Price LH (1994) Effects of tryptophan depletion in panic disorder. *Biol Psychiat*, **36**, 775–777.

Goddard AW, Charney DS, Germine M, Woods SW, Heninger GR, Krystal JH, Goodman WK, Price LH (1995) Effects of tryptophan depletion on responses to yohimbine in healthy human subjects. *Biol Psychiat*, **38**, 74–85.

Goetz RR, Klein DF, Gorman JM (1997) Symptoms essential to the experience of sodium lactate-induced panic. *Neuropsychopharmacology*, **14**, 355–366.

Goodall EM, Cowen PJ, Franklin M, Silverstone T (1993) Ritanserin attenuates anorectic, endocrine and thermic responses to d-fenfluramine in human volunteers. *Psychopharmacology*, **112**, 461–466.

Goodman WK, Price LH, Rasmussen SA, Delgado P, Heninger GR, Charney DS (1989) The efficacy of fluvoxamine in obsessive-compulsive disorder: a double-blind comparison with placebo. *Arch Gen Psychiat*, **46**, 36–42.

Goodman WK, Price LH, Woods SW, Charney DS (1991) Pharmacologic challenges in obsessive-compulsive disorder. In J Zohar, T Insel, S Rasmussen (eds) *The Psychobiology of Obsessive-Compulsive Disorder*. New York: Springer-Verlag, 162–186.

Goodman WK, McDougle CJ, Barr LC, Aronson SC, Price LH (1993) Biological approaches to treatment-resistant obsessive compulsive disorder. *J Clin Psychiat*, **54**, 16–26.

Goodman WK, McDougle C, Price LH, Barr LC, Hills OF, Caplik JF, Charney DS, Heninger GK (1995) *m*-Chlorophenylpiperazine in patients with obsessive compulsive disorder: absence of symptom exacerbation. *Biol Psychiat*, **38**, 138–149.

Goodwin GM, Austin MP, Dougall N, Ross M, Murray C, O'Carroll RE, Moffoot A, Prentice N, Ebmeier KP (1993) State changes in brain activity shown by the uptake of ^{99m}Tc-exametazime with single photon emission tomography in major depression before and after treatment. *J Affect Dis*, **29**, 243–253.

Greenwald BS, Kramer Ginsberg E, Krishnan RR, Ashtari M, Aupperle PM, Patel M (1996) MRI signal hyperintensities in geriatric depression. *Am J Psychiat*, **153**, 1212–1215.

Greenwald BS, Kramer Ginsberg E, Bogerts B, Ashtari M, Aupperle P, Wu H, Allen L, Zeman D, Patel M (1997) Qualitative magnetic resonance imaging findings in geriatric depression. Possible link between later-onset depression and Alzheimer's disease? *Psychol Med*, **27**, 421–431.

Griez EJ, Lousberg H, Van den Hout MA, van der Molen GM (1987) CO_2 vulnerability in panic disorder. *Psychiat Res*, **20**, 87–95.

Gurguis GNM, Uhde TW (1990) Plasma 3-methoxy-4-hydroxyphenylethylene glycol (MHPG) and growth hormone responses to yohimbine in panic disorder patients and normal controls. *Psychoneuroendocrinology*, **15**, 217–224.

Hamik A, Peroutka SJ (1989) 1-(*m*-Clorophenyl)-iperazine (*m*-CPP) interactions with neurotransmitter receptors in the human brain. *Biol Psychiat*, **25**, 569–575.

Harro J, Jossan SS, Oreland L (1992) Changes in cholecystokinin receptor binding in rat brain after selective damage of the locus coeruleus projections by DSP-4 treatment. *Arch Pharmacol*, **364**, 425–431.

Hartig PR (1992) Molecular biology of $5-HT_{1D}$ receptors. *Abstracts, 2nd International Symposium on Serotonin*. Houston: p. 1.

Hauser P, Altshuler LL, Berrettini W, Dauphinais ID, Gelernter J, Post RM (1989) Temporal lobe measurement in primary affective disorder by magnetic resonance imaging. *J Neuropsychiatry Clin Neurosci*, **1**, 128–134.

Heninger GR, Charney DS, Price LH (1988) α_2-Adrenergic receptor sensitivity in depression: the plasma MHPG, behavioral, and cardiovascular responses to yohimbine. *Arch Gen Psychiat*, **45**, 718–726.

Hewlett WA, Martin K (1993) Fenfluramine challenges and serotonergic functioning in obsessive-compulsive disorder. Presented at First International Obsessive-Compulsive Disorder Congress, Capri, Italy, 12–13 March.

Hickie I, Scott E, Mitchell P, Wilhelm K, Austin MP, Bennett B (1995) Subcortical hyperintensities on magnetic resonance imaging: clinical correlates and prognostic significance in patients with severe depression. *Biol Psychiat*, **37**, 151–160.

Hirono N, Mori E, Ishii K, Ikejiri Y, Imamura T, Shimomura T, *et al.* (1998) Frontal lobe hypometabolism and depression in Alzheimer's disease. *Neurology*, **50**, 380–383.

Hjorth S (1993) Serotonin 5-HT$_{1A}$ autoreceptor blockade potentiates the ability of the 5-HT reuptake inhibitor citalopram to increase nerve terminal output of 5-HT *in vivo*—a microdialysis study. *J Neurochem*, **60**, 776–779.

Hjorth S, Auerbach SB (1994) Lack of 5-HT$_{1A}$ autoreceptor desensitization following chronic citalopram treatment as determined by *in vivo* microdialysis. *Neuropharmacol*, **33**, 331–334.

Hoehn Saric R, Pearlson GD, Harris GJ, Machlin SR, Camargo EE (1991) Effects of fluoxetine on regional cerebral blood flow in obsessive-compulsive patients. *Am J Psychiat*, **148**, 1243–1245.

Hoehn Saric R, Mcleod DR, Hipsley A (1993) Effect of fluvoxamine on panic disorder. *J Clin Psychopharmacol*, **5**, 321–326.

Hollander E, Fay M, Cohen B, Campeas R, Gorman JM, Liebowitz MR (1988) Serotonergic and adrenergic sensitivity in obsessive-compulsive disorder: behavioral findings. *Am J Psychiat*, **145**, 1015–1017.

Hollander E, DeCaria C, Nitescu A, Cooper T, Sover B, Gully R, Klein DF, Liebowitz MR (1991a) Noradrenergic function in obsessive compulsive disorder: behavioral and neuroendocrine responses to clonidine and comparison to healthy controls. *Psychiat Res*, **37**, 161–177.

Hollander E, DeCaria C, Gully R *et al.* (1991b) Effects of chronic fluoxetine treatment on behavioral and neuroendocrine responses to *meta*-chlorophenylpiperazine in obsessive-compulsive disorder. *Psychiat Res*, **36**, 1–17.

Hollander E, DeCaria CM, Nitescu A *et al.* (1992) Serotonergic function in obsessive-compulsive disorder. *Arch Gen Psychiat*, **49**, 21–28.

Hollander E, Prohovnik I, Stein DJ (1995) Increased cerebral blood flow during *m*-CPP exacerbation of obsessive-compulsive disorder. *J Neuropsychiatry Clin Neurosci*, **7**, 485–490.

Ho-Pian KL, Westenberg HGM, Van Megen HJGM, Den Boer JA (1998a) Sumatriptan (5-HT$_{1D}$ receptor agonist) does not exacerbate symptoms in obsessive-compulsive disorder. *Psychopharmacology*, **140**, 365–370.

Ho Pian KL, Westenberg HGM, den Boer JA, de Bruin WI, van Rijk PP (1998b) Effects of *m*-chlorophenylpiperazine (*m*CPP) on cerebral blood flow in obsessive-compulsive disorder and controls. *Biol Psychiat*, **44**, 367–370.

Hoyer D, Middlemiss DN (1989) Species differences in the pharmacology of terminal 5-HT autoreceptors in mammalian brain. *TIPS*, **10**, 130–132.

Humphrey PPA, Hartig P, Hoyer D (1993) A proposed new nomenclature for 5-HT receptors. *TIPS*, **14**, 233–236.

Husain MM, McDonald WM, Doraiswamy PM, Figiel GS, Na C, Escalona PR, Boyko OB, Nemeroff CB, Krishnan KR (1991) A magnetic resonance imaging study of putamen nuclei in major depression. *Psychiat Res*, **40**, 95–99.

Innis RB, Charney DS, Heninger GR (1987) Differential ^{3}H-Imipramine platelet binding in patients with panic disorder and depression. *Psychiat Res*, **21**, 33–41.

Insel TR, Donnelly EF, Lalakea ML, Alterman IS, Murphy DL (1983) Neurological and neuropsychological studies of patients with obsessive-compulsive disorder. *Biol Psychiat*, **18**, 741–751.

Insel TR, Mueller EA, Alterman I, Linnoila M, Murphy DL (1985) Obsessive-compulsive disorder and serotonin: is there a connection? *Biol Psychiat*, **20**, 1174–1188.

Invernizzi R, Belli S, Samanin R (1992) Citalopram's ability to increase the extracellular concentrations of serotonin in the dorsal raphe prevents the drug's effect in the frontal cortex. *Brain Res*, **584**, 322–324.

Isaac MT (1997) Can we identify subgroups for targeted adjunctive treatment? Abstract S.11.04 Vienna: ECNP.

Isaac MT, Tome MB (1997) Selective serotonin reuptake inhibitors plus pindolol (letter). *Lancet*, **350**, 288–289.

Jenike MA, Breiter HC, Baer L, Kennedy DN, Savage CR, Olivares MJ, O'Sullivan RL, Shera DM, Rauch SL, Keuthen N, Rosen BR, Caviness VS, Filipek PA (1996) Cerebral structural abnormalities in obsessive-compulsive disorder. A quantitative morphometric magnetic resonance imaging study. *Arch Gen Psychiat*, **53**, 625–632.

Jeste DV, Lohr JB, Goodwin FK (1988) Neuroanatomical studies of major affective disorders. A review and suggestions for further research. *Br J Psychiat*, **153**, 444–459.

Kahn RS, Wetzler S (1991) *m*-Chlorophenylpiperazine as a probe of serotonin function. *Biol Psychiat*, **30**, 1139–1166.

Kahn RS, Asnis GM, Wetzler S, Van Praag HM (1988a) Neuroendocrine evidence for serotonin hypersensitivity in panic disorder. *Psychopharmacology*, **96**, 360–364.

Kahn RS, Welzer S, Van Praag HM, Asnis GM (1988b) Behavioral indications for serotonin receptor hypersensitivity in panic disorder. *Psychiat Res*, **25**, 101–104.

Kaschka W, Feistel H, Ebert D (1995) Reduced benzodiazepine receptor binding in panic disorders measured by iomazenil SPECT. *J Psychiat Res*, **29**, 427–434.

Kellner CH, Rubinow DR, Post RM (1986) Cerebral ventricular size and cognitive impairment in depression. *J Affect Dis*, **10**, 215–219.

Kellner CH, Jolley RR, Holgate RC, Austin L, Lydiard RB, Laraia M, Ballenger JC (1991) Brain MRI in obsessive-compulsive disorder. *Psychiat Res*, **36**, 45–49.

Klein E, Zohar J, Geraci F, Murphy DL, Uhde TW (1991) Anxiogenic effects of *m*CPP in patients with panic disorder: comparison to caffeine's anxiogenic effects. *Biol Psychiat*, **30**, 973–984.

Koran LM, Mueller K, Maloney A (1996) Will pindolol augment the response to a serotonin reuptake inhibitor in obsessive-compulsive disorder? (letter). *J Clin Psychopharmacol*, **16**, 253–254.

Koszycki D, Zacharko RM, Le Melledo JM, Young SN, Bradwejn J (1996) Effect of acute tryptophan depletion on behavioral, cardiovascular, and hormonal sensitivity to cholecysto-kinin-tetrapeptide challenge in healthy volunteers. *Biol Psychiat*, **40**, 648–655.

Kramer MS, Cutler NR, Ballenger JC, Patterson WM, Mendels J, Chenault A, Shrivastava R, Matzura-Wolfe D, Lines C, Reines S (1995) A placebo controlled trial of L-365,260, a CCKB antagonist, in panic disorder. *Biol Psychiat*, **37**, 462–466.

Kraus RP (1996) Rapid cycling triggered by pindolol augmentation of paroxetine, but not with desipramine. *Depression*, **4**, 92–94.

Kraus RP (1997) Pindolol augmentation of tranylcypromine in psychotic depression (letter). *J Clin Psychopharmacol*, **17**, 225–226.

Kreiss DS, Lucki I (1993) Repeated administration of the antidepressant fluoxetine, but not desipramine or mianserin, produces desensitization of 5-HT$_{1A}$ autoreceptors. *Soc Neurosci Abstr*, **19**, (abstr no 763.10).

Krishnan KR, Hays JC, Blazer DG (1997) MRI-defined vascular depression. *Am J Psychiat*, **154**, 497–501.

Krishnan KR, Doraiswamy PM, Figiel GS, Husain MM, Shah SA, Na C, Boyko OB, McDonald WM, Nemeroff CB, Ellinwood EH Jr (1991) Hippocampal abnormalities in depression. *J Neuropsychiat Clin Neurosci*, **3**, 387–391.

Kuikka JT, Pitkanen A, Lepola U, Partanen K, Vainio P, Bergstrom KA, Wieler HJ, Kaiser KP, Mittelbach L, Koponen H et al. (1995) Abnormal regional benzodiazepine receptor uptake in the prefrontal cortex in patients with panic disorder. Nucl Med Commun, 16, 273–280.

Kumar A, Newberg A, Alavi A, Berlin J, Smith R, Reivich M (1993) Regional cerebral glucose metabolism in late-life depression and Alzheimer disease: a preliminary positron emission tomography study. Proc Natl Acad Sci USA, 90, 7019–7023.

Kumar A, Schweizer E, Jin Z, Miller D, Bilker W, Swan LL, Gottlieb G (1997) Neuroanatomical substrates of late-life minor depression. A quantitative magnetic resonance imaging study. Arch Neurol, 54, 613–617.

Lam RW, Zis AP, Grewal A, Delgado PL, Charney DS, Krystal JH (1996) Effects of rapid tryptophan depletion in patients with seasonal affective disorder in remission after light therapy. Arch Gen Psychiat, 53, 41–44.

Langer SZ, Moret C, Raisman R (1980) High affinity ^{3}H-imipramine binding in rat hypothalamus: association with uptake of serotonin but not norepinephrine. Science, 210, 1133–1135.

Lee MA, Cameron OG, Garguis GNM, Glitz D, Smith CB, Hariharan M, Abelson JL, Curtis GC (1990) Alpha$_2$-adrenoceptor status in obsessive compulsive disorder. Biol Psychiat, 27, 1083–1093.

Lee MA, Nash JF, Barnes M, Meltzer HY (1991) Inhibitory effect of ritanserin on the 5-hydroxytryptophan-mediated cortisol, ACTH and prolactin secretion in humans. Psychopharmacology, 103, 258–264.

Lenze E, Cross D, McKeel D, Neuman RJ, Sheline YI (1999) White matter hyperintensities and gray matter lesions in physically healthy depressed subjects. Am J Psychiat, 156, 1602–1607.

Lepola U, Nousiainen U, Puranen M, Riekkinen P, Rimon R (1990) EEG and CT findings in patients with panic disorder. Biol Psychiat, 28, 721–727.

Lesch KP, Mayer S, Disselkamp-Tietze J, Hoh A, Wiesmann M, Osterheider M, Schulte HM (1990) 5-HT$_{1A}$ receptor responsivity in unipolar depression. Evaluation of ipsapirone-induced ACTH and cortisol secretion in patients and controls. Biol Psychiat, 28, 620–628.

Lesch KP, Hoh A, Disselkamp-Tietze J, Weismann M, Osterheider M, Schulte HM (1991a) 5-Hydroxytryptamine$_{1A}$ (5-HT$_{1A}$) receptor responsivity in obsessive-compulsive disorder: comparison of patients and controls. Arch Gen Psychiat, 48, 540–547.

Lesch KP, Hoh A, Osterheider M, Schulte HM, Muller T (1991b) Long-term fluoxetine treatment decreases 5-HT$_{1A}$ receptor responsivity in obsessive-compulsive disorder. Psychopharmacology, 105, 415–420.

Lesch KP, Wiesmann M, Hoh A, Muller T, Disslekamp-Tietze T, Osterheider M, Schulte HM (1992) 5-HT$_{1A}$ receptor-effector system responsivity in panic disorder. Psychopharmacology, 106(2), 111–117.

Lichtenberg P, Shapira B, Gillon D et al. (1992a) Hormone responses to fenfluramine and placebo challenge in endogenous depression. Psychiat Res, 43, 137–146.

Lichtenberg P, Shapiro B, Blacker M, Gropp C, Calev A, Lerer B (1992b) Effect of fenfluramine on mood: a double blind placebo controlled trial. Biol Psychiat, 31, 351–356.

Liebowitz MR, Fyer AJ, Gorman JM (1984) Lactate provocation of panic attacks. I. Clinical and behavioral findings. Arch Gen Psychiat, 41, 764–770.

Liebowitz MR, Gorman JM, Fyer AJ, Levitt M, Dillon D, Levy G, Appleby IL, Anderson S, Palij M, Davies SO, Klein DF (1985) Lactate provocation of panic attacks. II. Biochemical and physiological findings. Arch Gen Psychiat, 42, 709–719.

Liebowitz MR, Gorman JM, Fyer A, Dillon D, Levitt M, Klein DF (1986) Possible mechanisms for lactate induction of panic. Am J Psychiat, 143, 495–502.

Lines C, Reines S (1995) A placebo-controlled trial of L-365,260, a CCKB antagonist, in panic disorder. Biol Psychiat, 37, 462–466.

Lines C, Challenor J, Traub M (1995) Cholecystokinin and anxiety in normal volunteers: an investigation of the anxiogenic properties of pentagastrin and reversal by cholecystokinin receptor subtype B antagonist L-365,260. *Br J Pharmacol*, **39**, 235–242.

Lowy MT, Meltzer HY (1988) Stimulation of serum cortisol and prolactin secretion in humans by MK-212. *Biol Psychiat*, **23**, 818–828.

Lucey JV, Barry S, Webb MGT, Dinan TG (1992a) The desipramine-induced growth hormone response and the DST in obsessive compulsive disorder. *Acta Psychiat Scand*, **86**, 367–370.

Lucey JV, O'Keane V, Butcher G, Dinan GT (1992b) Cortisol and prolactin responses to D-fenfluramine in normotensive obsessive compulsive disorder, a comparison with depressed and healthy controls. *Br J Psychiat*, **161**, 517–521.

Lucey JV, Butcher G, Clare AW, Dinan TG (1992c) Buspirone-induced prolactin responses in obsessive compulsive disorder. *Int J Psychopharmacol*, **7**, 45–49.

Lucey JV, Costa DC, Busatto G, Pilowsky LS, Marks IM, Ell PJ, Kerwin RW (1997) Caudate regional cerebral blood flow in obsessive-compulsive disorder, panic disorder and healthy controls on single photon emission computerised tomography. *Psychiat Res Neuroimag*, **74**, 25–33.

Luxenberg JS, Swedo SE, Flament MF, Friedland RP, Rapoport J, Rapoport SI (1988) Neuroanatomical abnormalities in obsessive-compulsive disorder detected with quantitative X-ray computed tomography. *Am J Psychiat*, **145**, 1089–1093.

Machlin SR, Harris GJ, Pearlson GD, Hoehn Saric R, Jeffery P, Camargo EE (1991) Elevated medial-frontal cerebral blood flow in obsessive-compulsive patients: a SPECT study. *Am J Psychiat*, **148**, 1240–1242.

Maes M, Dierckx R, Meltzer HY, Ingels M, Schotte C, Vandewoude M, Calabrese J, Cosyns P (1993) Regional cerebral blood flow in unipolar depression measured with Tc-99m-HMPAO single photon emission computed tomography: negative findings. *Psychiat Res*, **50**, 77–88.

Maes M, Vandoolaeghe E, Desnyder R (1996) Efficacy of treatment with trazodone in combination with pindolol or fluoxetine in major depression. *J Affect Dis*, **41**, 201–210.

Malizia, AL, Nutt DJ (1997) Obsessive-compulsive disorder and the brain: what do imaging techniques tell us? In: JA den Boer, HGM Westenberg (eds) *Obsessive Compulsive Spectrum Disorders*. Amsterdam: Syn-thesis Publishers, 107–122.

⁂Malizia AL, Cunningham VJ, Bell CJ, Liddle PF, Jones T, Nutt DJ (1998) Decreased brain GABA(A)-benzodiazepine receptor binding in panic disorder—preliminary results from a quantitative PET study. *Arch Gen Psychiat*, **55**, 715–720.

Mann JJ, Stanley M, McBride PA, McEwen BS (1986) Increased serotonin-2 and beta-adrenergic receptor binding in the frontal cortices of suicide victims. *Arch Gen Psychiat*, **43**, 954–959.

Martinez D, Mawlawi O, Hwang DR, Kent J, Simpson N, Parsey RV, Hashimoto T, Slifstein M, Huang YY, Van Heertum R, Abi Dargham A, Caltabiano S, Malizia A, Cowley H, Mann JJ, Laruelle M (2000a) Positron emission tomography study of pindolol occupancy of 5-HT$_{1A}$ receptors in humans: preliminary analyses. *Nucl Med Biol*, **27**, 523–527.

Martinez D, Broft A, Laruelle M (2000b) Pindolol augmentation of antidepressant treatment: recent contributions from brain imaging studies. *Biol Psychiat*, **48**, 844–853.

Martinot JL, Hardy P, Feline A, Huret JD, Mazoyer B, Attar Levy D, Pappata S, Syrota A (1990a) Left prefrontal glucose hypometabolism in the depressed state: a confirmation. *Am J Psychiat*, **147**, 1313–1317.

Martinot JL, Allilaire JF, Mazoyer BM, Hantouche E, Huret JD, Legaut Demare F, Deslauriers AG, Hardy P, Pappata S, Baron JC *et al.* (1990b) Obsessive-compulsive disorder: a clinical, neuropsychological and positron emission tomography study. *Acta Psychiat Scand*, **82**, 233–242.

Matthes H, Boschert U, Amlaiky N, Grailkhe R, Plassat JL, Muscatelli F, Mattei MG, Hen R, (1993) Mouse 5-hydroxytryptamine$_{2A}$ and 5-hydroxytryptamine$_{5B}$ define a new family of serotonin receptors: cloning, functional expression, and chromosomal localization. *Mol Pharmacol*, **129**, 333–337.

Mayberg HS, Lewis PJ, Regenold W, Wagner HN Jr (1994a) Paralimbic hypoperfusion in unipolar depression. *J Nucl Med*, **35**, 929–934.

Mayberg HS (1994b) Frontal lobe dysfunction in secondary depression. *J Neuropsychiat Clin Neurosci*, **6**, 428–442.

Mayberg HS, Brannan SK, Mahurin RK, Jerabek PA, Brickman JS, Tekell JL, Silva JA, McGinnis S, Glass TG, Martin CC, Fox PT (1997) Cingulate function in depression: a potential predictor of treatment response. *Neuroreport*, **8**, 1057–1061.

McBride PA, DeMeo MD, Sweeney JA, Halper J, Mann JJ, Shear MK (1992) Neuroendocrine and behavioral responses to challenge with the indirect serotonin agonist D-fenfluramine in adults with obsessive compulsive disorder. *Biol Psychiat*, **164**, 19–34.

McAllister-Williams RH, Young AH (1998) Pindolol augmentation of antidepressant therapy. *Br J Psychiat*, **173**, 536–537.

McAskill R, Mir S, Taylor D (1998) Pindolol augmentation of antidepressant therapy. *Br J Psychiat*, **173**, 203–208 (published erratum in *Br J Psychiat*, **173**, 443).

McCann UD, Thorne D, Hall M, Popp K, Avery W, Sing H, Thomas M, Belenky G (1995) The effects of L-dihydroxyphenylalanine on alertness and mood in α-methyl-*p*-tyrosine-treated healthy humans. *Neuropsychopharmacology*, **13**, 41–52.

McGuire PK, Bench CJ, Frith CD, Marks IM, Frackowiak RS, Dolan RJ (1994) Functional anatomy of obsessive-compulsive phenomena. *Br J Psychiat*, **164**, 459–468.

McHugh PR (1990) The basal ganglia: the region, the integration of its systems and implications for psychiatry and neurology. In: AJ Franks (ed) *Function and Dysfunction of the Basal Ganglia*. Manchester: Manchester University Press, 259–269.

Meltzer HY, Maes M (1994) Effect of pindolol on the L-5-HTP-induced increase in plasma prolactin and cortisol concentrations in man. *Psychopharmacology*, **114**, 635–643.

Meltzer HY, Lowy M, Robertson A, Goodnick P, Perline R (1984) Effect of 5-hydroxytryptophan on serum cortisol level in major affective disorders. *Arch Gen Psychiat*, **41**, 391–397.

Meltzer H, Bastani B, Jayathilake K, Maes M (1997) Fluoxetine, but not tricyclic antidepressants, potentiates the 5-hydroxytryptophan-mediated increase in plasma cortisol and prolactin secretion in subjects with major depression or with obsessive compulsive disorder. *Neuropsychopharmacology*, **17**, 1–11.

Mendez MF, Adams NL, Lewandowski KS (1989) Neurobehavioral changes associated with caudate lesions. *Neurology*, **39**, 349–354 (abstr).

Mervaala E, Fohr J, Kononen M, Valkonen-Korhonen M, Vainio P, Partanen K, et al. (2000) Quantitative MRI of the hippocampus and amygdala in severe depression. *Psychol Med*, **30**, 117–125.

Miller HL, Delgado PL, Salomon RM, Heninger GR, Charney DS (1996) Effects of α-methyl-*p*-tyrosine (AMPT) in drug-free depressed patients. *Neuropsychopharmacology*, **14**, 151–157.

Monteleone P, Catapano F, Bortolotti F, Maj M (1997a) Plasma prolactin response to D-fenfluramine in obsessive-compulsive patients before and after fluvoxamine treatment. *Biol Psychiat*, **42**, 175–180.

Monteleone P, Catapano F, Tortorella A, Maj M (1997b) Cortisol response to D-fenfluramine in patients with obsessive-compulsive disorder and in healthy subjects: evidence for a gender-related effect. *Neuropsychobiology*, **36**, 8–12.

Moret C, Briley M (1990) Serotonin autoreceptor subsensitivity and antidepressant activity. *Eur J Pharmacol*, **180**, 351–356.

Morley JE (1990) Appetite Regulation by Gut Peptides. *Ann Rev Nutr*, **10**, 383–395.

Murphy DL, Mueller EA, Hill JL, Tolliver TJ, Jacobsen FM (1989) Comparative anxiogenic, neuroendocrine, and other physiologic effects of *m*-chlorophenylpiperazine given intravenously or orally to healthy volunteers. *Psychopharmacology*, **98**, 275–282.

Nasrallah HA, Coffman JA, Olson SC (1989) Structural brain-imaging findings in affective disorders: an overview. *J Neuropsychiatry Clin Neurosci*, **1**, 21–26.

Nesse RM, Cameron OG, Cuirtis GC *et al.* (1984) Adrenergic function in patients with panic anxiety. *Arch Gen Psychiat,* **41**, 771–776.

Newman ME, Shapira B, Lerer B (1992) Effects of lithium and desimipramine on second messenger responses in rat hippocampus: relation to G protein effects. *Neuropharmacology,* **30**, 1297–1302.

Nordahl TE, Semple WE, Gross M, Mellman TA, Stein MB, Goyer P, King AC, Uhde TW, Cohen RM (1990) Cerebral glucose metabolic differences in patients with panic disorder. *Neuropsychopharmacology,* **3**, 261–272.

Norman TR, Judd FK, Gregory M, James RH, Kimber NM, McIntyre IM, Burrows GD (1986) Platelet serotonin uptake in panic disorder. *J Affect Dis,* **11**, 69–72.

Norman TR, Kimber NM, Judd FK *et al.* (1987) Platelet 3H-rauwolscine binding in patients with panic attacks. *Psychiat Res,* **22**, 43–48.

Norman TR, Sartor DM, Judd FK, Burrows GD, Gregory MS, McIntrye IM (1989) Platelet serotonin uptake and 3H-Imipramine binding in panic disorder. *J Affect Dis,* **17**, 77–81.

Norman TR, Judd FK, Staikos V, Burrows GD, McIntyre IM (1990) High-affinity platelet [3H]LSD binding is decreased in panic disorder. *J Affect Dis,* **19**, 119–123.

Nutt DJ (1989) Altered α_2-adrenoceptor sensitivity in panic disorder. *Arch Gen Psychiat,* **46**, 165–169.

Nutt DJ, Fraser S (1987) Platelet binding studies in panic disorder. *J Affect Dis,* **12**, 7–11.

O'Connor JJ, Kruk ZL (1994) Effects of 21 days treatment with fluoxetine on stimulated endogenous 5-hydroxytryptamine overflow in the rat dorsal raphe and suprachiasmatic nucleus studied using fast cyclic voltammetry *in vitro. Brain Res,* **640**, 328–335.

Ontiveros A, Fontaine R, Breton G, Elie R, Fontaine S, Dery R (1989) Correlation of severity of panic disorder and neuroanatomical changes on magnetic resonance imaging. *J Neuropsychiat Clin Neurosci,* **1**, 404–408.

Park SBG, Cowen PJ (1995) Effect of pindolol on the prolactin response to D-fenfluramine. *Psychopharmacology,* **18**, 471–474.

Park SBG, Williamson DJ, Cowen PJ (1996) 5-HT neuroendocrine function in major depression: prolactin and cortisol responses to D-fenfluramine. *Psychol Med,* **26**, 1191–1196.

Paul SM, Rehavi M, Skolnick P, Goodwin FK (1980) Demonstration of high-affinity binding sites for 3H-Imipramine on human platelets. *Life Sci,* **26**, 953–959.

Paul SM, Rehavi M, Skolnick KP, Ballenger JC, Goodwin FK (1981) Depressed patients have decreased binding of tritiated imipramine to platelet serotonin transporter. *Arch Gen Psychiat,* **38**, 1315–1317.

Pecknold JC, Suranyi-Cadotte B, Chang H, Nair NPV (1988) Serotonin uptake in panic disorder and agoraphobia. *Neuropsychopharmacology,* **39**, 917–928.

Perani D, Colombo C, Bressi S, Bonfanti A, Grassi F, Scarone S, Bellodi L, Smeraldi E, Fazio F (1995) [F-18] FDG PET study in obsessive-compulsive disorder a clinical/metabolic correlation study after treatment. *Br J Psychiat,* **166**, 244–250.

*Perez V, Gilaberte I, Faries D, Alvarez E, Artigas F (1997) Randomised, double-blind, placebo-controlled trial of pindolol in combination with fluoxetine antidepressant treatment. *Lancet,* **349**, 1594–1597.

*Perez V, Soler J, Puigdemont D, Alvarez E, Artigas F (1999) A double-blind, randomized, placebo-controlled trial of pindolol augmentation in depressive patients resistant to serotonin reuptake inhibitors. *Arch Gen Psychiat,* **56**, 375–379.

Perse TL, Greist JH, Jefferson JW (1987) Fluvoxamine treatment of obsessive-compulsive disorder. *Am J Psychiat,* **144**, 1543–1548.

Phillips ML, Marks IM, Senior C, Lythgoe D, O'Dwyer AM, Meehan O, *et al.* (2000) A differential neural response in obsessive-compulsive disorder patients with washing compared with checking symptoms to disgust. *Psychol Med,* **30**, 1037–1050.

Pigott TA, Yoney TH, L'Heureux F (1990) Serotonergic responsivity to m-CPP in OCD patients during clomipramine and fluoxetine treatment. *Biol Psychiat*, 27, 4A–17A.

Pigott TA, Zohar J, Hill JL, *et al.* (1991) Metergoline blocks the behavioral and neuroendocrine effects of orally administered m-chlorophenylpiperazine in patients with obsessive-compulsive disorder. *Biol Psychiat*, 29, 418–426.

Pigott TA, Hill JL, Grady TA *et al.* (1993a) A comparison of the behavioral effects of oral versus intravenous mCPP administration in OCD patients and the effect of metergoline prior to i.v. mCPP. *Biol Psychiat*, 33, 3–14.

Pigott TA, Murphy DL, Brooks A (1993b) Pharmacological probes in OCD: support for selective 5-HT dysregulation. Presented at the First International Obsessive Compulsive Disorder Congress, Capri, Italy, 12–13 March 1993.

Pillay SS, Yurgelun Todd DA, Bonello CM, Lafer B, Fava M, Renshaw PF (1997) A quantitative magnetic resonance imaging study of cerebral and cerebellar gray matter volume in primary unipolar major depression: relationship to treatment response and clinical severity. *Biol Psychiat*, 42, 79–84.

Plassat JL, Boschert U, Amlaiky N, Hen R (1992) The mouse 5-HT$_5$ receptor reveals a remarkable heterogeneity within the 5-HT$_{1D}$ receptor family. *EMBO J*, 11, 4779–4786.

Pohl R, Rainey JM, Ortiz A *et al.* (1985) Isoproterenol-induced anxiety states. *Psychopharmacol Bull*, 21, 424–427.

Pohl R, Yeragani VK, Balon R *et al.* (1988) Isoproterenol-induced panic attacks. *Biol Psychiat*, 24, 891–902.

✳ Pohl R, Yeragani VK, Balon R (1990) Effects of isoproterenol in panic disorder patients after antidepressant treatment. *Biol Psychiat*, 28, 203–214.

Post RM, DeLisi LE, Holcomb HH, Uhde TW, Cohen R, Buchsbaum MS (1987) Glucose utilization in the temporal cortex of affectively ill patients: positron emission tomography. *Biol Psychiat*, 22, 545–553.

Power AC, Cowen PJ (1992) Neuroendocrine challenge tests: assessment of 5-HT function in anxiety and depression. *Mol Aspects Med*, 13, 205–220.

Pratt J, Lenner P, Reynolds EH, Marsden CD (1979) Clonazepam induces decreased serotonergic activity in the mouse brain. *Neuropharmacology*, 18, 791–799.

Price LH, Charney DS, Delgado PL, Anderson GM, Heninger GR (1989) Effects of desipramine and fluvoxamine treatment on the prolactin response to tryptophan: Serotonergic function and the mechanism of antidepressant action. *Arch Gen Psychiat*, 46, 625–631.

Rabiner EA, Gunn RN, Wilkins MR, Sargent PA, Mocaer E, Sedman E, Cowen PJ, Grasby PM (2000a) Drug action at the 5-HT$_{1A}$ receptor in vivo: autoreceptor and postsynaptic receptor occupancy examined with PET and [carbonyl-11C]WAY-100635. *Neuropsychopharmacology*, 23, 285–293.

Rabiner EA, Gunn RN, Castro ME, Sargent PA, Cowen PJ, Koepp MJ, Meyer JH, Bench CJ, Harrison PJ, Pazos A, Sharp T, Grasby PM (2000b) β-Blocker binding to human 5-HT$_{1A}$ receptors in vivo and in vitro: implications for antidepressant therapy. *Nucl Med Biol*, 27, 509–513.

Rabins PV, Pearlson GD, Aylward E, Kumar AJ, Dowell K (1991) Cortical magnetic resonance imaging changes in elderly inpatients with major depression [see comments]. *Am J Psychiat*, 148, 617–620.

Rainey M Jr, Ettedgui E, Pohl B *et al.* (1984) The α-receptor: isoproterenol anxiety states. *Psychopathology*, 17, 40–51.

Raisman R, Sechter D, Briley MS (1981) High affinity ^{3}H-imipramine binding in platelets from untreated and treated depressed patients compared to healthy controls. *Psychopharmacology*, 75, 368–371.

Rasmussen SA, Goodman WK, Woods SW *et al.* (1987) Effects of yohimbine in obsessive-compulsive disorder. *Psychopharmacology*, **93**, 308–373.

Rauch SL, Jenike MA, Alpert NM, Baer L, Breiter HC, Savage CR, Fischman AJ (1994) Regional cerebral blood flow measured during symptom provocation in obsessive-compulsive disorder using oxygen 15-labeled carbon dioxide and positron emission tomography [see comments]. *Arch Gen Psychiat*, **51**, 62–70.

Rausch JL, Stahl SM, Hauger R (1990) Cortisol and growth hormone responses to the 5-HT$_{1A}$ agonist gepirone in depressed patients. *Biol Psychiat*, **28**, 73–78.

Redmond DE (1987) Studies of the nucleus locus coeruleus in monkeys and hypotheses for neuropsychopharmacology. In: HY Meltzer (ed) *Psychopharmacology: The third generation of Progress.* New York: Raven, 967–975.

Rehfeld JF (1978) Immunohistochemical studies on cholecystokinin. II. Distribution and molecular heterogenity in central nervous system and small intestine of man and dog. *J Biol Chem*, **253**, 4022–4030.

Reiman EM (1987) The study of panic disorder using positron emission tomography. *Psychiat Dev*, **5**, 63–78.

Reiman EM, Raichle ME, Butler FK, Herscovitch P, Robins E (1984) A focal brain abnormality in panic disorder, a severe form of anxiety. *Nature*, **310**, 683–685.

Reiman EM, Raichle ME, Robins E, Butler FK, Herscovitch P, Fox P, Perlmutter J (1986) The application of positron emission tomography to the study of panic disorder. *Am J Psychiat*, **143**, 469–477.

Reiman EM, Raichle ME, Robins E, Mintun MA, Fusselman MJ, Fox PT, Price JL, Hackman KA (1989) Neuroanatomical correlates of a lactate-induced anxiety attack. *Arch Gen Psychiat*, **46**, 493–500.

Robinson DS, Alms DR, Shrotriya RC, Messina M, Wickramaratne P (1989) Serotonergic anxiolytics and treatment of depression. *Psychopathology*, **22** (suppl 1), 27–36.

Robinson D, Wu HW, Munne RA, Ashtari M, Alvir JMJ, Lerner G, Koreen A, Cole K, Bogerts B (1995) Reduced caudate nucleus volume in obsessive-compulsive disorder. *Arch Gen Psychiat*, **52**, 393–398.

Romero L, Celada P, Artigas F (1994) Reduction of in vivo striatal 5-hydroxytryptamine release by 8-OH-DPAT after inactivation of Gi/Go proteins in dorsal raphe nucleus. *Eur J Pharmacol*, **265**, 103–106.

Romero L, Bel N, Artigas F, De Montigny C, Blier P (1996) Effect of pindolol on the function of pre- and postsynaptic 5-HT$_{1A}$ receptors: *in vivo* microdialysis and electrophysiological studies in the rat brain. *Neuropsychopharmacology*, **15**, 349–360.

Rosenbaum JF, Biederman J, Hirshfeld DR, Bolduc EA, Chaloff J (1991) Behavioral inhibition in children: a possible precursor to panic disorder or social phobia. *J Clin Psychiat*, **52** (11, suppl), 5–9.

Rosenberg DR, Keshavan MS (1998) Toward a neurodevelopmental model of obsessive-compulsive disorder. *Biol Psychiat*, **43**, 623–640.

Roy A, Everett D, Pickar D, Paul SM (1987) Platelet tritiated imipramine binding and serotonin uptake in depressed patients and controls: relationship between plasma cortisol levels before and after dexamethasone administration. *Arch Gen Psychiat*, **44**, 320–327.

Rubin RT, Villanueva Meyer J, Ananth J, Trajmar PG, Mena I (1992) Regional xenon-133 cerebral blood flow and cerebral technetium-99m HMPAO uptake in unmedicated patients with obsessive-compulsive disorder and matched normal control subjects. Determination by high-resolution single-photon emission computed tomography [see comments]. *Arch Gen Psychiat*, **49**, 695–702.

Rubin RT, Ananth J, Villanueva Meyer J, Trajmar PG, Mena I (1995) Regional [133]xenon cerebral blood flow and cerebral ^{99m}Tc-HMPAO uptake in patients with obsessive-compulsive disorder before and during treatment. *Biol Psychiat*, **38**, 429–437.

Rutter JJ, Gundlah C, and Auerbach SB (1994) Increase in extracellular serotonin produced by uptake inhibitors is enhanced after chronic treatment with fluoxetine. *Neurosci Lett*, **171**, 183–186.

Sackeim HA, Prohovnik I, Moeller JR, Brown RP, Apter S, Prudic J, Devanand DP, Mukherjee S (1990) Regional cerebral blood flow in mood disorders. I. Comparison of major depressives and normal controls at rest. *Arch Gen Psychiat*, **47**, 60–70.

Salloway S, Price LH, Charney DS, Shapiro M (1988) Multiple sclerosis presenting as major depression: a diagnosis suggested by MRI scan but not CT scan. *J Clin Psychiat*, **49**, 364–366.

Saxena S, Rauch SL (2000) Functional neuroimaging and the neuroanatomy of obsessive-compulsive disorder. *Psychiatr Clin North Am*, **23**, 563–586.

Saxena S, Brody AL, Maidment KM, Dunkin JI, Colgan M, Alborzian S, *et al.* (1999) Localized orbitofrontal and subcortical metabolic changes and predictors of response to paroxetine treatment in obsessive-compulsive disorder. *Neuropsychopharmacology*, **21**, 683–693.

Schechter LE, Bolanos FJ, Gozlan H, Lanfumay L, Haj-Dahmane S, Laporte AM, Fattaccini M, Hamon M (1990) Alterations of central serotonergic and dopaminergic transmission in rats chronically treated with ipsapirone: biochemical and electrophysiological studies. *J Pharmacol Exp Ther*, **255**, 1335–1347.

Schildkraut JJ, Orsulak PJ, Gudeman JE (1977) Recent studies of the role of catecholamines in the pathophysiology and classification of depressive disorders. In: R Usdin (ed) *Neuroregulators and Psychiatric Disorders*. New York: Oxford University Press, 122–128.

Schlegel S, Maier W, Philipp M, Aldenhoff JB, Heuser I, Kretzschmar K, Benkert O (1989a) Computed tomography in depression: association between ventricular size and psychopathology. *Psychiat Res*, **29**, 221–230.

Schlegel S, Aldenhoff JB, Eissner D, Lindner P, Nickel O (1989b) Regional cerebral blood flow in depression: associations with psychopathology. *J Affect Dis*, **17**, 211–218.

Schlegel S, Steinert H, Bockisch A, Hahn K, Schloesser R, Benkert O (1994) Decreased benzodiazepine receptor binding in panic disorder measured by IOMAZENIL-SPECT. A preliminary report. *Eur Arch Psychiat Clin Neurosci*, **244**, 49–51.

Schneider LS, Munjack D, Severson JA, Palmer R (1987) Platelet [^{3}H]Imipramine binding in generalized anxiety disorder, panic disorder and agoraphobia with panic attacks. *Biol Psychiat*, **22**, 59–66.

Schneier FR, Jihad BS, Campeas R, Fallon BA, Hollander E, Coplan J, Liebowitz MR (1993) Buspirone in social phobia. *J Clin Psychopharmacol*, **13**, 251–56.

Schwartz JM, Stoessel PW, Baxter LR Jr, Martin KM, Phelps ME (1996) Systematic changes in cerebral glucose metabolic rate after successful behavior modification treatment of obsessive-compulsive disorder. *Arch Gen Psychiat*, **53**, 109–113.

Schweizer EE, Amsterdam J, Rickels K, Kaplan M, Droba M (1986) Open trial of buspirone in the treatment of major depressive disorder. *Psychopharmacol Bull*, **22**, 183–185.

Seibyl JP, Krystal JH, Price LH, Woods SW, D'Amico C, Heninger GR, Charney DS (1991) Effects of ritanserin on the behavioral, neuroendocrine and cardiovascular responses to *m*-chlorphenylpiperazine in healthy subjects. *Psychiat Res*, **38**, 227–236.

Shear MK, Fyer AJ, Ball G, Josephson S, Fitzpatrick M, Gitlin B, Frances A, Gorman JM, Liebowitz MR, Klein DF (1991) Vulnerability to sodium lactate in panic disorder patients given cognitive-behavioral therapy. *Am J Psychiat*, **148**, 795–797.

Sheehan DV, Raj BA, Trehan RR, Knapp EL (1993) Serotonin in panic disorder and social phobia. *Int Clin Psychopharmacol*, **8** (suppl 2), 63–77.

Shima S, Shikano T, Kitamura T, Masuda Y, Tsukumo T, Kanba S, Asai M (1984) Depression and ventricular enlargement. *Acta Psychiat Scand*, **70**, 275–277.

Shopsin B, Gershon S, Goldstein M, Friedman E, Wilk S (1975) Use of synthesis inhibitors in defining a role for biogenic amines during imipramine treatment in depressed patients. *Psychopharmacol Comm*, **1**, 239–249.

Shopsin B, Friedman E, Gershon S (1976) Parachlorophenylalanine reversal of tranylcypromine effects in depressed patients. *Arch Gen Psychiat*, **33**, 811–819.

Siever LJ, Murphy DL, Slater S, de la Vega E, Lipper S (1984) Plasma prolactin changes following fenfluramine in depressed patients compared to controls: an evaluation of central serotonergic responsivity in depression. *Life Sci*, **34**, 1029–1039.

Sleight AJ, Smith RJ, Marsden CA, Palfreyman MG (1989) The effects of chronic treatment with amitriptyline and MDL 72394 on the control of 5-HT release *in vivo*. *Neuropharmacol*, **28**, 477–480.

Smeraldi E, Diaferia G, Erzegovesi S, Lucca A, Bellodi L, Moja EA (1996) Tryptophan depletion in obsessive-compulsive patients. *Biol Psychiat*, **40**, 398–402.

Smith GS, Reynolds CF III, Pollock B, Derbyshire S, Nofzinger E, Dew MA, *et al.* (1999) Cerebral glucose metabolic response to combined total sleep deprivation and antidepressant treatment in geriatric depression. *Am J Psychiat*, **156**, 683–689.

Smith KA, Cowen PJ (1997) Serotonin and depression. In: A Honig, HM van Praag (eds) *Depression: Neurobiological, Psychopathological and Therapeutic Advances*. Chichester: Wiley, 129–146.

Smith KA, Morris JS, Friston KJ, Cowen PJ, Dolan RJ (1999) Brain mechanisms associated with depressive relapse and associated cognitive impairment following acute tryptophan depletion. *Br J Psychiat*, **174**, 525–529.

Southwick SM, Krystal J, Morgan CA *et al.* (1993) Abnormal noradrenergic function in post-traumatic stress disorder. *Arch Gen Psychiat*, **50**, 266–274.

Stahl SM, Ciaranello RD, Berger PA (1982) Platelet serotonin in schizophrenia and depression. In: BT Ho (ed) *Serotonin in Biological Psychiatry*. New York: Raven, 182.

Stein DJ, Hollander E, Cohen L, Simeon D, Aronowitz B (1995) Serotonergic responsivity in trichotillomania: neuroendocrine effects of *m*-chlorophenylpiperazine. *Biol Psychiat*, **37**, 414–416.

Stewart RS, Devous MD Sr, Rush AJ, Lane L, Bonte FJ (1988) Cerebral blood flow changes during sodium-lactate-induced panic attacks. *Am J Psychiat*, **145**, 442–449.

Swedo SE, Schapiro MB, Grady CL, Cheslow DL, Leonard HL, Kumar A, Friedland R, Rapoport SI, Rapoport JL (1989) Cerebral glucose metabolism in childhood-onset obsessive-compulsive disorder. *Arch Gen Psychiat*, **46**, 518–523.

Swedo SE, Pietrini P, Leonard HL, Schapiro MB, Rettew DC, Goldberger EL, Rapoport SI, Rapoport JL, Grady CL (1992) Cerebral glucose metabolism in childhood-onset obsessive-compulsive disorder. Revisualization during pharmacotherapy. *Arch Gen Psychiat*, **49**, 690–694.

Targum SD, Marshall LE (1989) Fenfluramine provocation of anxiety in patients with panic disorder. *Psychiat Res*, **28**, 295–306.

Terao T (1997) Selective serotonin reuptake inhibitors plus pindolol (letter). *Lancet*, **350**, 289.

Thomas P, Bordet R, Alexandre JY, Catteau, Cyran C, Danel T, Debieve J, Dumon JP, Dumont P, Dutoit D, Duthoit D, Geraud C, Lalaux N, Lanviv F, Lebert F, Louvrier J, Maix JP, Plumecocq C, Scottez B, Servant D, Trinh E, Vaiva G, Vignau J, Thomas CE, Dupuis B (1997) Pindolol addition shorten delay of action of paroxetine in major depression: a double blind controlled trial. Abstract P.1.121. Vienna: ECNP.

Thoren P, Asberg M, Bertilsson L, Mellstrom B, Sjoqvist F, Traskmah L (1980) Clomipramine treatment of obsessive compulsive disorder. II. Biochemical aspects. *Arch Gen Psychiat*, **37**, 1289–1294.

Tome MB, Cloninger CR, Watson JP, Isaac MT (1997a) Serotonergic autoreceptor blockade in the reduction of antidepressant latency: personality variables and response to paroxetine and pindolol. *J Affect Dis*, **44**, 101–109.

Tome MB, Isaac MT, Harte R, Holland C (1997b) Paroxetine and pindolol: a randomized trial of serotonergic autoreceptor blockade in the reduction of antidepressant latency. *Int Clin Psychopharmacol,* **12,** 81–89.

Tuomisto J, Tukiainen E (1976) Depressed uptake of 5-hydroxytryptamine in blood platelets from depressed patients. *Nature,* **262,** 596–598.

Turner SM, Jacob RG, Beidel DC (1985) Fluoxetine in the treatment of obsessive compulsive disorder. *J Clin Psychopharmacol,* **5,** 207–212.

Tyrer P, Candy J, Kelly D (1973) A study of the clinical effects of phenelzine and placebo in the treatment of phobia anxiety. *Psychopharmacologia,* **32,** 237–254.

Uchitomi Y, Yamawaki S (1993) Chronic lithium treatment enhances the postsynaptic 5-HT$_{1A}$ receptor-mediated 5-HT behavioral syndrome induced by 8-OH-DPAT in rats via catecholaminergic systems. *Psychopharmacology,* **112,** 74–79.

Uhde TW, Kellner CH (1987) Cerebral ventricular size in panic disorder. *J Affect Dis,* **12,** 175–178.

Uhde TW, Vittone BJ, Siever LJ *et al.* (1986) Blunted growth hormone response to clonidine in panic disorder patients. *Biol Psychiat,* **21,** 1077–1081.

Uhde TW, Berrettini WH, Boy-Byrne PP, Bordenger JP, Post RM (1987) [3H]Imipramine binding in patients with panic disorder. *Biol Psychiat,* **22,** 52–58.

Upadhyaya AK, Pennel I, Cowen PJ, Deakin JFK (1991) Blunted growth hormone and prolactin responses to L-tryptophan in depression: a state-dependent abnormality. *J Affect Dis,* **21,** 213–218.

van den Hout MA, Griez E (1984) Panic symptoms after inhalation of carbondioxide. *Br J Psychiat,* **144,** 503–507.

van Megen HJGM, den Boer JA, Westenberg HGM (1992) Single blind dose response study with cholecystokinin (CCK-4) in panic disorder patients. *Clin Neuropharm,* **15** (suppl 1), 532B.

van Megen HJGM, den Boer JA, Westenberg HGM, Bradwejn J (1994a) On the significance of cholecystokinin receptors in panic disorder. *Prog Neuropsychopharmacol,* **18,** 1235–1246.

van Megen HJGM, den Boer JA, Westenberg HGM (1994b) Pentagastrin induced panic attacks: enhanced sensitivity in panic disorder patients. *Psychopharmacology,* **114,** 449–455.

van Megen HJGM, Westenberg HGM, den Boer JA (1994c) Effect of the cholecystokinin-B (CCK-B) receptor antagonist L-365,260 on lactate induced panic attacks (PA). *Biol Psychol,* **40,** 804–860.

van Megen HJGM, Westenberg HGM, den Boer JA, Kahn RS (1996) Cholecystokinin in panic disorder. In: HGM Westenberg, JA den Boer, DL Murphy (eds) *Advances in the Neurobiology of Anxiety Disorders.* Chichester: Wiley, 197–227.

van Megen HJGM, Westenberg HGM, den Boer JA, Slaap B, Scheepmakers A (1997a) Effect of the selective serotonin reuptake inhibitor fluvoxamine on CCK-4 induced panic attacks. *Psychopharmacology,* **129,** 357–364.

van Megen HJGM, Westenberg HGM, den Boer JA, Slaap BR (1997b) The cholecystokinin-B receptor antagonist CI-988 failed to affect CCK-4 induced symptoms in panic disorder patients. *Psychopharmacology,* **129,** 243–248.

van Praag HM (1997) Demoralization and melancholy; concerning the biological interface between traumatic life experiences and depression. In: A Honig, HM van Praag (eds) *Depression: Neurobiological, Psychopathological and Therapeutic Advances.* Chichester: Wiley, 251–276.

van Praag HM, Lemus C, Kahn RS (1987) Hormonal probes of central serotonergic activity: do they really exist?. *Biol Psychiat,* **22,** 86–98.

van Vliet IM, Slaap BR, Westenberg HGM, den Boer JA (1996) Behavioral, neuroendocrine and biochemical effects of different doses of 5-HTP in panic disorder. *Eur Neuropsychopharmacol,* **6,** 103–110.

van Vliet IM, Westenberg HGM, Slaap BR, den Boer JA, Ho Pian KL (1997) Anxiogenic effects of pentagastrin in patients with social phobia and healthy controls. *Biol Psychiat*, **42**, 76–78.

Videbech P (2000) PET measurements of brain glucose metabolism and blood flow in major depressive disorder: a critical review. *Acta Psychiat Scand*, **101**, 11–20.

Vythilingam M, Anderson ER, Goddard A, Woods SW, Staib LH, Charney DS, *et al.* (2000) Temporal lobe volume in panic disorder—a quantitative magnetic resonance imaging study. *Psychiat Res*, **99**, 75–82.

Wang XJ, Wang XH, Han S (1990) Cholecystokinin octapeptide antagonized opioid analgesia mediated by μ- and τ- but not δ-receptors in the spinal cord of the rat. *Brain Res*, **523**, 5–10.

Westenberg HGM, and Verhoeven WMA (1988) CSF monoamine metabolites in patients and controls: support for a bimodal distribution in major affective disorders. *Acta Psychiat Scand*, **78**, 541–549.

Winokur G (1982) The development and validity of familial subtypes in primary unipolar depression. *Pharmacopsychiatry*, **15**, 142–146 (abstr).

Woods SW, Charney DS, McPherson CA *et al.* (1987) Situational panic attacks: behavioral, physiological, and biochemical characterization. *Arch Gen Psychiat*, **44**, 365–375.

Woods SW, Hoffer PB, McDougle CJ, Charney DS (1991) Effects of yohimbine on regional cerebral blood flow in panic disorder. *Soc Neurosci Abstr*, **17**, 293.8.

Wu JC, Gillin JC, Buchsbaum MS, Hershey T, Johnson JC, Bunney WE Jr (1992) Effect of sleep deprivation on brain metabolism of depressed patients. *Am J Psychiat*, **149**, 538–543.

Yaksh TL, Furui T, Kanawati IS, Go VLW (1987) Release of cholecystokinin from rat cerebral cortex *in vivo*: role of GABA and glutamate receptor systems. *Brain Res*, **406**, 207–214.

Yazici KM, Kapucu O, Erbas B, Varoglu E, Gulec C, Bekdik CF (1992) Assessment of changes in regional cerebral blood flow in patients with major depression using the ^{99m}Tc-HMPAO single photon emission tomography method. *Eur J Nucl Med*, **19**, 1038–1043.

Young SN (1994) The use of diet and dietary components in the study of factors controlling affect in humans: a review. *J Psychiat Neurosci*, **18**, 235–244.

Young SN, Smith SE, Pihl RO, Ervin FR (1985) Tryptophan depletion causes a rapid lowering of mood normal males. *Psychopharmacology*, **87**, 173–177.

Zanardi R, Artigas F, Franchini L, Sforzini L, Gasperini M, Smeraldi E, Perez J (1997) How long should pindolol be associated with paroxetine to improve the antidepressant response? *J Clin Psychopharmacol*, **17**, 446–450.

Zandbergen J, Pols H, Fernandez I, Griez E (1991) An analysis of panic symptoms during hypercarbia compared to hypocarbia in patients with panic attacks. *J Affect Dis*, **23**, 131–136.

Zitrin CM, Klein DF, Woerner MG, Ross DC (1983) Treatment of phobias: comparison of imipramine and placebo. *Arch Gen Psychiat*, **40**, 125–138.

Zitterl W, Wimberger D, Demal U, Hofer E, Lenz G (1994) [Nuclear magnetic resonance tomography findings in obsessive-compulsive disorder] Kernspintomographische Befunde bei der Zwangserkrankung. *Nervenarzt*, **65**, 619–622.

Zohar J (1996) Is 5-HT$_{1D}$ involved in obsessive compulsive disorder? In: 6, suppl. 4 edition, pp. S4–54.

Zohar J, Insel TR (1987) Obsessive-compulsive disorder: psychobiological approaches to diagnosis, treatment, and pathophysiology. *Biol Psychiat*, **22**, 667–687.

Zohar J, Mueller EA, Insel TR (1987) Serotonin responsivity in obsessive compulsive disorder. *Arch Gen Psychiat*, **44**, 946–951.

Zohar J, Insel TR, Zohar-Kadoush RC, Hill JL, Murphy DL (1988) Serotonergic responsivity in obsessive-compulsive disorder: effects of clomipramine treatment. *Arch Gen Psychiat*, **45**, 167–172.

Zohar J, Insel TR, Berman KF, Foa EB, Hill JL, Weinberger DR (1989) Anxiety and cerebral blood flow during behavioral challenge. Dissociation of central from peripheral and subjective measures. *Arch Gen Psychiat*, **46**, 505–510.

3

Comorbidity of depression and anxiety disorders

Ronald C. Kessler

Studies of diagnostic patterns in both treatment samples (Ross *et al.*, 1988; Wolf *et al.*, 1988; Mezzich *et al.*, 1990; Rounsaville *et al.*, 1991) and community samples (Robins *et al.*, 1991; Wittchen *et al.*, 1992; WHO International Consortium in Psychiatric Epidemiology, 2000) show that depression and anxiety often co-occur with each other as well as with other psychiatric disorders. Indeed, comorbidity appears to be the norm, with up to two-thirds of those having a lifetime history of major depression in general population samples also having a history of at least one other psychiatric disorder, and an even higher proportion of those with anxiety having multiple disorders (Robins *et al.*, 1991). Furthermore, the majority of people in an episode of either depression or anxiety also meet criteria for at least one other current psychiatric disorder if diagnostic hierarchy rules are relaxed (Kessler, 1997). By far the strongest comorbidities in both these cases are between depression and anxiety disorders.

There is controversy about these results relating to the possibility that they are, at least in part, artifacts of changes in the DSM diagnostic system that has been used in most recent studies of comorbidity (First *et al.*, 1990, Frances *et al.*, 1990; 1992). These changes included, beginning with DSM-III (American Psychiatric Association [APA], 1980) and continuing with DSM-III-R (APA, 1987) and DSM-IV (APA, 1994), a dramatic increase in the number of diagnostic categories and a reduction in the number of exclusion criteria in an effort to retain potentially important differentiating information (First *et al.*, 1990). As a result of these changes, many

SSRIs in Depression and Anxiety, Second Edition. Edited by S.A. Montgomery and J.A. den Boer.
© 2001 John Wiley & Sons Ltd.

patients who would have previously received only a single diagnosis, received multiple diagnoses. An argument could be made that this had the undesirable consequence of artificially increasing the estimated prevalence of comorbidity and introducing distinctions among cases that are not clinically useful (Frances *et al.*, 1990). However, it is impossible to judge this without making the distinctions and investigating whether they are useful. The disaggregation successively introduced into recent versions of the DSM system allows this to be done using established criteria for determining the validity of diagnostic distinctions (Robins and Guze, 1970; Cloninger, 1989). Although this work is still in progress, it is likely to result in the conclusion that some of the diagnostic distinctions currently in vogue are useful, while others are not.

The bulk of work in this area is being done in treatment samples, including longitudinal and family genetic studies and biological studies aimed at improving our understanding of the underlying pathogenesis of pure and comorbid disorders as well as treatment studies aimed at determining whether a target symptom approach to treatment can be enhanced by introducing evidence about comorbidity. These studies are the focus of the present volume. However, it is important that these results be interpreted against the backdrop of descriptive general population data on the distributions and associations among sets of diagnostic criteria. General population data of this sort provide a context in which clinical results can be interpreted, as well as an external validity check to guard against the selection biases that exist in clinical samples.

The present chapter presents an overview of recent general population epidemiologic research of this sort, with a special focus on results from the US National Comorbidity Survey (NCS; Kessler *et al.*, 1994), a large nationally representative survey of the US household population designed explicitly to study the epidemiology of comorbid psychiatric disorders. We begin by examining basic patterns of comorbidity between depression and anxiety disorders in the general population. We next consider temporal priorities in the predictive relationships between comorbid depression and anxiety disorders. And we close by presenting data on the consequences of comorbidity for course and severity.

Basic patterns of morbidity and comorbidity

Epidemiologic studies consistently find that mood disorders are both less prevalent and less persistent than anxiety disorders (Orn *et al.*, 1988; Canino, *et al.*, 1987; Lépine *et al.*, 1989; Wittchen *et al.*, 1992; Faravelli *et al.*, 1989; Hwu *et al.*, 1989; Lee *et al.*, 1990; Wells *et al.*, 1989; Oakley-Browne, *et al.*, 1989). In the NCS, for example, we estimated that 17.1% of the 8098 respondents met DSM-III-R criteria for a major depressive episode (MDE) at some time in their life and 14.9% a nonbipolar major depressive disorder (MDD) at some time in their life compared to 28.7% who met lifetime criteria for one or more anxiety disorders, including panic disorder, phobia, generalized anxiety disorder, or post-traumatic stress disorder (Kessler and Zhao,

1999). In addition, we found that the persistence of major depression, roughly estimated as the ratio of recent prevalence to lifetime prevalence, was approximately 15% less than the persistence of overall anxiety disorders (Kessler & Zhao, 1999).

Basic patterns of bivariate comorbidity between MDD and NCS/DSM-III-R anxiety disorders are reported in Table 3.1. The results in the first four columns concern lifetime (LT) comorbidity. As shown there, 58.0% of the NCS respondents with lifetime depression also had a lifetime anxiety disorder, while 29.5% of respondents with a lifetime anxiety disorder also had lifetime MDD. The odds-ratios (ORs) reported in the next column are all significant at the 0.05 level and greater than 1.0. The strongest ORs are associated with the relationships of depression with generalized anxiety disorder (6.0), panic disorder (4.0) and post-traumatic stress disorder (4.0).

The results in the last four columns concern 12-month comorbidity. As shown there, 51.2% of the respondents with 12-month MDD also experienced at least one other NCS/DSM-III-R anxiety disorder during this same period of time, while 22.1% of those with a 12-month anxiety disorder also had 12-month depression. The ORs in the next column are all significant and greater than 1.0 and consistently larger than the LT ORs. This means that the tendency for episodes of anxiety and depression to co-occur is more powerful than the tendency for people with one of these lifetime disorders to have the other lifetime disorder.

Temporally primary and secondary disorders

The results in Table 3.1 are cross-sectional. This means that they do not provide any insights into the temporal priorities between comorbid conditions. An international task force found consistent evidence that respondents with comorbid depression and anxiety retrospectively report that their anxiety started at an earlier age than their depression (Merikangas *et al.*, 1996). These retrospective reports are confirmed in long-term longitudinal studies (Angst *et al.*, 1990; Dohrenwend, 1990; Hagnell and Grasbeck, 1990; Murphy, 1990).

As shown in Table 3.2, similar results are found in the NCS. More than two-thirds of those with a lifetime history of both MDD and anxiety retrospectively reported that the first onset of at least one anxiety disorder occurred at an earlier age than first onset of depression. Only 15.4% reported that their MDD started before their first anxiety disorder and the remaining 16.0% that their depression and anxiety started in the same year.

It is noteworthy that there is considerable variation in these patterns across the different anxiety disorders assessed in the NCS. The most dramatic distinction is between panic disorder (PD) and generalized anxiety disorder (GAD), on the one hand, compared with all other anxiety disorders. The vast majority of respondents with a history of comorbidity between MDD and either PD (83.3%) or GAD (75.9%) reported that their depression occurred either before or in the same year as these anxiety disorders. Depression was much less likely to be primary, in comparison,

Table 3.1 Comorbidities between DSM-III-R MDD and NCS/DSM-III-R anxiety disorders.

Anxiety disorder	Lifetime MDD				12-Month MDD			
	A/M (%)*	M/A (%)*	OR	(95% CI)	A/M (%)*	M/A (%)*	OR	(95% CI)
Generalized anxiety disorder	17.2	47.8	6.0**	(4.2–8.6)	15.4	41.3	8.2**	(5.0–13.5)
Agoraphobia	16.3	33.3	3.4***	(2.5–4.6)	12.6	26.5	4.4***	(2.8–6.9)
Simple phobia	24.3	31.3	3.1***	(2.5–3.8)	23.7	22.9	3.7***	(2.8–4.8)
Social phobia	27.1	29.4	2.9***	(2.3–3.6)	20.0	21.1	3.3***	(2.4–4.5)
Panic disorder	9.9	40.8	4.0***	(2.7–6.1)	8.6	32.3	5.0**	(3.1–8.0)
Post-traumatic stress disorder	19.5	39.0	4.0***	(3.1–5.2)	15.2	32.4	6.0**	(4.1–8.6)
Any anxiety disorder	58.0	29.5	4.2**	(3.4–5.2)	51.2	22.1	5.1**	(4.3–6.0)

*The first column (A/M%) shows the percentage of respondents with lifetime MDD who also reported the anxiety disorder in the row. The second column (%M/A) shows the percent of respondents with lifetime anxiety who also reported a history of generalized anxiety disorder. For example, 17.2% of those with lifetime MDD also reported a history of generalized anxiety disorder. For example, 47.8% of those with lifetime generalized anxiety disorder also reported a history of MDD. The odds-ratio (OR) between the two disorders is reported in the third column, with the 95% confidence interval (CI) of the OR in the fourth column. The results in the fifth through eighth columns are similar, but refer to comorbidity between episodes of depression and anxiety during the 12 months prior to interview. **$p < 0.05$. Reproduced, in part, from Kessler et al. (1996) with permission.

Table 3.2 The distribution of temporally primary and secondary DSM-III-R MDD among NCS respondents with a lifetime history of both MDD and one or more NCS/DSM-III-R anxiety disorder.

Anxiety disorder	MDD is temporally:					
	Primary		Secondary		Same year	
	(%)	(se)	(%)	(se)	(%)	(se)
Generalized anxiety disorder	28.5	(3.5)	24.0	(5.0)	47.4	(4.4)
Agoraphobia	26.7	(4.6)	50.7	(4.9)	22.6	(3.7)
Simple phobia	15.5	(2.9)	75.0	(3.6)	9.4	(2.0)
Social phobia	18.8	(2.2)	72.0	(3.0)	9.1	(1.8)
Panic disorder	49.4	(5.6)	16.6	(3.2)	33.9	(5.6)
Post-traumatic stress disorder	36.6	(4.0)	51.9	(4.0)	11.5	(2.7)
Any anxiety disorder	15.4	(1.7)	68.6	(2.1)	16.0	(1.5)

se = Standard error.

among respondents with a history of comorbidity between MDD and the other anxiety disorders.

It is also noteworthy that same-year onsets are quite common for comorbidities of MDD with either PD or GAD. This is part of a larger pattern seen in Table 3.3 for a shorter time lag between the onset of primary PD or GAD and secondary MDD than between any other primary anxiety disorder and secondary MDD. It is noteworthy that no such differentiation can be seen in the comparative time lags of comorbidity between primary MDD and secondary anxiety disorders, indirectly suggesting that the

Table 3.3 Time lag (in years) between the ages of onset of primary and secondary disorders among NCS respondents with a history of both DSM-III-R MDD and one or more NCS/DSM-III-R anxiety disorder.

Anxiety disorder	Temporally primary depression		Temporally primary depression	
	With a time lag of one year (%)	Median time lag (years)	With a time lag of one year (%)	Median time lag (years)
Generalized anxiety disorder	11.0	6	28.1	3
Agoraphobia	22.1	7	14.8	9
Simple phobia	21.0	3	8.6	12
Social phobia	16.6	5	9.2	11
Panic disorder	6.5	6	15.3	6
Post-traumatic stress disorder	14.1	5	8.6	10
Any anxiety disorder	19.2	4	9.3	13

large concentration of same-year onsets of MDD-PD and MDD-GAD are likely to involve the anxiety disorders occurring somewhat earlier than the depression.

The effects of earlier anxiety on risk of secondary MDD

Theoretical discussions of the causal pathways linking anxiety and depression have usually been based on the assumption that the anxiety is primary (Akiskal, 1990; Klein and Gorman, 1987). This assumption, in turn, is based largely on the fact that age of onset comparisons of the sort presented in Table 3.2 consistently find anxiety to occur at an earlier age than depression among patients with comorbid depression and anxiety. However, there is a flaw in the logic of these comparisons because they exclude information on the relative sizes and age of onset distributions of pure versus comorbid cases (Lavori, 1990). The problem can be illustrated with a simple example (Kessler and Price, 1993). Imagine two disorders, A and B, with a lifetime odds-ratio of 2.3, having equal lifetime prevalences and equal temporal priorities (i.e. 50% A before B and 50% B before A). This does not mean that the two disorders are equally powerful in predicting each other. Indeed, it is a simple matter to generate these observed results from an underlying process in which disorder A has no effect in predicting B but B has a strong effect in predicting A. One such process is as follows: 80% of lifetime cases of A have onsets at birth; 100% of lifetime cases of B have onsets at age 10 for reasons that are totally unrelated to prior A; and the remaining 20% of lifetime cases of A have onsets at age 20 that are powerfully influenced by prior history of B (odds-ratio of 20). This set of processes will yield a cross-sectional odds-ratio of 2.3 between the two lifetime disorders among people older than age 20.

This example illustrates the general point that a rigorous evaluation of temporal priority requires the researcher to go beyond a simple comparison of onset ages to examine reciprocal conditional risks in a way that takes into consideration the relative prevalences and age of onset distributions of both pure and comorbid cases. Such an analysis can more accurately be carried out in a general population sample than a clinical sample. This is true because age of onset distributions are biased in clinical samples because of a significant association between age of onset and probability of seeking treatment (Kessler, et al., 1998a).

The most elegant way to examine temporal priority is by means of reciprocal survival analysis in which each disorder in a comorbid pair is treated as a time-varying covariate to predict the first onset of the other disorder in the pair. This was done in the NCS by estimating a series of survival models to study the extent to which temporally primary anxiety disorders predict the subsequent first onset of depression and vice versa. Results show that these reciprocal effects are generally quite similar in magnitude in bivariate models that assume constant effects. Indeed, the differences between the reciprocal effects are less than their standard errors in all models other than those for comorbidity between depression and PTSD. In the latter, the predicted effect of depression on PTSD (OR = 6.7) is significantly greater than the predicted effect of PTSD on depression (OR = 2.7) (Kessler, 1997).

These results deal with metric effects—the relative odds of an onset of the outcome disorder depending on the prior existence of the predictor disorder. It is possible to have very large metric effects that explain only a trivial part of the variance in an outcome if the predictor is rare. For example, the relative odds of depressive episodes subsequent to the onset of schizophrenia is very high, but this accounts for only a trivial proportion of all depressive episodes due to the fact that schizophrenia is much more rare than depression. When we analyze the reciprocal survival data to evaluate explained variance, we find that the effects of prior anxiety on subsequent depression are generally larger than the effects of prior depression on subsequent anxiety. This is due to the fact that early-onset anxiety disorders are more common than early-onset depression.

All of the models described so far assumed constant effects. That is, they assumed that the relative odds of the onset of the secondary disorder do not vary as a function of time since onset of the primary disorder. This is an implausible assumption for at least two reasons. First, one would expect that people who do not develop a secondary disorder after a number of years are somehow more resilient than others. This should lead to a decrease in the ORs over time. Second, clinical investigators have observed that secondary depression often occurs only many years after a chronic primary psychiatric disorder (Cloninger *et al.*, 1990) or in the context of a chronic and seriously impairing physical illness (Hong *et al.*, 1987). This observation leads to the suggestion that secondary depression is often a response to the exhaustion and demoralization created by chronic intractable stress (Akiskal, 1985, 1990), which implies that ORs of primary anxiety disorders predicting subsequent depression should increase over time.

The results in Table 3.4 investigate the time lag issue for the effects of earlier anxiety disorders predicting secondary depression. The bivariate model used to generate these results stipulated that the onset of MDD within a given year is related to onset of anxiety disorders in the same year (cross-section association), onset of the anxiety disorders in earlier years (time-lagged effect), and a linear term for change in the time-lagged effect depending on the number of years since the onset of the earlier disorder (time-trend effect). As shown in the table, same-year associations are generally quite large, especially those associated with PD and GAD. We cannot interpret these as predictive because they are based on cross-sectional associations. However, the time-lagged effects are predictive and these, too, are consistently significant. By far the largest of the time-lagged effects is associated with GAD, with an OR of 7.6. It is noteworthy that the effect of PD (OR = 2.4) is lower than that of any other anxiety disorder (2.5–4.2) despite the large cross-sectional association.

The time-trend effects, finally, are insignificant with the exception of GAD. This means that OR magnitude generally does not change with time; that the elevated risk of MDD associated with an earlier onset of these anxiety disorders persists for many years without any significant change. The situation is different for GAD, whose effects decay with time. As shown in Figure 3.1, the decline in the time-lagged effects of GAD (reported as log-odds rather than odds-ratios) is linear and fairly gradual after the first year. It is noteworthy that despite the decline, the estimated effect of GAD remains greater than zero for more than a decade after onset.

Table 3.4 The effects (exponentiated discrete-time survival coefficients)* of prior NCS/DSM-III-R anxiety disorders on first onset of DSM-III-R MDD.

Anxiety disorders	Cross-sectional association		Time-lagged effect		Time-trend effect	
	OR	(95% CI)	OR	(95% CI)	OR	(95% CI)
Generalized anxiety disorder	62.0**	(37.1–103.9)	7.6**	(3.6–16.3)	0.85**	(0.8–0.9)
Agoraphobia	15.7**	(9.7–25.6)	2.5**	(1.0–6.1)	1.02	(0.9–1.1)
Simple phobia	9.1**	(5.8–14.4)	4.2**	(2.2–7.7)	0.95	(0.9–1.0)
Social phobia	6.5**	(3.7–11.4)	3.0**	(1.9–4.8)	0.98	(0.9–1.0)
Panic disorder	28.0**	(15.7–49.8)	2.4**	(1.1–5.5)	0.91	(0.8–1.1)
Post-traumatic stress disorder	9.2**	(4.7–17.8)	3.0**	(1.7–5.4)	0.97	(0.9–1.0)
Any anxiety disorder	12.0**	(8.9–16.0)	2.7**	(1.7–4.4)	0.99	(0.9–1.0)

* Coefficients are from a series of discrete-time survival equations in which first onset of MDD was predicted from the onset of one anxiety disorder in the same year as MDD (cross-sectional association), prior onset of this disorder (time-lagged effect), and a time-trend term for number of years since the onset of the anxiety disorder, controlling for age, sex and race. **$p \leqslant 0.05$. Reproduced from Kessler *et al.* (1996) with permission.

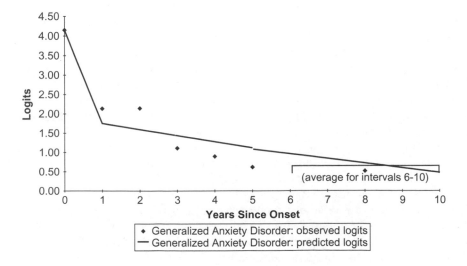

Figure 3.1. Logits for depression by time since onset of generalized anxiety disorder. Reproduced from Kessler *et al.* (1990) with permission.

Similar results hold when we reverse the investigation to look at the effects of temporally primary MDD in predicting first onset of anxiety disorders. The time-lagged effects are generally significant and the time-trend effects are generally not significant. And in those cases where the time-trend effects are significant, the trends are consistently negative. That is, to the extent that the predictions change over time, recent-onset depression is more powerful than persistent or recurrent depression in predicting the subsequent onset of anxiety.

One important specification of this general pattern of results is that the effects of primary disorders are largely confined to those that are active rather than in remission. This means that respondents with a history of disorder A are at elevated risk of the first onset of disorder B only if disorder A is active at the time of onset of B. This finding implies that the primary disorders are risk factors rather than merely markers of risk. An important exception, though, is the effect of temporally primary panic in predicting the subsequent first onset of MDD. Significantly elevated risk of MDD exists among all respondents with a lifetime history of panic, whether their most recent panic attack occurred a few days ago or many years ago (Kessler *et al.*, 1998b). This finding suggests that prior panic is a marker of some more fundamental risk factor for MDD. Another result consistent with this interpretation is that no dose–response relationship exists between primary panic (i.e. number of attacks) and subsequent depression.

The effects of comorbidity on disorder persistence

Other than the results reported above, there has been little previous epidemiologic research on the effects of temporally primary anxiety or depression on the subsequent first onset of secondary anxiety or depression. However, there has been a good deal of research on the relationship between anxiety-depression comorbidity and illness course (Bronisch and Hecht, 1990; Joffe *et al.*, 1993; Keitner *et al.*, 1991). Results show consistently that comorbid anxiety-depression is more persistent than either pure anxiety or pure depression. We have already seen an indication of this same pattern in Table 3.1, where episode comorbidity was found to be stronger than lifetime comorbidity. This finding means that anxiety and depression covary over time, a result that has previously been documented in treatment samples (e.g. Uhde *et al.*, 1985) and is linked to the fact that comorbid disorders tend to be recurrent.

A more direct evaluation of the relationship between comorbidity and persistence is reported in Table 3.5, where we show the results of logistic regression analyses in which the lifetime co-occurrence of either anxiety or depression is used to predict the persistence (12-month prevalence among lifetime cases) of the other disorder. The ORs have been adjusted for the effects of demographic variables (age, sex and race), age of onset of the outcome disorder, and time since onset of the outcome disorder. The results in the first column show that comorbid anxiety is associated with a significant increase in the persistence of depression. Panic is the only anxiety disorder here that is not associated with an elevated OR of depression persistence. The results in the third

Table 3.5 The effects of lifetime comorbidity on the persistence of DSM-III-R MDD and NCS/DSM-III-R anxiety disorders.*

Anxiety disorder	Persistence of MDD		Persistence of anxiety	
	OR	(95% CI)	OR	(95% CI)
Generalized anxiety disorder	1.4	(1.0–2.1)	0.8	(0.5–1.4)
Agoraphobia	2.1**	(1.3–3.6)	1.0	(0.6–1.7)
Simple phobia	1.8**	(1.3–2.7)	1.1	(0.7–1.6)
Social phobia	1.6**	(1.1–2.2)	1.2	(0.8–1.7)
Panic disorder	1.1	(0.7–1.7)	1.1	(0.6–1.8)
Post-traumatic stress disorder	1.6**	(1.2–2.1)	1.1	(0.7–1.8)
Any anxiety disorder	1.9**	(1.4–2.6)	1.2	(1.0–1.5)

*Coefficients are from a series of logistic regression equations in which 6-month prevalence of the outcome disorder in the subsample of respondents with a lifetime history of that disorder was predicted by comorbidity with the other disorders considered here, controlling for age of onset of the outcome disorder, time since onset of the outcome disorder, sex and race. **$p \leqslant 0.05$.

row, in comparison, show that comorbid depression is not associated with a significantly increased persistence of anxiety.

Comorbidity and severity

Previous research has found that comorbidity is associated with illness severity (Weissman *et al.*, 1989; Marshall, 1996; Kessler, 1995). As shown in Table 3.6, the NCS results are consistent with this finding. Among respondents with a lifetime history of MDD there is a significant association between comorbid anxiety and serious role impairment due to depression (OR = 1.9). This association is non-specific in the sense that each of the six different types of anxiety considered in the survey is a significant predictor of role impairment due to depression, with ORs ranging between 1.3 for simple phobia and 2.6 for panic disorder. In addition, comorbid PD (OR = 2.1) and PTSD (OR = 5.0) are associated with significantly increased risk of suicide attempts among respondents with lifetime MDD.

In addition, among respondents with a lifetime history of anxiety there is a significant association between comorbid depression and serious role impairment due to anxiety (OR = 2.3). However, this association is not consistent across all anxiety disorders. Depression significantly predicts serious role impairment associated with GAD (OR = 1.8) and social phobia (OR = 2.4), but not with any of the other anxiety disorders considered here. There is a more consistent association of comorbid depression with suicide attempts. This association is found among respondents with a history of simple phobia (OR = 1.6), social phobia (OR = 1.9) PD (OR = 1.9), and PTSD (OR = 2.6).

A related type of analysis looks at pure (i.e. noncomorbid) disorders in an effort to investigate whether they have any effects on severity or impairment that cannot be

Table 3.6 The effects of lifetime comorbidity on the severity of DSM-III-R MDD and NCS/DSM-III-R anxiety disorders. *

Anxiety disorder	Severity of MDD				Severity of anxiety			
	Role impairment		Suicide attempt		Role impairment		Suicide attempt	
	OR	(95% CI)	OR	(95% CI)	OR	(95% CI)	OR	(95% CI)
Agoraphobia	2.0	(1.4–2.8)	1.3	(0.8–2.2)	1.2	(0.6–2.5)	1.3	(0.8–2.3)
Generalized anxiety disorder	2.0	(1.4–3.0)	1.6	(1.0–2.9)	1.8	(1.2–2.8)	0.8	(0.4–1.6)
Simple phobia	1.3	(1.0–1.7)	1.2	(0.7–2.0)	1.0	(0.6–1.5)	1.6	(1.0–2.6)
Social phobia	1.5	(1.1–2.2)	1.2	(0.8–1.9)	2.4	(1.7–3.3)	1.9	(1.2–3.0)
Panic disorder	2.6	(1.6–4.3)	2.1	(1.1–4.0)	1.7	(0.9–3.0)	1.9	(1.2–3.4)
Post-traumatic stress disorder	1.9	(1.3–2.7)	5.0	(3.2–7.8)	—**	(—)	2.6	(1.7–4.0)
Any anxiety disorder	1.9	(1.4–2.5)	2.7	(1.6–4.5)	2.3	(1.9–2.8)	2.3	(1.7–3.1)

* Coefficients are from a series of logistic regression equations in which either a self-report that the outcome disorder "interfered a lot with your life or activities" (role impairment) or a self-reported suicide attempt in the subsample of respondents with a lifetime history of the outcome disorder was predicted by comorbidity with the other disorders considered here, controlling for age, sex and race. **Role impairment was not assessed for this disorder.

accounted for by comorbid conditions. This type of work has been of special interest in studies of GAD due to the fact that the extremely high comorbidity of GAD with MDD in clinical samples has led some commentators to argue that GAD should be conceptualized as a prodrome or residual or severity marker of MDD rather than as an independent disorder (Gorman, 1996; Roy-Byrne, 1996). If this is the case, though, then we would not expect to find that GAD without MDD is associated with high severity or high impairment. Analysis of the NCS shows clearly that pure GAD is associated with levels of impairment that are comparable to the impairments found among respondents with pure MDD (Kessler *et al.*, 1999a). Furthermore, these high impairments cannot be explained by other comorbid conditions. These results argue that GAD is an independent disorder (Kessler, 2000).

DISCUSSION

The epidemiologic literature reviewed above has two important limitations. One is that it provides no way of assessing the extent to which failure to report lifetime disorders distorts the results concerning patterns and correlates of comorbidity. We know very little about the cognitive processes involved in forgetting, but we do know from a number of prospective studies that it occurs with alarmingly high frequency in population surveys (Bromet *et al.*, 1986; McLeod *et al.*, 1990; Wilhelm and Parker, 1994). A complicating factor is that there are now two separate studies which have documented that forgetting depression is more common among men than women (Angst and Dobler-Mikola, 1984a, b; Wilhelm and Parker, 1994). This factor could lead to an artificial increase in the estimated comorbidity between depression and anxiety and a related decrease in the estimated comorbidity between depression and substance use disorders, due to the fact that anxiety disorders are much more common among women and substance disorders among men (Kessler *et al.*, 1994). Based on this evidence, caution is needed in interpreting any results concerning comorbidity based on cross-sectional lifetime recall data such as those generated in most general population epidemiologic studies.

A related limitation is that the distinction between primary and secondary disorders is based on retrospective reports concerning age of onset that are subject to memory error. This is true not only in epidemiologic samples but also in clinical samples. There is some evidence in the cognitive psychological literature that first experiences have a special place in autobiographical memory (Pillemer *et al.*, 1988; Robinson, 1992), but the extent to which this is true varies as a function of a number of factors. Our analysis of responses to the question "Can you remember your *exact* age the *very* first time" (emphasis in the original) disorders of particular types occurred documented clearly that vivid memories are much more likely to exist for acute-onset disorders such as panic and PTSD than for disorders with insidious onsets such as depression (Kessler *et al.*, 1999b). This difference could lead to incorrect recall of the temporal priority of anxiety over depression in retrospective studies. Long-term longitudinal studies of representative community samples beginning in childhood are needed to resolve this problem of recall bias and arrive at a clear description of the natural history and correlates of pure, primary and secondary comorbid depression and anxiety.

Within the context of these limitations, the results reported above show that depression and anxiety are prevalent and highly comorbid disorders in the general population. Most lifetime cases of comorbid MDD are temporally secondary to prior anxiety disorders. However, the increased relative odds of the subsequent onset of an anxiety disorder associated with prior MDD are equally as large as the relative odds of subsequent MDD associated with prior anxiety. These time-lagged effects generally persist for many years without change. Some forms of secondary MDD are more persistent than pure or temporally primary MDD, but there is no relationship between comorbidity and the persistence of anxiety disorders. Comorbid depression–anxiety is generally more severe than either pure depression or pure anxiety. Whether these results hold cross-nationally is unclear, although collaborative cross-national comparative studies aimed at answering this question are currently under way.

In making sense of the finding that the majority of cases of lifetime depression and anxiety are comorbid, it is important to keep in mind that this finding is based on DSM-III-R, a diagnostic system that encourages multiple diagnoses. For example, while DSM-III did not allow the diagnosis of panic disorder in the presence of MDD, DSM-III-R does. As noted at the beginning of this paper, there is currently a good deal of controversy concerning whether cases of this sort should be conceived of as representing multiple comorbid disorders or a single disorder with a complex phenomenological expression. It is too early to know how this controversy will be resolved. Until we do, it is important to continue carrying out research with a diagnostic scheme that encourages multiple diagnoses while avoiding the reification of the notion of comorbidity in favor of an empirical approach which allows us to learn more about which clusters of narrowly defined comorbid disorders do and do not matter (Frances *et al.*, 1990).

The analysis of same-year and time-lagged associations between MDD and prior anxiety disorders was motivated by the results of an earlier investigation of comorbid PTSD in the NCS, where we found that many of the people who experienced a traumatic event such as rape or assault responded not only by developing PTSD but also by experiencing their first episodes of depression, panic, agoraphobia or substance abuse (Kessler *et al.*, 1995, 1999c). This result led us to speculate that a similar sort of within-year clustering or 1-year lagged effect of other disorders on MDD might exist. Consistent with our earlier PTSD work, the time-trend analysis documented a tendency for the ORs associated with comorbidity to be much higher for same-year onsets of MDD and anxiety disorders than for time-lagged onsets.

We suspect that this finding is, at least in part, due to the effects of precipitating life experiences. Not only is this interpretation consistent with our own findings concerning same-year onset of PTSD and other disorders in the wake of a traumatic life experience, but it is also consistent with Monroe's (1990) review of the literature on stressful life experiences and episode onset of depression and anxiety. The latter documented a number of common precipitating stresses associated with the two types of disorders. Furthermore, a small number of epidemiologic studies have shown that there is specificity in the stresses associated with episodes of pure depression, pure anxiety, and mixed anxiety-depression, with stresses that involve interpersonal conflict and a mixture of danger and loss more powerfully predicting mixed anxiety-depression than pure forms of either disorder (Cooke, 1981; Finlay-Jones and Brown, 1981; Prudo *et al.*, 1984; Torgersen, 1990).

It is relevant in this regard to note that clinical researchers have suggested that certain primary psychiatric disorders, if they are sufficiently impairing, can also operate as stressors that promote secondary depression (Akiskal, 1985; Cloninger *et al.*, 1990). The NCS results concerning same-year comorbidities of depression and anxiety are consistent with this thinking in that these ORs are much larger than for other psychiatric disorders (Kessler, 1995), a pattern of results that conforms with clinical evidence that anxiety disorders are more likely than other disorders to lead to a rapid-onset stress-related secondary depression (Akiskal, 1990).

It is also important to note that there is evidence from the Virginia twin sample that at least some forms of comorbidity between depression and anxiety may be due to genetic influences rather than to precipitating life experiences. This is most clear in the case of comorbidity between depression and GAD (Kendler *et al.*, 1992; Kendler, 1996), where the best-fitting genetic model suggests that the genes for these two disorders are identical and the environmental precipitants distinct. This raises the possibility that an underlying genetic vulnerability might interact with stressful experiences of various sorts to determine whether high-risk people manifest exclusively with depression, exclusively with anxiety, or with a combination of depression and anxiety.

This kind of underlying genetic diathesis could explain the finding reported above that the time-lagged effects of earlier anxiety on temporally secondary depression persist for many years without change. This could be because the earlier disorder represents a marker for an enduring genetic vulnerability. This result appears at first glance to be inconsistent with the observations of clinical investigators that secondary depression often occurs only many years after a chronic primary psychiatric disorder (Cloninger et al., 1990) or in the context of a chronic and seriously impairing physical illness (Hong et al., 1987), an observation that has been the basis of an argument that secondary depression is often a response to the exhaustion and demoralization created by chronic intractable stress (Akiskal, 1985; 1990).

This inconsistency, however, is more apparent than real because a constant time-lagged effect will lead to a preponderance of cases where the secondary depression does not occur until many years after the primary disorder. Furthermore, as noted by Akiskal (1990), the response of exhaustion or demoralization can occur as quickly as several months after the onset of the primary disorder, rather than invariably requiring years of unremitting prior exposure to the primary disorder. More detailed analysis is likely to show that the speed of onset of the secondary disorder is a joint function of the persistence and impairment caused by the primary disorder and the coping resources that characterize the person confronting the challenges imposed by the primary disorder. In the case of comorbidity of MDD with the anxiety disorders, recent family and genetic studies suggest that common genetic predisposition may also play a part (Kendler, 1996; Kendler et al., 1993; Merikangas, 1990; Torgersen, 1990; Weissman, 1990).

Although our current understanding of these processes is only partial, one clear conclusion is that same-year and time-lagged comorbidities are quite different in the sense that the ORs for same-year comorbidities are much larger than those for time-lagged comorbidities. Each of these two types is quite common in the general population. It would be informative to know whether the same-year and time-lagged forms differ in other important ways such as age of onset and course. These issues have not yet been investigated comprehensively, although there is preliminary evidence that comorbid panic–depression with same-year onsets has a stronger pattern of family aggregation than comorbid panic–depression with time-lagged onsets (Kessler et al., 1998).

It would be informative, in light of the above results, to determine whether same-year comorbidities are more likely than time-lagged comorbidities invariably to co-occur in recurring episodes of disorder. For example, in cases where the first onset of MDD occurs a few months after the first onset of panic, is the invariable co-occurrence of subsequent episodes of panic and depression throughout the life course more likely than in cases where the first onset of MDD occurred many years after the onset of a persistent panic disorder? This question cannot be answered with the baseline NCS data because information was not obtained about either the consistency of syndrome co-occurrence throughout the life course or about the chronicity of primary disorders. A second wave of the NCS is planned, however, in which this additional information will be collected along with prospective data that can help resolve some of the current uncertainties in the cross-sectional data.

Most previous research on the consequences of comorbidity has focused on the predictors of episode recovery and relapse in treatment samples (e.g. Bronisch and Hecht, 1990; Joffe *et al.*, 1993; Keitner *et al.*, 1991) and has generally found that patients with comorbidity have a poorer prognosis than those with pure disorders (e.g. Coryell *et al.*, 1988; Fawcett and Kravitz, 1983; Keitner *et al.*, 1991). In contrast, the focus of our analysis was on lifetime consequences. We found that comorbid anxiety is consistently associated with the persistence of depression, while comorbid depression is not associated with the persistence of any of the anxiety disorders considered. This asymmetry is inconsistent with a purely genetic hypothesis, but is consistent with the notion, mentioned earlier, that secondary depression is often a severity marker of chronic anxiety linked to exhaustion and demoralization (Akiskal, 1985; 1990). This interpretation would explain the fact that most types of anxiety predict the persistence of depression. This observation raises the possibility that genetic influences are more important in accounting for lifetime comorbidity than episode co-occurrence among people with a history of both depression and anxiety, while the opposite is true for environmental influences.

It is unclear from these results whether comorbidity has implications for treatment. As reviewed elsewhere in this volume, there is a good deal of evidence to suggest that the treatment of depression with modern medications is equally effective whether or not the patient presents with co-occurring anxiety, and that some treatment strategies for anxiety disorders are equally effective whether or not the patient also suffers from depression. Epidemiologic data of the sort presented here are not able to shed much light on this matter.

Epidemiologic data are more useful, however, in raising questions about the implications of comorbidity for prevention. It is clear from the results reviewed in this chapter that comorbid disorders are more severe than pure disorders. Furthermore, it is clear from studies of service use that most people with comorbid depression and anxiety do not come into contact with the treatment system until after they have had onsets of both types of disorder (Kessler *et al.*, 1996). The question could be raised, then, whether more aggressive early outreach and treatment of people with pure temporally primary (mostly anxiety) disorders could be successful in preventing the onset of temporally secondary comorbid (mostly depression) disorders and, if so, whether success in this secondary prevention could help reduce the severity and persistence of the primary disorders.

The science of prevention is too underdeveloped to provide answers to any of these questions. Furthermore, clinical research on comorbidity is not yet advanced enough to tell us much about the etiology of comorbidity. If depression and anxiety are both manifestations of a common underlying genetic vulnerability, then there is no reason to think that the successful treatment of primary anxiety will prevent the subsequent onset of secondary depression. If, on the other hand, primary disorders are either causal or in a causal pathway linked to risk of the secondary disorders, early interventions aimed at treatment of primary disorders could well be effective in preventing secondary disorders. Furthermore, if primary disorders are early warnings of risk that are amenable to environmental intervention, early interventions aimed at preventing secondary disorders among people who already have primary disorders might prove to be effective. Given the enormous complexities involved in sorting out contending causal hypotheses about the reasons for comorbidity with non-experimental data, experimental interventions of these types might be the most promising way to study the etiology of comorbidity as well as to deal with its implications (Kessler and Price, 1993).

ACKNOWLEDGMENT

Preparation of this report was supported by a Research Scientist Award from the US National Institute of Mental Health (Grant MH00507). The data reported here from the National Comorbidity Survey were collected and analyzed with the support of Grants MH46376, MH49098, and RO1 MH52861) with supplemental support from the National Institute of Drug Abuse (through a supplement to MH46376) and the W.T. Grant Foundation (Grant 90135190). Parts of this chapter appeared previously in the *British Journal of Psychiatry* and are reproduced here with the permission of the *British Journal of Psychiatry*. A complete list of all NCS publications along with abstracts, study documentation, interview schedules, and the raw NCS public-use data files can be obtained directly from the NCS Homepage by using the URL: http:// www.hcp.med.harvard.edu/ncs/.

REFERENCES

Akiskal HS (1985) Anxiety: definition, relationship to depression, and proposal for an integrative model. In: AH Tuma, JD Maser (eds) *Anxiety and the Anxiety Disorders*. Hillsdale, NJ: Erlbaum, 787–797.

Akiskal HS (1990) Toward a clinical understanding of the relationship of anxiety and depressive disorders. In: JD Maser, CR Cloninger (eds) *Comorbidity of Mood and Anxiety Disorders*. Washington, DC: American Psychiatric Press, 597–607.

American Psychiatric Association (1980) *Diagnostic and Statistical Manual of Mental Disorders*, 3rd edn. Washington, DC: American Psychiatric Press.

American Psychiatric Association (1987) *Diagnostic and Statistical Manual of Mental Disorders*, revised 3rd edn. Washington, DC: American Psychiatric Press.

American Psychiatric Association. (1994) *Diagnostic and Statistical Manual of Mental Disorders*, 4th edn. Washington, DC: American Psychiatric Press.

Angst J, Dobler-Mikola A (1984a) Do the diagnostic criteria determine the sex ratio in depression? *J Affect Dis*, **7**, 189–198.

Angst J, Dobler-Mikola A (1984b) The definition of depression. *Psychiat Res*, **18**, 401–406.

Angst J, Vollrath M, Merikangas KR, Ernst C (1990) Comorbidity of anxiety and depression in the Zurich Cohort Study of young adults. In: JD Maser, CR Cloninger (eds) *Comorbidity of Mood and Anxiety Disorders*. Washington, DC: American Psychiatric Press, 123–137.

Bromet EJ, Dunn LO, Connell MM, Dew MA, Schulberg HC (1986) Long-term reliability of diagnosing lifetime major depression in a community sample. *Arch Gen Psychiat*, **43**, 435–440.

Bronisch T, Hecht H (1990) Major depression with and without a coexisting anxiety disorder: social dysfunction, social integration, and personality features. *J Affect Dis*, **20**, 151–157.

Canino GJ, Bird HR, Shrout PE, Rubio-Stipec M, Bravo M, Martinez R *et al.* (1987) The prevalence of specific psychiatric disorders in Puerto Rico. *Arch Gen Psychiat*, **44**, 727–735.

Cloninger CR (1989) Establishment of diagnostic validity in psychiatric illness: Robins and Guze's method revised. In: LN Robins, J Barrett (eds) *Validity of Psychiatric Diagnosis*. New York: Raven Press, 9–18.

Cloninger CR, Martin RL, Guze SB, Clayton PJ (1990) The empirical structure of psychiatric comorbidity and its theoretical significance. In: JD Maser, CR Cloninger (eds) *Comorbidity of Mood and Anxiety Disorders*. Washington, DC: American Psychiatric Press, 439–462.

Cooke DJ (1981) Life events and syndrome of depression in the general population. *Soc Psychiat*, **16**, 181–186.

Coryell W, Endicott J, Andreasen NC, Keller MB, Clayton PJ, Hirschfeld RMA, Scheftner WA, Winokur G (1988) Depression and panic attacks: the significance of overlap as reflected in follow-up and family study data. *Am J of Psychiat*, **145**, 293–300.

Dohrenwend BP (1990) Notes on some epidemiologic studies of comorbidity. In: JD Maser, CR Cloninger (eds) *Comorbidity of Mood and Anxiety Disorders*. Washington, DC: American Psychiatric Press, 177–185.

Faravelli C, Degl'Innocenti BG, Aiazzi L, Incerpi G, Pallanti S (1989) Epidemiology of anxiety disorder in Florence. *J Affect Dis*, **19**, 1–5.

Fawcett J, Kravitz HM (1983) Anxiety syndromes and their relationship to depressive illness. *J Clin Psychiat*, **44**, 8–11.

Finlay-Jones R, Brown GW (1981) Types of stressful life events and the onset of anxiety and depressive disorders. *Psychol Med*, **11**, 803–815.

First MB, Spitzer RL, Williams JBW (1990) Exclusionary principles and the comorbidity of psychiatric diagnoses: a historical review and implications for the future. In: JD Maser, CR Cloninger (eds) *Comorbidity of Mood and Anxiety Disorders*. Washington, DC: American Psychiatric Press, 139–152.

Frances A, Widiger T, Fyer MR (1990) The influence of classification methods on comorbidity. In: JD Maser, CR Cloninger (eds) *Comorbidity of Mood and Anxiety Disorders*. Washington, DC: American Psychiatric Press, 139–152.

Frances A, Manning D, Marin D, Kocsis J, McKinney K, Hall W, Kline M (1992) Relationship of anxiety and depression. *Psychopharmacology*, **106**, S82–S86.

Gorman JM (1996) Comorbid depression and anxiety spectrum disorders. *Depression Anxiety*, **4**, 160–168.

Hagnell O, Grasbeck A (1990) Comorbidity of Anxiety and Depression in the Lundby 25-Year Prospective Study: the pattern of subsequent episodes. In: JD Maser, CR Cloninger (eds) *Comorbidity of Mood and Anxiety Disorders*. Washington, DC: American Psychiatric Press, 139–152.

Hong B, Smith MD, Robson AM, Wetzel RD (1987) Depressive symptomatology and treatment in patients with end-stage renal disease. *Psychol Med,* 17, 185–190.

Hwu HG, Yeh EK, Chang LY (1989) Prevalence of psychiatric disorders in Taiwan defined by the Chinese diagnostic interview schedule. *Acta Psychiat Scand,* 79, 136–147.

Joffe RT, Babgy RM, Levitt A (1993) Anxious and nonanxious depression. *Am J Psychiat,* 150, 1257–1258.

Keitner GI, Ryan CE, Miller IW, Kohn R, Epstein NB (1991) 12-month outcome of patients with major depression and comorbid psychiatric or medical illness (compound depression). *Am J Psychiat,* 148, 345–350.

Kendler KS (1996) Major depression and generalized anxiety disorder: same genes (partly) different environments—revisited. *Br J Psychiat,* 168, 68–75.

0 Kendler KS, Neale MC, Kessler RC, Heath AC, Eaves LJ (1992) Major depression and generalized anxiety disorder: same genes (partly) different environments? *Arch Gen Psychiat,* 49, 716–722.

Kendler KS, Neale MC, Kessler RC, Heath AC, Eaves LJ (1993) Major depression and phobias: the genetic and environmental sources of comorbidity. *Psychol Med,* 23, 361–371.

Kessler RC (1995) The epidemiology of psychiatric comorbidity. In: M Tsuang, M Tohen, G Zahner (eds) *Textbook of Psychiatric Epidemiology.* New York: Wiley, 23–48.

⚹ Kessler, RC (1997) The prevalence of psychiatric comorbidity. In: S Wetzler, WC Sanderson (eds) *Treatment Strategies for Patients with Psychiatric Comorbidity.* New York: Wiley, 23–48.

Kessler RC (2000) The epidemiology of pure and comorbid generalized anxiety disorder: a review and evaluation of recent research. *Acta Psychiat Scand,* 102 (suppl 406), 7–13.

Kessler RC, Price RH (1993) Primary prevention of secondary disorders: a proposal and agenda. *Am J Comm Psychol,* 21, 607–634.

Kessler RC, Zhao S (1999) The prevalence of mental illness. In: AV Horwitz, TL Scheid (eds) *Sociology of Mental Health and Illness.* New York: Cambridge University Press, 58–78.

Kessler RC, McGonagle KA, Zhao S, Nelson CB, Hughes M, Eshleman S, Wittchen H-U, Kendler KS (1994) Lifetime and 12-month prevalence of DSM-III-R psychiatric disorders in the United States: results from the National Comorbidity Survey. *Arch Gen Psychiat,* 51, 8–19.

Kessler RC, Sonnega A, Bromet E, Hughes M, Nelson CB (1995) Post-traumatic stress disorder in the National Comorbidity Survey. *Arch Gen Psychiat,* 52, 1048–1060.

Kessler RC, Nelson CB, McGonagle KA, Liu J, Swartz M, Blazer DG (1996) Comorbidity of DSM-III-R major depressive disorder in the general population: results from the US National Comorbidity Survey. *Br J Psychiat,* 168, 17–30.

Kessler RC, Olfson M, Berglund P (1998a) Patterns and predictors of treatment contact after first onset of a psychiatric disorder. *Am J Psychiat,* 155, 62–69.

Kessler RC, Stang P, Wittchen H-U, Ustun TB, Roy-Byrne PP, Walters EE (1998b) Lifetime panic-depression comorbidity in the National Comorbidity Survey. *Arch Gen Psychiat,* 55, 801–808.

Kessler RC, DuPont RL, Berglund P, Wittchen H-U. (1999a) Impairment in pure and comorbid generalized anxiety disorder and major depression at 12 months in two national surveys. *Am J Psychiat,* 156, 1915–1923.

Kessler RC, Mroczek DK, Belli RF (1999b). Retrospective adult assessment of childhood psychopathology. In: D Shaffer, C Lucas, J Richters (eds) *Assessment in Child Psychopathology.* New York: Guilford Press.

Kessler RC, Sonnega A, Bromet E, Hughes M, Nelson CB, Breslau N (1999c) Epidemiologic risk factors for trauma and PTSD. In: R Yehuda (ed) *Risk Factors for Post Traumatic Stress Disorder.* Washington, DC: American Psychiatric Press.

Klein DF, Gorman JM (1987) A model of panic and agoraphobic development. *Acta Psychiat Scand,* 76, 87–95.

Lavori PW (1990) Double diagnosis: the role of the prior odds on each disorder. In JD Maser, CR Cloninger (eds) *Comorbidity of Mood and Anxiety Disorders*. Washington, DC: American Psychiatric Press, 681–692.

Lee CK, Kwak YS, Yamamoto J, Rhee H, Kim YS, Han JH *et al*. (1990) Psychiatric epidemiology in Korea: Part I: Gender and age differences in Seoul. *J Nerv Mental Dis*, **178**, 242–246.

Lépine JP, Lellouch J, Lovell A, Teherani M, Ha C, Verdier-Taillefer MH *et al*. (1989) Anxiety and depressive disorders in a French population: methodology and preliminary results. *Psychiatr Psychobiol*, **4**, 267–274.

Marshall JR (1996) Comorbidity and its effects on panic disorder. *Bull Menninger Clin*, **60**, A39–A53.

McLeod JD, Turnbull JE, Kessler RC, Abelson JM (1990) Sources of discrepancy in the comparison of a lay-administered diagnostic instrument with clinical diagnosis. *Psychiat Res*, **31**, 145–159.

Merikangas KR (1990) Comorbidity for anxiety and depression: review of family and genetic studies. In: JD Maser, CR Cloninger (eds) *Comorbidity of Mood and Anxiety Disorders*. Washington, DC: American Psychiatric Press, 331–348.

Merikangas KR, Angst J, Eaton W, Canino G (1996) Comorbidity and boundaries of affective disorders with anxiety disorders and substance misuse: results of an international task force. *Br J Psychiat*, **168**, 58–67.

Mezzich JE, Ahn CW, Fabrega H Jr, Pilkonis PA (1990) Patterns of psychiatric comorbidity in a large population presenting for care. In: JD Maser, CR Cloninger (eds) *Comorbidity of Mood and Anxiety Disorders*. Washington, DC: American Psychiatric Press, 189–204.

Monroe SM (1990) Psychosocial factors in anxiety and depression. In: JD Maser, CR Cloninger (eds) *Comorbidity of Mood and Anxiety Disorders*. Washington, DC: American Psychiatric Press, 463–497.

Murphy JM (1990) Diagnostic comorbidity and symptom co-occurrence: the Stirling County Study. In: JD Maser, CR Cloninger (eds) *Comorbidity of Mood and Anxiety Disorders*. Washington, DC: American Psychiatric Press, 153–176.

Oakley-Browne MA, Joyce PR, Wells JE, Bushnell JA, Hornblow AR (1989) Christchurch psychiatric epidemiology study. Part II: Six month and other period prevalences for specific psychiatric disorders. *Aust NZ J Psychiat*, **23**, 327–340.

Orn H, Newman SC, Bland RC (1988) Design and field methods of the Edmonton survey of psychiatric disorders. *Acta Psychiat Scand.*, **77**, 17–23.

Pillemer DB, Goldsmith LR, Panter AT, White SH (1988) Very long-term memories of the first year in college. *J Exp Psychol Learning, Memory Cognit*, **14**, 709–714.

Prudo R, Harris T, Brown GW (1984) Psychiatric disorder in a rural and an urban population, 3: Social integration and the morphology of affective disorder. *Psychol Med*, **14**, 327–345.

Robins LN, Guze SB (1970) Establishment of diagnostic validity in psychiatric illness: its application to schizophrenia. *Am J Psychiat*, **126**, 983–987.

Robins LN, Locke BZ, Regier DA (1991) Overview: psychiatric disorders in America. In: LN Robins, DA Regier (eds) *Psychiatric Disorders in America*. New York: Free Press, 328–366.

Robinson JA (1992) First experience memories: Contexts and functions in personal histories. In MA Conway, DC Rubin, H Spinnler, WA Wagennar (eds) *Theoretical Perspectives on Autobiographical Memory*. Boston: Kluwer Academic, 223–239.

Ross HE, Glaser FB, Germanson T (1988) The prevalence of psychiatric disorders in patients with alcohol and other drug problems. *Arch Gen Psychiat*, **45**, 1023–1031.

Rounsaville BJ, Anton SF, Carroll K, Budde D, Prusoff BA, Gawin F (1991) Psychiatric diagnosis of treatment-seeking cocaine abusers. *Arch Gen Psychiat*, **48**, 43–51.

Roy-Byrne PP (1996) Generalized anxiety and mixed anxiety-depression: association with disability and health care utilization. *J Clin Psychiat*, **57**, 86–91.

Torgersen S (1990) A twin-study perspective of the comorbidity of anxiety and depression. In: JD Maser, CR Cloninger (eds) *Comorbidity of Mood and Anxiety Disorders.* Washington, DC: American Psychiatric Press, 367–378.

Uhde TW, Boulenger JP, Roy-Byrne PP, Geraci M, Vittone J, Post RM (1985) Longitudinal course of panic disorder: clinical and biologic considerations. *Prog Neuropsychopharmacol Biol Psychiatry,* **9**, 39–51.

Weissman, MM (1990) Evidence for comorbidity of anxiety and depression: family and genetic studies of children. In: JD Maser, CR Cloninger (eds) *Comorbidity of Mood and Anxiety Disorders.* Washington, DC: American Psychiatric Press, 349–365.

Weissman MM, Klerman GL, Markowitz J, Ouellette R (1989) Suicidal ideation and attempts in panic disorder. *N Eng J Medicine,* **321**, 1209–1214.

Wells JE, Bushnell JA, Hornblow AR, Joyce PR, Oakley-Browne MA (1989) Christchurch psychiatric epidemiology study. Part I: Methodology and lifetime prevalence for specific psychiatric disorders. *Aust NZ J Psychiat,* **23**, 315–326.

WHO International Consortium in Psychiatric Epidemiology (2000) Cross-national comparisons of the prevalences and correlates of mental disorders. *Bull World Health Organ,* **78** 413–426.

Wilhelm K, Parker G (1994) Sex differences in lifetime depression rates: fact or artefact? *Psych Med,* **24**, 97–111.

Wittchen H-U, Essau CA, Von Zersen D, Krieg J-C, Zaudig M (1992) Lifetime and six-month prevalence of mental disorders in the Munich Follow-up Study. *Eur Arch Psychiat Clin Neurosci,* **241**, 247–258.

Wolf AW, Schubert DSP, Patterson MB, Marion B, Grande TP (1988) Associations among major psychiatric diagnoses. *J Consult Clin Psychol,* **56**, 292–294.

4

Utility of SSRIs in anxious depression

William Boyer and John P. Feighner

INTRODUCTION

Most patients suffering from major depression have anxiety symptoms as well as depressive symptoms and these commonly occurring anxiety symptoms are normally regarded as part of the depressive disorder. The presence of anxiety symptoms does not lead necessarily to a separate diagnosis of an anxiety disorder and indeed widely used depression rating scales include a large number of items devoted to anxiety symptoms, which contribute to the assessment of overall severity of the depression.

The large epidemiological studies that have been carried out in recent years have drawn attention to the high rates of comorbidity of psychiatric disorders in the general community (Robins and Regier, 1990; Kessler *et al.*, 1994). Major depression is known to have a high comorbidity with separate anxiety disorders and a problem can arise in attributing certain anxiety symptoms as part of either the depression or the anxiety disorder. The overlap of major depression and an anxiety disorder where both conditions satisfy the full diagnostic criteria is perceived as comorbidity. In this case separate diagnoses may be considered. The overlap of major depression and anxiety disorders, where neither disorder satisfies the full criteria, has come to be known as mixed anxiety depression (MAD). This chapter attempts to address the degree of overlap which is so confusing for the clinician and to assess the data relating the role of selective serotonin reuptake inhibitors (SSRIs) in treatment.

SSRIs in Depression and Anxiety, Second Edition. Edited by S.A. Montgomery and J.A. den Boer.
© 2001 John Wiley & Sons Ltd.

ANXIOUS DEPRESSION OR COMORBID ANXIETY AND DEPRESSION

Mixed anxiety depression is a common but poorly defined condition with multiple possible aetiologies. Both anxiety and depression may occur as a symptom of or reaction to a primary psychiatric or medical disorder. The concept of major depression includes a variety of subgroups, including the more severe (psychotic features, melancholia) and chronic subtypes. Anxiety disorders are classified according to whether and how the anxiety is limited to particular situations (phobias, compulsions), thoughts (obsessions) or times (panic attacks). Generalized anxiety disorder (GAD) may be thought of as chronic anxiety which is not limited to any of these dimensions. Some basic researchers believe that anxiety and depression exist on a continuum and that depression may represent under-activity of serotonergic pathways while anxiety results from over-activity in serotonergic neurones (Eison, 1990).

There are two general meanings for mixed anxiety depression. One is the depressed patient who has signs or symptoms of an anxiety disorder which does not meet the threshold for a separate diagnosis, such as the patient with panic attacks which do not occur often enough or with the requisite number of symptoms to be diagnosed as panic disorder. The other is the patient with GAD who intermittently fulfils criteria for major depression. MAD also appears as an experimental diagnosis in DSM-IV (Table 4.1). Its anxiety symptom criteria are very similar, and in some cases identical,

Table 4.1. Research criteria for mixed anxiety depressive disorder (DSM-IV, 1994).

A   Persistent or recurrent dysphoric mood lasting at least 1 month
B   The dysphoric mood is accompanied by at least 1 month of four (or more) of the following symptoms:
 1. Difficulty concentrating or mind going blank
 2. Sleep disturbance (difficulty falling or staying asleep, or restless unsatisfying sleep)
 3. Fatigue or low energy
 4. Irritability
 5. Worry
 6. Being easily moved to tears
 7. Hypervigilance
 8. Anticipating the worst
 9. Hopelessness (pervasive pessimism about the future)
 10. Low self-esteem or feelings of worthlessness
C   The symptoms cause clinically significant distress or impairment in social, occupational or other important areas of functioning
D   The symptoms are not due to the direct physiological effects of a substance (e.g. a drug of abuse, a medication) or a general medical condition
E   All of the following:
 1. Criteria have never been met for major depressive disorder, dysthymic disorder, panic disorder, or generalized anxiety disorder
 2. Criteria are not currently met for any other anxiety or mood disorder (including an anxiety or mood disorder in partial remission)
 3. The symptoms are not better accounted for by any other mental disorder

to those for GAD. However, DSM-IV requires that the disorder does not meet, and *never has met*, criteria for GAD, major depression, dysthymic disorder and/or panic disorder. This is a problem, especially because the symptom threshold for dysthymic disorder is so low (requiring only two symptoms) that chronically depressed and anxious patients will almost never meet criteria for MAD. One might summarize this by saying that MAD, as it is currently regarded, is an admixture of a subsyndromal depressive disorder with a subsyndromal anxiety disorder. In a sense it is a testament to the importance of MAD that it has received as much research attention as it has despite this lack of satisfactory diagnostic criteria.

ANXIETY SYMPTOMS IN DEPRESSION

The scales employed for rating the severity of depression reflect the nature of these anxiety symptoms as integral to the depression. The scores on these anxiety items are seen to reduce as the depression improves and the items have good face validity in depression. For example, the Hamilton Scale for Depression (Hamilton, 1960) includes items to measure agitation, somatic anxiety and psychic anxiety. Three items that measure sleep disturbance and an item to assess the phenomenon of depersonalization feelings also form part of the scale. Moreover, it can be argued that the items for assessing obsessional symptoms and hypochondriasis also register anxiety symptoms. Most studies of the efficacy of various treatments for depression have shown that the symptoms measured by these anxiety items in the scales improve at the same rate as other symptoms of depression.

Some of the items in the Hamilton Rating Scale are more sensitive to treatment change than others and Hamilton himself recognized that the depersonalization and obsessional items, which are less sensitive, should be used more appropriately for diagnostic purposes only (Hamilton, 1967).

SSRI IN THE TREATMENT OF ANXIETY SYMPTOMS WITHIN DEPRESSION

Some treatments are acknowledged to be more effective than others in treating particular anxiety symptoms that occur with depression. The items that measure disturbed sleep improve more rapidly in response to sedative antidepressants with marked histaminergic receptor properties such as the sedative tricyclic antidepressants or mianserin. This has been shown in a number of comparisons with non-sedative antidepressants such as the SSRIs. However, the advantage seen with the sedative antidepressants, which is more evident at the start of treatment, tends to diminish as the sleep improves as part of the general improvement of the depression in response to SSRIs. By the end of the acute treatment period, the advantage of the sedative antidepressants on sleep is no longer evident. On the other hand, the negative effects on psychomotor function of the histaminergic activity become apparent with daytime drowsiness and the need to desist from driving cars or operating heavy machinery.

The early effect of anxiolytic drugs on disturbed sleep and certain other anxiety, symptoms in depression has been reported but an antidepressant effect cannot be attributed to these drugs merely on these grounds. The studies of benzodiazepines in the treatment of depression show their effects on improving the sleep items and anxiety but also show that they are less effective, or not effective at all, in improving other features of depression, and it is for this reason that, independently of the associated long-term problems of tolerance and dependence, benzodiazepines are not licensed or recommended for the treatment of major depression. Some studies have reported an increase in paradoxical aggression with benzodiazepines, possibly mediated by a mechanism involving disinhibition, and this characteristic makes these drugs unsuitable for depression, where there is an elevated risk of suicide attempts.

The selective advantages of SSRIs in treating the anxiety symptoms of depression compared with sedative tricyclic antidepressants came as a surprise. Zimelidime, an early non-sedative SSRI that was withdrawn from the market, was found to be more effective than amitriptyline in treating the anxiety symptoms of depression in a 6-week treatment study (Montgomery *et al.*, 1981). This finding raised the possibility that serotonin reuptake might have a special beneficial effect on the symptoms of anxiety within depression. Subsequent analysis for paroxetine and fluvoxamine have confirmed this hypothesis (Dunbar and Fuell, 1992; Wakelin, 1988), with a differential advantage in treating anxiety symptoms in depression reported for the SSRIs compared with reference tricyclic antidepressants. These observations led to the hypothesis that SSRIs might have particular advantages in treating separate anxiety disorders, such as panic disorder and social phobia.

The first generation of antidepressant medication included tricyclics (TCAs) and monoamine oxidase inhibitors. A number of investigators have shown these drugs to be helpful in the treatment of anxious depression (Paykel, 1987; Coplan *et al.*, 1993; Joyce and Paykel, 1989). Several trials have also shown TCAs to be equivalent or even superior to benzodiazepines in the treatment of this syndrome (Kahn *et al.*, 1986; Haskell *et al.*, 1978; Hoehn-Saric *et al.*, 1988). SSRIs improved over TCAs and MAOIs in two main areas: tolerability and safety. However, anxiety and agitation have been reported as occasional side effects with all SSRIs, which might lead to reluctance to use these agents in anxious depression. A review of the available data concerning the use of SSRIs in anxious depression, especially relating to whether baseline anxiety is a poor prognostic sign, is therefore timely.

The first line of evidence is indirect. It stems from the observation that patients with anxiety disorders often have concomitant depressive symptoms. There is considerable direct evidence of the efficacy of the SSRIs in anxiety disorders. All four SSRIs approved for marketing in the USA have shown sufficient efficacy to garner an official indication for at least one anxiety disorder, obsessive-compulsive disorder (OCD). Paroxetine and sertraline are also indicated for the treatment of panic disorder (PD). While patients with bona-fide major depression are usually excluded from trials of an antidepressant in an anxiety disorder, it is likely that a substantial number of the subjects in OCD and PD trials had clinically significant depressive symptoms.

Filteau and colleagues analysed data from 10 studies of SSRIs (sertraline; zimelidine; fluvoxamine; fluoxetine; selective noradrenergic uptake inhibitors—desipramine, maprotiline, oxaprotiline; mixed uptake inhibitors—amitriptyline, imipramine; and partial 5-HT$_2$ antagonists—ritanserin, trazodone, nefazodone. The data showed no differences between the efficacy of these classes in agitated or retarded depression. In a subsequent analysis the same investigators found that SSRI responders tended to be initially more anxious and agitated than non-responders (Filteau *et al.*, 1995).

Fluoxetine

The efficacy of fluoxetine in anxious depression was reported by Montgomery (1989) in an analysis of the pooled data of those patients who entered studies with moderate or severe degrees of agitation. In a small study, Jouvent and colleagues (1989) reported that fluoxetine was more effective in anxious-impulsive patients than in those with a blunted affect. Several large-scale meta-analyses of fluoxetine data have reported findings supporting the efficacy of fluoxetine in anxious depression.

Tollefson and co-workers (1998) reported that fluoxetine was significantly ($p < 0.05$) more effective than placebo in treating both anxious and non-anxious depression ($N = 3183$). Fluoxetine was also significantly more effective than placebo in reducing the Hamilton Depression and Anxiety (HAMD) scales anxiety/somatization factor score. The efficacy of fluoxetine and TCAs was comparable on all measures and in all groups (Tollefson *et al.*, 1998). Furthermore, fluoxetine-treated patients were less likely to drop out of treatment due to anxiety than those given a TCA. This was true whether or not the patient was considered "anxious" at baseline.

A similar analysis examined the effect of fluoxetine on psychomotor agitation. These data came from double-blind trials involving 4737 patients with major depression randomly assigned to fluoxetine, a comparison antidepressant or placebo. Item 9 of the Hamilton Depression Rating Scale was used to assess psychomotor agitation. Agitation occurred at a similar incidence across treatment groups. The rate of *increased* agitation (after starting treatment) was comparable between fluoxetine, placebo and TCAs. Improvement in agitation occurred significantly more often among fluoxetine-treated than placebo-treated patients (Blomgren *et al.*, 1997).

The previous two studies primarily concerned patients treated with average doses of fluoxetine (20 mg/day). Higher doses are often used for non-responsive or partially responsive patients. There is also evidence that high-dose fluoxetine is also associated with anxiety reduction. In the earliest clinical trials, fluoxetine was typically prescribed at a dose of 60–80 mg/day. Beasley and colleagues reviewed data from 706 outpatients with DSM-III major depression treated with either high-dose fluoxetine (median 80 mg/day) or imipramine (median 200 mg/day). Imipramine and fluoxetine were comparable in overall antidepressant effect as well as in reduction of sleep disturbance and scores on the anxiety/somatization factor. Reduction in sleep disturbance and anxiety was again independent of baseline psychomotor agitation or retardation. Baseline psychomotor state predicted activation-sedation side effects only for imipramine, which caused more sedation in patients with baseline psychomotor retardation. There was a non-significant trend ($p = 0.92$) for more drug discontinuations due to activation for fluoxetine than imipramine (Beasley *et al.*, 1991). Such a small difference, however, is unlikely to be clinically significant given the very large sample size.

Prospective data support this pattern of findings. Three hundred and thirty-six primary care patients with major depression were randomly assigned to fluoxetine or imipramine in one study. Improvement was essentially identical in the two groups. Neither baseline anxiety nor insomnia scores predicted group differences. Patients assigned to fluoxetine were again significantly less likely to change or discontinue medication (Simon *et al.*, 1997).

These findings contrast with those reported by Fava and colleagues (1997). These investigators studied 294 outpatients with major depressive disorder who were treated with fluoxetine 20 mg/day for 8 weeks. They found that non-anxious patients improved slightly but significantly more during treatment than anxious depressives on all outcome measures. However, this study was not strictly comparable to the others reviewed here, since anxious depression was defined as meeting *full* criteria for a comorbid anxiety disorder. As a general rule the presence of one or more comorbid disorders is associated with poorer outcome across a variety of psychiatric conditions.

Paroxetine

Paroxetine has produced some of the most striking data showing superior efficacy on anxiety symptoms within depression compared with other antidepressants. It has been perceived as one of the more "anxiolytic of the SSRIs" and this has been recognized in the granting of specific labelling for both depression and depression and anxiety in some countries, including the UK. More recently the granting of licenses for OCD, panic disorder, social anxiety disorder, GAD and PTSD (see Chapter 6) are further evidence of this profile of activity.

The evidence of the effect of paroxetine on anxiety symptoms within depression comes from several sources including meta-analysis of studies in depression, from a large study in patients with depression and anxiety symptoms, and from investigation of the effect of paroxetine on coexistent symptoms of anxiety in studies of depressed patients.

Meta-analyses have been conducted on paroxetine data similar to those reported on fluoxetine. Dunbar and Fuell (1992) compared a database of 2963 paroxetine-treated patients with 554 who received placebo and 1151 given a comparison antidepressant (most often a TCA). Paroxetine and active control both reduced baseline psychic anxiety more effectively than placebo. Both pharmacological treatments were effective in treating somatic anxiety with paroxetine, demonstrating an earlier onset of activity. Neither paroxetine nor active control induced new anxiety symptoms. Paroxetine was superior to placebo in the treatment of agitation at weeks 4 and 6 and to active control at week 4 only. Both paroxetine and active control were more protective against new-onset agitation than placebo. Finally, there was no difference between the three groups in the incidence of spontaneously reported adverse events indicative of anxiety.

Two large reference controlled studies have been carried out in patients with anxiety and depression. Ravindran and colleagues (1996) conducted a 12-week, double-blind, parallel-group comparison of paroxetine 20–40 mg/day with clomipramine 75–150 mg/day. This was a large study that included 1002 patients. Inclusion criteria were drafted so as to recruit patients with moderate levels of both anxiety and depression as defined by the Montgomery–Asberg Depression Rating Scale (MADRS) score and Clinical Anxiety Score (CAS). Both paroxetine and clomipramine reduced the MADRS and CAS ratings at 2, 6 and 12 weeks and at endpoint, with no significant differences between treatment groups at any time point. The Clinical Global Improvement (CGI) severity of illness score and CGI improvement ratings were also similar throughout the trial. However, there was a statistically significant difference in the CGI efficacy index at 6 weeks and at endpoint, which favoured paroxetine. There were also significantly fewer adverse events and study dropouts due to adverse effects among paroxetine-treated patients.

Paroxetine has also been compared to amitriptyline in patients with a diagnosis of depression with anxiety in an 8-week comparison that included 505 patients (Stott *et al.*, 1993). Both treatments showed similar reduction in mean total MADRS, CAS and CGI scores during the study. However, paroxetine was better tolerated and significantly more anticholinergic events were reported in the amitriptyline group than in patients treated with paroxetine (30% vs. 17%).

In addition to these studies designed to select patients with depression and anxiety, further evidence of the efficacy of paroxetine on the anxiety symptoms in depression comes from a large comparison of paroxetine, imipramine, and placebo in outpatients. A significantly better effect was reported with paroxetine than imipramine at week 2 on the anxiety somatization factor of the Hamilton Depression Rating Scale (Dunbar *et al.*, 1991). This early improvement of the anxiety symptoms with paroxetine was also registered on the Covi scale as early as the second week of treatment, whereas imipramine was effective only at the end of treatment. Meta-analysis of the large paroxetine comparator and placebo database confirmed this finding with paroxetine, showing a significant advantage over the comparators in treating the psychic anxiety, measured on the Hamilton Depression Scale, at weeks 2, 4 and 6. A similar result was seen in a separate analysis of the US data (where a five-point scale was used for the agitation item) with an advantage for paroxetine on the agitation scores compared with comparators antidepressants at weeks 2, 4 and 6 (Dunbar and Fuell, 1992).

There have been very few studies comparing individual SSRIs, so that it is difficult to draw conclusions on possible differences between them. Paroxetine has been compared with fluoxetine in two comparator studies, both relatively small. In one (Gagiano, 1993), 90 patients suffering from moderate to severe depression were treated with either paroxetine 20 mg/day or fluoxetine 20 mg/day, increasing to paroxetine 30 mg/day or fluoxetine 40 mg/day after a week and then flexible dosing according to efficacy and tolerability. In this study there were no significant differences between the two treatments at any time points. The anxiety scores measured on the Hamilton Anxiety Scale were significantly reduced in both treatment groups during the study. The study of de Wilde and colleagues (1993) compared paroxetine and fluoxetine in a 6-week double-blind trial of 100 patients. There were no significant differences between treatment groups in reduction of either depression or anxiety scores. However, both depression and anxiety were significantly reduced in the paroxetine group earlier (week 3) than among patients treated with fluoxetine.

Sertraline

Carrasco and colleagues (1997) treated 36 patients with mixed anxiety-depression (ICD-10) with sertraline in an open trial. Concomitant benzodiazepines were not allowed during the study. Twenty-seven patients (75%) were rated as marked or moderate responders by the end of the 8-week study period.

A meta-analysis compared the efficacy of sertraline ($N = 218$), amitriptyline ($N = 214$), and placebo ($N = 214$) in two outpatient studies. The results showed similar efficacy of sertraline and amitriptyline in reducing both depression and anxiety. Amitriptyline was not tolerated as well as sertraline and had a greater overall incidence of side effects. There was a higher incidence of anxiety and agitation with amitriptyline in the high anxiety subgroup, and a higher incidence of agitation associated with amitriptyline in the low anxiety subgroup (Berti et al., 1995).

Sertraline has also been compared with newer antidepressants in MAD. Sertraline and nefazodone were studied in 41 patients with anxious depression. All subjects met DSM-III-R criteria for major depression, had minimum Hamilton Depression Rating scores of 18 and Hamilton Anxiety Scale scores of 21 at baseline. Twenty-one also met DSM-III-R criteria for panic disorder. The patients were treated with flexible doses of nefazodone (200–600 mg/day) or sertraline (50–200 mg/day) for 6 weeks. There were no significant differences in outcome between drugs and no significant treatment differences between patients with or without concomitant panic disorder (Targum et al., 1997). Aguglia and colleagues (1993) conducted an 8-week multi-centre comparison of sertraline and fluoxetine in 108 patients with DSM-III-R major depression. Again there were no significant differences in efficacy between the two treatment groups in either anxiety or depression.

Fluvoxamine

Houck and Stankovic (1997) performed an 8-week open-label trial of fluvoxamine in 15 outpatients diagnosed as having MAD. Baseline scores on the HAMD indicated moderate degrees of both anxiety and depression prior to treatment. The patients experienced significant improvement in both areas ($p < 0.001$).

Fluvoxamine has also been compared with benzodiazepines in several relevant clinical trials. Laws and colleagues (1990) conducted a 6-week, multi-centre double-blind comparison of fluvoxamine and lorazepam in the treatment of mixed anxiety depression in 112 outpatients treated by general practitioners. Dosage could range up to 300 mg/day of fluvoxamine and 6 mg/day of lorazepam. Six patients in the fluvoxamine group and four treated with lorazepam dropped out of the study because of intolerance. The majority of these dropouts occurred during the first week. The average final daily doses indicated that treatment was adequate; 163 mg/day of fluvoxamine and 2.96 mg/day for lorazepam. The investigators found equal and significant reductions in depression and anxiety ratings in both groups.

Chabannes and Douge (1989) reported two comparative trials of fluvoxamine and benzodiazepines. In the first they treated 60 outpatients with "low mood and anxiety" with either fluvoxamine or diazepam for 6 weeks. The average initial HAMD score was 23.4, which is consistent with a moderate or greater severity of depression. Fluvoxamine and diazepam reduced anxiety to an equivalent degree. In a second study they treated 130 outpatients described as having major depression plus anxiety with fluvoxamine, prazepam or the combination for 6 weeks. Here there was a trend for a greater decrease in Hamilton Anxiety Scores in patients receiving fluvoxamine alone or fluvoxamine plus prazepam than those treated with prazepam alone.

Citalopram

Shaw and Crimmins (1989) compared citalopram and amitriptyline in a 6-week trial of 59 in- and outpatients suffering from major depression. No differences in antidepressant effectiveness were observed, and the drugs were equally effective in reducing anxiety despite the greater sedative action of amitriptyline. The large clinical trial database shows that the anxiety symptoms seem to respond with the depression but the full analyses have not yet been adequately published.

SUMMARY

A considerable body of evidence has been accumulated supporting the efficacy of the SSRIs in treating anxiety symptoms in depression. It is clear that the SSRIs are at least as effective as the TCAs in treating these symptoms and several studies have shown either an overall advantage for the SSRIs compared with TCAs in treating the anxiety symptoms, or else an earlier effect.

Transient increases in anxiety have been reported from time to time during treatment with some SSRIs; however, extensive investigation of large clinical trial databases of the SSRIs as well as specific studies in depressed/anxious patients have shown that SSRIs are effective across the range of depression, including both depressive and anxious symptoms. Significant pretreatment anxiety or agitation does *not* predict the subsequent development of either of these side effects with an SSRI. All the evidence points to the fact that SSRIs are particularly effective in the treatment of anxiety symptoms associated with depression. There is some evidence to suggest that anxious–depressed patients may respond better to an SSRI than those with more psychomotor retardation (Filteau *et al.*, 1995; Berti *et al.*, 1995).

The investigation of mixed anxiety depression is to some extent hampered by the imprecise diagnostic criteria currently available. Improvement is needed to facilitate serious study of this category in the future. We have already alluded to the unsatisfactory criteria contained in DSM-IV, which requires the presence of four or more symptoms from a list of 10 as well as the absence of current or previous episodes of major depression, dysthymic disorder, GAD and/or panic disorder. Yet the symptoms used for diagnosis are nearly the same as those used for the "exclusionary" disorders. If one considers only dysthymic disorder and GAD, then at least 86% of the possible combinations of four or more symptoms are eliminated.

It might be more useful to conceptualize mixed anxiety depression in a way analogous to that adopted for schizoaffective disorder, which requires that symptoms of schizophrenia and an affective disorder always coexist. If applied to mixed anxiety depression it would require that symptoms of a depressive and anxiety disorder always be present at the same time at either a full or a nearly syndromal level.

In spite of these diagnostic difficulties an increasing number of studies are being carried out on the treatment of mixed anxiety depression. The studies reviewed in this chapter have shown that the SSRIs are at least as effective as TCAs in relieving symptoms of anxiety and depression. They are also better tolerated, as would be expected from their neuropharmacologic profile. It also appears they may be as effective as benzodiazepines in reducing anxiety.

The extensive research and clinical experience with the SSRIs in the treatment of anxious depressed patients supports their efficacy as well as tolerability and safety. It is our opinion that they are now the treatment of choice for this condition, especially when long-term treatment is indicated.

REFERENCES

Aguglia E, Casacchia M, Cassano GB, Faravelli C, Ferrari G, Giordano P *et al.* (1993) Double-blind study of the efficacy and safety of sertraline vs. fluoxetine in major depression. *Int Clin Psychopharmacol*, **8**, 197–202.

Beasley CM, Sayler ME, Bosomworth JC, Wernicke JF (1991) High-dose fluoxetine: efficacy and activating-sedating effects in agitated and retarded depression. *J Clin Psychiat*, **11**, 166–174.

Berti C, Doogan DP, Scott NR, Dinan TG (1995) Sertraline in the treatment of depressive disorders with associated anxiety. *J Serotonin Res*, **2**(3), 151–170.

Blomgren S, Tollefson GD, Sayler ME (1997) *The Course of Psychomotor Agitation during Pharmarcotherapy of Depression: Analysis from Double-blind Controlled Trials.* San Diego, CA: American Psychiatric Association.

Carrasco JL, Diaz-Marsa M, Saiz J (1997) Sertraline in the treatment of mixed anxiety and depression disorder. *Actos Lus-Espanolas de Neurologica, Psiquiatria y Ciencias Afines*, **25**(3), 141–145.

Chabannes SF, Douge R (1989) Efficacy on anxiety of fluvoxamine vs. prazepam, diazepam with anxiodepressed patients. In: CN Stefanis, CR Soldatos, AD Rabavilas (eds) *Psychiatry Today: VIII World Congress of Psychiatry Abstracts.* New York; Elsevier, 282.

Coplan J, Tiffon L, Gorman JM (1993) Therapeutic strategies for the patient with treatment-resistant anxiety. *J Clin Psychiat*, **54**, 69–74.

de Wilde J, Spiers R, Mertens C, Bartholome F, Schotte G, Leyman S (1993) A double-blind, comparative, multicentre study comparing paroxetine with fluoxetine in depressed patients. *Acta Psychiat Scand*, **87**, 141–145.

Diagnostic and Statistical Manual of Mental Disorders, 4th edn (DSM-IV) (1994) Washington, DC: American Psychiatric Association.

Dunbar GC, Cohn JB, Fabre LF, Feighner JP, Fieve RR, Mendels J, Shrivastava RK (1991) A comparison of paroxetine, imipramine and placebo in depressed out-patients. *Br J Psychiat*, **159**, 394–398.

Dunbar GC, Fuell DL (1992) The anti-anxiety and anti-agitation effects of paroxetine in depressed patients. *Int Clin Psychopharmacol*, **6**(S4), 81–90.

Eison MS (1990) Azapirones: clinical uses of serotonin partial agonists. *Drugs Therapeut*, (suppl), 1–7.

Fava M, Uebelacker LA, Alpert JE, Nierenberg AA, Pava JA, Rosenbaum JF (1997) Major depressive subtypes and treatment response. *Biol Psychiat*, **42**, 568–576.

Filteau MJ, Baruch P, Lapierre Y, Bakish D, Blanchard A (1995) SSRIs in anxious-agitated depression: a post-hoc analysis of 279 patients. *Int Clin Psychopharmacol*, **10**, 51–54.

Gagiano GA (1993) A double-blind comparison of paroxetine and fluoxetine in patients with major depression. *Br J Clin Res*, **4**, 145–152.

Hamilton M (1960) A rating scale for depression. *J Neurol Neurosurg Psychiat*, **23**, 56–62.

Hamilton M (1967) Development of rating scale for primary depressive illness. *Br J Soc Clin Psychol*, **6**, 278–296.

Haskell DS, Gambill JD, Gardos G, McNair DM, Fisher S (1978) Doxepin or diazepam for anxious and anxious-depressed outpatients? *J Clin Psychiat*, **39**, 135–139.

Hoehn-Saric R, McLeod DR, Zimmerli WD (1988) Differential effects of alprazolam an imipramine in generalized anxiety disorder: somatic vs. psychic symptoms. *J Clin Psychiat*, **49**, 293–301.

Houck C, Stankovic S (1997) An open-label study of fluvoxamine in outpatients with mixed-anxiety depressive disorder. *Psychopharmacol Bull*, **33**(3), S30–31.

Jouvent R, Baruch P, Ammar S, Montreuil M, Beuzen JN, Widlocher D (1989) Fluoxetine efficacy in depressives with impulsitivity vs. blunted affect. In: CN Stefanis, CR Soldatos, AD Rabavilas (eds) *Psychiatry Today: VIII World Congress of Psychiatry Abstracts.* New York: Elsevier, 398.

Joyce PR, Paykel ES (1989) Predictors of drug response in depression. *Arch Gen Psychiat*, **46**, 89–99.

Kahn RJ, McNair DM, Lipman RS, Covi L, Rickels K, Downing R *et al.* (1986) Imipramine and chlordiazepoxide in depressive and anxiety disorders. II. Efficacy in anxious outpatient. *Arch Gen Psychiat*, **43**, 79–85.

Kessler RC, McGonagle KA, Zhao S, Nelson CB, Hughes M, Eshelman S *et al.* (1994) Life-time and 12-month prevalence of DSM-III-R psychiatric disorders in the United States. Results from the National Comorbidity Survey. *Arch Gen Psychiat*, **51**, 8–19.

Laws D, Ashford JJ, Anstee JA (1990) A multicentre double-blind comparative trial of fluvoxamine vs. lorazepam in mixed anxiety and depression treated in general practice. *Acta Psychiat Scand*, **81**, 185–189.

Montgomery SA, McAulay R, Rani SJ, Roy D, Montgomery DB (1981) A double-blind comparison of zimelidine and amitriptyline in endogenous depression. *Acta Psychiat Scand*, **63**(suppl 290), 314–327.

✴Montgomery SA (1989) The efficacy of fluoxetine as an antidepressant in the short and long term. *Int Clin Psychopharmacol*, **4**(suppl 1), 113–119.

✦Paykel ES (1987) Depression, anxiety and antidepressant response. In: G Racagni, E Smeraldi (eds) *Anxious Depression: Assessment and Treatment*. New York: Raven, 171–179.

Ravindran AV, Judge R, Hunter BN, Bray J, Hunter NH (1996) A double-blind, multicenter study in primary care comparing paroxetine and clomipramine in patients with depression and associated anxiety. *J Clin Psychiat*, **58**, 112–118.

Robins LN, Regier DA (1990) *Psychiatric Disorders in America: The Epidemiological Catchment Area Study*. New York: Free Press.

Shaw DM, Crimmins R (1989) A multicentre trial of citalopram and amitriptyline in major depressive illness. In: SA Montgomery (ed) *Citalopram: The New Antidepressant from Lundbeck Research*. Amsterdam: Excerpta Medica, 43–49.

✴ Simon GE, Heiligenstein JH, Katon WJ (1997) *Anxiety, Insomnia and Antidepressant Selection*. San Diego: American Psychiatric Association.

Stott PC, Aitken CA (1993) A double blind comparison of paroxetine and amitriptyline in community patients with depression and associated anxiety. 146th Annual Meeting, America Psychiatric Association, San Francisco, CA, 1993.

Targum SD, Muthu P, Marcus R (1997) Serotonergic treatment of concomitant panic and major depressive disorder. Presented at the 1996 NCDEU meeting, Boca Raton, FL.

✗Tollefson GD, Holman SL, Sayler ME, Potvin JH (1998) Fluoxetine, placebo, and tricyclic antidepressants in major depression with and without anxious features. *J Clin Psychiat*, **55**, 59.

✴Wakelin JS (1988) The role of serotonin in depression and suicide: do serotonin reuptake inhibitors provide a key? *Adv Biol Psychiat*, **17**, 70–83.

5

SSRIs in panic disorder

James C. Ballenger

INTRODUCTION

Over the past 25 years, there has been continuous evolution in the psychological and pharmacological treatments for panic disorder (PD). Initially, pharmacotherapies involved imipramine and many of the tricyclic antidepressants (TCAs), phenelzine and the monoamine oxidase inhibitor (MAOI) antidepressants, and the high-potency benzodiazepines (BZs), particularly alprazolam and clonazepam. These three classes were found to be approximately equal in efficacy, with differences primarily in their side effects and the BZs' rapid onset of action. Treatment focus in PD has recently shifted to the use of serotonin reuptake inhibitors (SSRIs) due to their low side-effects profile. In 1995, an expert panel at the National Institutes of Mental Health (NIMH) Algorithm Development Meeting concluded that the SSRIs had become the first choice for pharmacotherapeutic treatment of PD (Jobson and Potter, 1995). SSRIs are at least as effective as the previous pharmacological treatments and are better tolerated (Boyer, 1995; Ballenger, 1998; Ballenger, 1999). Most of the SSRIs have been demonstrated to be effective and include paroxetine (Ballenger *et al.*, 1998b), fluvoxamine (den Boer, 1998), citalopram (Wade *et al.*, 1997), fluoxetine (Michelson *et al.*, 1998), and sertraline (Pohl *et al.*, 1998). There is increasing scientific evidence to confirm that the SSRIs are very effective and should generally be considered first-line treatment of PD for most patients worldwide (Ballenger *et al.*, 1998a).

In the studies reviewed in this chapter, "efficacy" of the SSRIs refers to how effective the treatment is in resolving the entire clinical picture, including not only panic

SSRIs in Depression and Anxiety, Second Edition. Edited by S.A. Montgomery and J.A. den Boer.
© 2001 John Wiley & Sons Ltd.

attacks, but also anticipatory anxiety, avoidance behavior, depression, and dysfunction in the patient's social, family, and occupational life. Many early studies utilized the complete disappearance of attacks ("zero panic attacks") as the primary or only outcome criteria. However, this has been shown to be both an unreliable measure of improvement and not always representative of clinically significant change which involves improvement in these other symptom domains as well. Most recent trials use multidomain measures of improvement (Shear *et al.*, 1997).

SSRI TREATMENT OF PANIC DISORDER

With the introduction of the serotonergic tricyclic clomipramine, medications with principal actions on the serotonin neuron became available for use in Europe about 25 years ago. Zimelidine was available in the early 1980s in Europe and was shown to be effective in PD, but it was taken off the market because of adverse side effects. The more widely used SSRIs have been developed over the last 10 years. These include fluvoxamine, fluoxetine, paroxetine, sertraline, and citalopram.

Clomipramine

Although clomipramine (CMI) is considered a TCA, it is included in this discussion because its primary effects are on serotonin (5-HT), and it has been extensively researched. Although it is only relatively recently that CMI has become available in the United States, it was considered the "gold standard" for treatment of PD in Europe due to its positive results in long-term use.

Early studies conducted in the 1980s by Gloger and colleagues demonstrated that CMI was effective in 75% of patients with either PD or agoraphobia with panic attacks, and beneficial effects were observed by the end of the second week with most patients having either mild symptoms or no symptoms at all after treatment (Gloger *et al.*, 1981).

Although a standard dose has not yet been determined, dosage ranges of 100–150 mg/day are usual for most patients. However, some studies have shown that lower dosages (10–30 mg/day) can be effective (Gloger *et al.*, 1981; Lesser *et al.*, 1992; Mavissakalian and Perel, 1995). In a 1989 follow-up study by Gloger and colleagues, 13 of the 17 patients receiving less than 25 mg/day of CMI became panic-free, and the remaining subjects showed improvement in the frequency of their panic attacks. These lower dosages are probably not effective in most patients. For example, these researchers did observe that higher dosages were needed when agoraphobia was present. This specific finding also was found with alprazolam and imipramine (LeCrubier *et al.*, 1997a,b; Mavissakalian and Perel, 1989). In a study conducted by Feet and Gotestam (1994), there was a positive correlation between overall clinical responses and serum concentration of CMI as has been observed with other effective agents (Lesser *et al.*, 1992; Mavissakalian and Perel, 1995; Ballenger, 1999).

It was Johnston and colleagues who designed one of the first studies that examined a diagnostically homogeneous PD group with a placebo control (Johnston *et al.*, 1988). This 8-week, double-blinded study of 108 agoraphobic women provided conclusive evidence documenting the clinical effectiveness of CMI in reducing not only panic attacks but also agoraphobia and depression.

Several studies led to CMI becoming the treatment of choice for PD in Europe. Cassano and colleagues compared CMI to imipramine, which was thought to be the best treatment for PD at the time. Both drugs were proven to be effective, but CMI was shown to be more effective on some outcome measures, with its beneficial effects seen by the end of the second week (Cassano *et al.*, 1988).

In a subsequent trial, Modigh and colleagues again compared imipramine and CMI to placebo in a 12-week trial (Modigh *et al.*, 1992). Despite the lower dosages of CMI, the effects on all major outcome measures, such as panic attacks and anticipatory anxiety, were significantly greater in the CMI group in a shorter period of time. In a recent trial comparing CMI and desipramine, CMI was again superior in efficacy (Sasson *et al.*, 1999).

Fluvoxamine

Numerous studies over a long period of time have confirmed fluvoxamine's efficacy in treating PD symptoms such as anxiety, panic attacks, phobia, and depression. In one 6-week trial, den Boer and colleagues (1987) compared CMI and fluvoxamine in 58 anxiety patients (38 having agoraphobia with panic attacks). Doses were increased progressively over a 2-week period to a maximum dosage of 150 mg/day of CMI or 100 mg/day of fluvoxamine. Both drugs were found to be equal in efficacy with approximately 60% of both patient groups experiencing almost complete alleviation of panic-like symptoms. There was some suggestion on the Symptom Checklist (SCL-90) that CMI's effects were superior to those of fluvoxamine, although this could have been due to the fact that higher doses of CMI were given to the patients (150 mg/day vs. 100 mg/day of fluvoxamine). Although no average dosage range has yet been determined for fluvoxamine, the dosages used to treat patients in most of the studies range from 100 to 300 mg/day.

Most of the fluvoxamine studies have shown the effectiveness of this SSRI over placebo, with the exception of one published trial. Nair and colleagues (1996) compared fluvoxamine, imipramine, and placebo in 148 patients with PD. Despite treatment with 171.4 mg/day fluvoxamine compared to 164.4 mg/day of imipramine, the study failed to demonstrate efficacy for fluvoxamine, although significant differences were observed for imipramine. There also was a high drop-out rate of patients who were taking the fluvoxamine (62%, compared to 32% on imipramine and 58% on placebo). Given the relatively large number of positive trials on fluvoxamine's efficacy, it is difficult to determine whether the failure of this trial to show a positive effect was due to the high drop-out rate or if it was because of the differences in baseline panic attack frequency. Because there have been very few negative fluvoxamine studies with PD, this large, seemingly well-performed trial may simply be an anomalous trial, or it may potentially imply something about fluvoxamine's potency.

Depression is a serious complication of PD. In fact, 60–80% of all PD patients develop depression at some point in their life (Ballenger, 1998). In a 12-month trial conducted by Spiegel and associates (1996), 17 patients with a prior diagnosis of PD and comorbid depression were treated with fluvoxamine. Symptoms such as panic attacks, anticipatory anxiety, depression, and disability all improved greatly, but the medication failed to improve agoraphobic avoidance at the doses employed. However, researchers in one recently published 2-year follow-up study did find that fluvoxamine combined with exposure therapy was effective in reducing agoraphobic avoidance (de Beurs *et al.*, 1999).

Citalopram

Although citalopram was introduced in Europe some time ago, there have been relatively few studies of its efficacy in PD. The first published open trial with this drug was conducted by Humble and colleagues (1989), who studied 20 PD patients with and without agoraphobia. After 8 weeks, 13 out of 17 patients treated with citalopram had positive responses, with decreases in anticipatory anxiety, agoraphobia, and the somatic symptomatology of PD. After this trial ended, 16 patients continued in a 15-month long-term maintenance trial; 11 patients completed this portion of the study. The earliest positive gains in the first trial were maintained throughout this longer period, with signs of further improvement in some patients, including two patients who had not responded in the initial 8-week trial.

Wade and Lepola reported results of the first controlled trial, an 8-week, double-blind, placebo-controlled, fixed-dose multi-center trial of citalopram and CMI in 475 PD patients (Wade *et al.*, 1997; Lepola *et al.*, 1998). Citalopram (20–60 mg/day) and CMI (60 or 90 mg/day) were significantly better than placebo in reducing panic attacks. The 20–30 mg dosage range for citalopram appeared to be the most effective. Interestingly, positive effects of citalopram were not observed until week 12. It remains to be seen whether citalopram has a slower onset of action than other SSRIs. A total of 279 of these patients on citalopram were followed for a full year and showed maintenance and extension of positive acute effects (Lepola *et al.*, 1998). Although this was one of the first long-term maintenance trials, positive clinical effects appear to be maintained with all effective medications, as long as the patient remains on the medication.

Paroxetine

The first publication of a placebo-controlled randomized trial of an actual SSRI other than fluvoxamine was a study conducted by Oehrberg and colleagues (1995). In this study, 60 patients were treated with paroxetine and 60 with placebo. In the paroxetine group, 75% of patients received either 40 or 60 mg/day of paroxetine (47% receiving 60 mg/day). Patients also received standard cognitive-behavioral treatment during this

12-week trial. Many of the patients were agoraphobic with moderate or severe avoidance behavior. The mean number of panic attacks per week in the paroxetine group fell from 21.2 to 5.2, compared to the placebo group, in which the decrease was from 26.4 to 16.6 over the final 3 weeks of the study. These differences in favor of paroxetine were statistically highly significant. Improvements in the secondary measures of outcome, which included the Hamilton Anxiety Rating Scale (HAM-A) and the Clinical Global Response (CGR), were all greater in the paroxetine group. Response began in the first 3 weeks and was statistically significant by week 6 and throughout the trial period. The study demonstrated that paroxetine was well tolerated, with a low drop-out rate. Side effects noted were those expected of the SSRI class and included nausea, sweating, headache, dizziness, asthenia, decreased libido, and dry mouth.

Additional definitive controlled evidence of paroxetine's efficacy was provided by a large multicenter trial of 367 patients randomized to receive paroxetine, CMI, or placebo (LeCrubier *et al.*, 1997a). The majority of patients (> 80%) had significant agoraphobic avoidance. At week 12, a higher percentage of patients (50.9%) in the paroxetine group had no panic attacks, compared to 36.7% of the CMI group and 31.6% of the placebo group ($p < 0.05$). In addition, anxiety, agoraphobia, and measures of interference with work, social, and family life were each reduced to a greater extent by paroxetine and CMI than by placebo. Effects of both drugs were similar, although paroxetine was effective earlier and was better tolerated than CMI.

In one of the initial long-term SSRI trials, paroxetine, CMI, and placebo responders ($N = 176$) were studied for a total of 1 year (LeCrubier *et al.*, 1997b). For the first time, the study carefully documented that both paroxetine and clomipramine reduced panic attacks, anxiety, agoraphobia, and functional disability, with improvement continuing during the full year of treatment. Although both medications were effective, paroxetine was clearly better tolerated and more effective in terms of several secondary measures of efficacy.

To establish a clear target dose, Ballenger and colleagues (1998b) conducted a 10-week trial comparing 10, 20, and 40 mg/day of paroxetine to placebo in 70 PD patients. Compared to placebo, significant improvements in symptoms occurred only in the 40 mg/day paroxetine group. The other two dosages also provided greater improvements in patients, but failed to show significant difference from placebo.

In an unpublished study, Ballenger and colleagues (1999) conducted a follow-up to this trial. A double-blind continuation study evaluated the necessity of continued medication to prevent PD relapse in 138 patients. In 10 weeks, continued paroxetine treatment was found to be significantly more effective than switching to placebo in continuing to further reduce the number of panic attacks and/or the overall severity of the illness. Relapse developed at a significantly greater rate in the paroxetine-to-placebo group than in the paroxetine-to-paroxetine group (30% vs. 5%). The greatest relapse rate was seen in the highest-dosage group (40 mg/day), 54% of whom relapsed after discontinuing the paroxetine, compared to 17% of those who crossed over to placebo from the lower-dosage groups (10 and 20 mg/day). It was difficult to distinguish early relapse and withdrawal symptoms in some patients with abrupt discontinuation of the medication, but the higher relapse rate appeared clear.

Sertraline

Two large, identical, double-blind, placebo-controlled sertraline trials have recently been published (Londborg *et al.*, 1998; Pollack *et al.*, 1998). A total of 352 patients from 20 US and Canadian centers were randomized to receive either sertraline or placebo. Doses ranged from 50 to 200 mg/day. Panic attack frequency was reduced significantly more in the sertraline group, beginning in the second week, and was sustained throughout each week of the trial.

The trial employed a new measure entitled "panic attack burden," which utilizes a multiple of the frequency of panic attacks and their severity. This measure showed significant differences between sertraline and placebo in the first week. Overall, the percentage of patients who stopped having panic attacks on sertraline (59.3%) was greater than the percentage of those whose attacks ceased on placebo (46.3%). In fact, the reductions in panic attacks with sertraline were greater than those on placebo as early as the second and fourth weeks. The drug also was well tolerated, with only an 8.3% dropout rate, compared with 2.3% for placebo. In one of the first trials to study changes in the quality of life, the sertraline patients had a higher overall improvement in quality of life, with specific significant improvements in mood, work, and social, family, and leisure activities. There also was significantly greater improvement on measures of satisfaction with medication and overall satisfaction with life.

In the multicenter, 12-week, fixed-dose trial study directed by Londborg, patients were given 50, 100, or 200 mg/day of sertraline and experienced a 65% decrease in the number of panic attacks, compared to 39% of patients on placebo (Londborg *et al.*, 1998). There were also greater reductions in anticipatory anxiety and HAM-A anxiety scores. Because responses in the different dosage groups did not differ significantly from each other, this trial did not provide proof of a dose–response relationship in the 50–200 mg/day range. However, most experts recommend a dosage range of 100–150 mg/day.

Fluoxetine

One of the first fluoxetine studies was by Gorman and colleagues (1987), who studied 16 patients in an 18-week open trial. Dosages began at 10 mg/day and increased to 80 mg/day. Most patients had a significant reduction in their panic attacks within about 6 weeks, and seven of the 16 subjects were considered responders, with no panic attacks for at least 4 weeks in a row. On the other hand, eight of nine who did not respond actually discontinued the medication because of side effects, primarily the "jitteriness syndrome." This "jitterness" with initial dosages that are too high has been well recognized with all antidepressants and obviously does occur with the SSRIs as well. Researchers from this first trial subsequently gave 25 patients a low dose of fluoxetine (5 mg/day) with gradual increases. Results showed that 76% of the patients experienced moderate improvement or better in their PD symptoms and the initial jitteriness was markedly reduced (Schneier *et al.*, 1991).

Recent controlled studies with large samples also confirmed significant improvement in PD symptoms as early as the third week of treatment with fluoxetine, again with approximately 70% of patients responding (Michelson *et al.*, 1998). In a recent trial, there also was evidence of continued improvement over a full year of fluoxetine treatment (Michelson *et al.*, 1999).

Although there are no reliable data documenting a particular target dosage for fluoxetine, an average of 20–80 mg/day was given to most patients in these studies. Some authors suggest 20 mg should be the target dosage, beginning with 5–10 mg/day. A recent trial documented that in stabilized patients once-a-week dosing does maintain the initial improvement, probably because of fluoxetine's long half-life (Emmanuel *et al.*, 1999).

EMERGENCE OF DEPRESSION

Despite the obvious efficacy of the SSRIs as antidepressants and anti-anxiety agents, there are reports that SSRIs might cause depressive symptoms in some patients. Fux and colleagues (1993) reported that seven out of 80 PD patients treated with fluvoxamine (50–200 mg/day) developed symptoms of depression during treatment, even though they had a positive response in terms of their anxiety symptoms. Five of the patients were treated with 20 mg fluoxetine and experienced ongoing depression, which actually became worse in four of them. Because depression is very common in PD, it is unclear whether the depression observed in this study was related to the SSRI or simply emergence of depression which was not prevented by the antidepressant.

COMPARISONS BETWEEN SSRIs

To date, there are very few trials comparing SSRIs in PD patients. As mentioned, paroxetine and CMI have been directly compared, both in short-term and long-term treatment (LeCrubier *et al.*, 1997a,b). Although both were effective, there was some evidence that paroxetine's effects were seen more rapidly, and greater reductions were seen in the ancillary symptoms of PD (anxiety, depression, functional disability) during the long-term maintenance trial on paroxetine. The other major difference was in side effects, paroxetine again having significantly fewer side effects than CMI.

As mentioned above, den Boer and colleagues compared CMI and fluvoxamine. Although both drugs were essentially equal in the trial, CMI was shown to be more effective than fluvoxamine in terms of reducing anxiety symptoms and depression (den Boer *et al.*, 1987). Other studies have suggested that the two agents are approximately equal (Wade, 1995). In the trial comparing citalopram and CMI, both drugs were effective, with few reported differences (Wade 1995; Wade et al., 1997).

Because scientifically valid direct comparisons are limited, it is difficult to compare these agents even in terms of side effects. While it appears that CMI probably has more side effects than the traditional SSRIs, the latter seem to share most side effects such as nausea and asthenia. Whether lower rates of these various symptoms are associated with one agent or another still needs to be further researched.

Certainly, the most important clinical comparison has been between the SSRIs and the TCAs. As a class, the TCAs produce certain problematic side effects, such as weight gain, anticholinergic side effects, sedation, and potentially dangerous interactions with the cardiovascular system. Overall, the frequency of side effects with the SSRIs is probably as high as with the TCAs, but the side effects are not as severe and are better tolerated by patients. Nausea, diarrhea, insomnia, agitation, delayed orgasm, and headache are probably the most common. The SSRIs may therefore be regarded as milder than the TCAs in overall side effects, better tolerated by patients, and much safer in overdose (Baldwin and Birtwistle, 1998).

INTEGRATED TREATMENT

There is considerable evidence that exposure-based treatment of PD, especially with agoraphobia, is quite effective, with panic-free rates of approximately 75% (Ballenger et al., 1997). This rate is at least as high as that found in trials utilizing SSRIs (Ballenger et al., 1997). Meta-analysis of cognitive behavioral therapy (CBT) also suggests that it is at least as effective as pharmacological treatments (Clum, 1993; van Balkom, 1997). In general, there is a low relapse rate with CBT, suggesting a potential advantage of CBT over the SSRIs. Additionally, exposure in vivo, when coupled with CBT, has been shown to be a highly effective treatment (Ballenger et al., 1997; Telch et al., 1993; Chambliss and Gillis, 1993; Clark, 1986). However, a recent large trial failed to demonstrate an added benefit of combination therapy, probably because both treatments when delivered alone were so effective in and of themselves (Barlow et al., 1998). Additional studies of CBT are needed, especially in combination with the SSRIs.

REFERENCES

Baldwin DS, Birtwistle J (1998) The side effect burden associated with the drug treatment of panic disorder. J Clin Psychiat, 59(suppl 8), 39–44.
Ballenger JC, Lydiard RB, Turner SM (1997) Panic disorder and agoraphobia. In: GO Gabbard. (ed) Treatments of Psychiatric Disorders vol 2, 2nd edn. Washington, DC: American Psychiatric Press, 1421–1452.

Ballenger JC (1998) Comorbidity of panic and depression: Implications for clinical management. *Int Clin Psychopharmacol,* **13**(suppl 4), S75–81.

Ballenger JC, Davidson JR, Lecrubier Y, Nutt DJ, Baldwin DS, den Boer JA (1998a) Consensus statement on panic disorder from the International Consensus Group on Depression and Anxiety. *J Clin Psychiat,* **59**(suppl 8), 7–54.

Ballenger JC, Steiner M, Bushnell W, Gergel I (1998b) Double-blind, fixed-dose, placebo-controlled study of paroxetine in the treatment of panic disorder. *Am J Psychiat,* **155**, 36–42.

Ballenger JC (1999) Selective serotonin reuptake inhibitors (SSRIs) in panic disorder. In: D Nutt, JC Ballenger, J Lépine (eds) *Panic Disorder: Clinical Diagnosis and Management.* London: Martin Dunitz, 159–178.

Barlow D, Shear K, Woods S, Gorman JA (1998) A multicenter trial comparing cognitive behavior therapy, imipramine, their combination and placebo. Presented at the Annual Convention of the Anxiety Disorders Association of America, Boston, March 26–29, 1998.

Boyer W (1995) Serotonin uptake inhibitors are superior to imipramine and alprazolam in alleviating panic attacks: a meta-analysis. *Int Clin Psychopharmacol,* **10**, 45–49.

Cassano GB, Petracca A, Perugi G (1988) Clomipramine for panic disorder: I. The first 10 weeks of a long-term comparison with imipramine. *J Affect Dis,* **14**, 123–127.

Chambless DL, Gillis MM (1993) Cognitive therapy of anxiety disorders. *J Consult Clin Psychol,* **61**, 248–260.

Clark DM (1986) A cognitive approach to panic. *Behav Res Ther,* **24**, 461–470.

Clum GA, Clum GA, Surls R (1993) A meta-analysis of treatments for panic disorder. *J Consul Clin Psych,* **61**, 317–326.

de Beurs E, van Balkom A, Van Dyck R *et al.* (1999) Long-term outcome of pharmacological and psychological treatment for panic disorder with agoraphobia: a 2-year naturalistic follow-up. *Acta Psychiatr Scand,* **99**, 59–67.

den Boer JA, Westenberg HGM, Kamerbeek WDJ (1987) Effect of serotonin uptake inhibitors in anxiety disorders: a double-blind comparison of clorimipramine and fluvoxamine. *Int Clin Psychopharmacol,* **2**, 21–32.

den Boer JA (1998) Pharmacotherapy of panic disorder: differential efficacy from a clinical viewpoint. *J Clin Psychiat,* **59**, 30–36.

Emmanuel NT, Ware M, Brawman-Mintzer O (1999) Once weekly dosing of fluoxetine in the maintenance of remission in panic disorder. *J Clin Psychiat,* **69**, 299–301.

Feet PO, Gotestam KG (1994) Increased antipanic efficacy in combined treatment with clomipramine and dixtyrazine. *Acta Psychiat Scand,* **89**, 230–234.

Fux M, Taub M, Zohar J (1993) Emergence of depressive symptoms during treatment for panic disorder with specific 5-hydroxytryptophan reuptake inhibitors. *Acta Psychiat Scand,* **88**, 235–237.

Gloger S, Grunhaus L, Birmacher B (1981) Treatment of spontaneous panic attacks with clomipramine. *Am J Psychiat,* **138**, 1215–1217.

Gloger S, Grunhaus L, Gladic D (1989) Panic attacks and agoraphobia: low dose clomipramine treatment. *J Clin Psychopharmacol,* **9**, 28–32.

Gorman JM, Lieowitz MR, Fyer AJ (1987) An open trial of fluoxetine in the treatment of panic attacks. *J Clin Psychopharmacol,* **7**, 329–332.

Humble M, Koczkas C, Wistedt B (1989) Serotonin and anxiety: an open study of citalopram in panic disorder. In: CN Stefanis, CR Soldatos, AD Rabavilas (eds) *Psychiatry Today: VIII World Congress of Psychiatry Abstracts.* New York: Elsevier, 151.

Jobson KO, Potter WZ (1995) International psychopharmacology algorithm project report. *Psychopharmacol Bull,* **31**, 457–507.

Johnston DG, Troyer IE, Whitsett SF (1988) Clomipramine treatment of agoraphobic women: an eight week controlled trial. *Arch Gen Psychiat,* **45**, 453–459.

LeCrubier I, Bakker A, Judge R (1997a) A comparison of paroxetine, clomipramine, and placebo in the treatment of panic disorder. *Acta Psychiat Scand*, **95**, 145–152.

LeCrubier Y, Judge R, and the Collaborative Paroxetine Study Investigators (1997b) Long-term evaluation of paroxetine, clomipramine, and placebo in panic disorder. *Acta Psychiat Scand*, **95**, 153–160.

Lepola U, Wade AG, Leinonen EV (1998) A controlled prospective, 1-year study of citalopram in the treatment of panic disorder. *J Clin Psychiat*, **59**, 528–534.

Lesser JM, Lydiard RB, Antel E (1992) Alprazolam plasma concentrations and treatment response in panic disorder and agoraphobia. *Am J Psychiat*, **149**, 1556–1562.

Londborg PD, Wolkow R, Smith WT (1998) Sertraline in the treatment of panic disorder. *Br J Psychiat*, **173**, 54–60.

Mavissakalian MR, Perel JM (1995) Imipramine treatment of panic disorder with agoraphobia: dose ranging and plasma level response relationships. *Am J Psychiat*, **152**, 673–682.

Mavissakalian M, Perel JM (1989) Imipramine dose–response relationship in panic disorder with agoraphobia. *Arch Gen Psychiat*, **46**, 127–131.

Michelson D, Lydiard RB, Pollack MH, Tamura RN, Hoog SL, Tepner R (1998) Outcome assessment and clinical improvement in panic disorder: evidence from a randomized controlled trial of fluoxetine and placebo. *Am J Psychiat*, **155**, 1570–1577.

Michelson D, Pollack M, Lydiard R (1999) Continuing treatment of panic disorder after acute response: randomised, placebo-controlled trial with fluoxetine. *Br J Psychiat*, **172**, 213–218.

Modigh K, Westberg P, Eriksson E (1992) Superiority of clomipramine over imipramine in the treatment of panic disorder: a placebo-controlled trial. *J Clin Psychopharmacol*, **51**(4S): 53–58.

Nair NP, Bakish D, Saxena B (1996) Comparison of fluvoxamine, imipramine, and placebo in the treatment of outpatients with panic disorder. *Anxiety*, **2**, 192–198.

Oehrberg S, Christiansen PE, Behnek K (1995) Paroxetine in the treatment of panic disorder, a randomized double blind placebo controlled study. *Br J Psychiat*, **167**, 374–379.

Pohl RB, Wolkow RM, Clary CM (1998) Sertraline in the treatment of panic disorder: a double-blind multicenter trial. *Am J Psychiat*, **155**, 1189–1195.

Pollack MH, Otto MW, Worthington JJ (1998) Sertraline in the treatment of panic disorder: a flexible-dose multicenter trial. *Arch Gen Psychiat*, **55**, 1010–1016.

Sasson Y, Iancu I, Fux M (1999) A double-blind crossover comparison of clomipramine and desipramine in the treatment of panic disorder. *Eur Neuropsychopharmacol*, **9**, 191–196.

Schneier FR, Liebowitz MR, Davies SO (1991) Fluoxetine in panic disorder. *J Clin Psychopharmacol*, **10**, 119–121.

Shear MK, Brown TA, Barlow DH (1997) Multicenter collaborative Panic Disorder Severity Scale. *Am J Psychiat*, **154**, 1571–1575.

Spiegel DA, Saeed SA, Bruct TJ (1996) An open trial of fluvoxamine therapy for panic disorder complicated by depression. *J Clin Psychiat*, **57**(Suppl 8), 37–40.

Telch MJ, Lucas JA, Schmidt NB, Hanna HH, Jaimez TL, Lucas RA (1993) Group cognitive-behavioral treatment of panic disorder. *Behav Res Ther*, **31**, 279–287.

van Balkom AJ, Bakker A, Spinhoven P, Blaauw BM, Smeenk S, Ruesink B (1997) A meta-analysis of the treatment of panic disorder with or without agoraphobia: a comparison of psychopharmacological, cognitive-behavioral, and combination treatments. *J Nerv Ment Dis*, **185**, 510–516.

Wade AG (1995) The optimal therapeutical area for SSRIs: panic disorder. Presented at the VIII Annual European College of Neuropsychopharmacology, Venice, Italy, October 1995.

Wade AG, Lepola U, Koponen HJ (1997) The effect of citalopram in panic disorder. *Br J Psychiat*, **170**, 549–553.

6

Social anxiety disorder treatment: role of SSRIs

R. Bruce Lydiard

INTRODUCTION

Social anxiety disorder (SAD) is a common and potentially disabling psychiatric disorder. The key DSM-IV diagnostic features of SAD are shown in Table 6.1. SAD occurs twice as often in women as in men. Without effective treatment, individuals with SAD exhibit persistence of social anxiety symptoms over time. Because SAD often co-exists with other psychiatric disorders, it often remains undetected. Community studies and treatment-seeking patient samples suggest that there is a high rate of comorbidity in individuals with anxiety disorders, including SAD (Lecrubier and Weiller 1997; Lépine and Pélissolo 1996; Lydiard *et al.*, 1996; Magee *et al.*, 1996; Markowitz *et al.*, 1992; Merikangas and Angst 1995; Merikangas *et al.*, 1996, 1998). There is evidence that SAD and generalized anxiety disorder are almost always associated with one or more anxiety and/or depressive disorders (Goldenberg *et al.*, 1996). This review will focus on the comorbidity of SAD with major depressive disorder (MDD), panic disorder (PD), post-traumatic stress disorder and alcohol abuse/dependence. Because of the high rate of depression and other comorbid disorders, it is suggested that use of antidepressant medications with a broad range of efficacy—such as the serotonin-selective reuptake inhibitors (SSRIs)—should be considered as the first-line treatment.

SSRIs in Depression and Anxiety, Second Edition. Edited by S.A. Montgomery and J.A. den Boer.
© 2001 John Wiley & Sons Ltd.

Table 6.1. Key clinical features of social anxiety disorders/social phobia.

Clinical feature
Subject fears of embarrassment in one or more or social situations
Subject fears of negative evaluation
Exposure to the situation in question reliably causes anxiety, often with panic-like symptoms
The fear is recognized as excessive or unreasonable
The social situation in question is often avoided, or is endured with dread
Panic attacks are associated with social situations and do not occur unexpectedly
Significant distress or interference is caused with in one or more domains of functioning

Subtypes
Generalized (encompasses most social interactions)
Non-generalized (a few discrete situations such as public speaking, eating, writing, etc. in front of others, but not most social situations)

COMORBIDITY OF PSYCHIATRIC DISORDERS

The National Comorbidity Study (NCS) which was conducted in the early 1990s, surveyed a US population sample of 8098 non-institutionalized individuals aged 18–54 years. Subjects were examined for the presence of one or more psychiatric disorders via a structured interview (Kessler *et al.*, 1994). The survey was intended to assess the patterns of co-existence of psychiatric disorders (i.e. psychiatric comorbidity) in the US population. The authors found that psychiatric disorders are not randomly distributed, but rather that they aggregated in a small percentage of the population. "Highly comorbid" individuals—those with a 12-month prevalence of three or more psychiatric disorders—carried 59% of all psychiatric disorders and 88% of all serious disorders, but constituted only about 14% of the US population. Many of these individuals suffered from comorbid anxiety and depression. These highly comorbid patients exhibited greater limitations in social, family and occupational functioning. They also had a disproportionately high level of health care usage (Kessler *et al.*, 1996a). The comorbid states of anxiety disorders and MDD were more common, and were more often chronic than "pure" or uncomplicated anxiety or depression. Importantly, individuals with a current anxiety disorder were at the highest risk for subsequent development of MDD. The authors found that anxiety disorders tend to appear earlier in life than most other psychiatric disorders, and in addition to depression, they also constituted a risk factor for the development of other psychiatric disorders. Thus, as comorbidity occurs, the risk for additional disorders also increases. The public health implications of these findings are that early detection and treatment of psychiatric disorders may reduce the risk for developing subsequent disorders, thus reducing both the considerable financial (Greenberg *et al.*, 1999) and psychosocial burden imposed by comorbidity in the US population.

SAD is more frequently associated with secondary depression (22.4%) than any other anxiety disorder (Kessler *et al.*, 1996b). In those individuals with primary SAD, MDD occurred an average of 11.9 years after the onset of SAD; an average of 4.3 total disorders affected those with secondary MDD. Of the individuals identified as having SAD in the NCS, approximately 80% had more than one psychiatric disorder. The NCS estimates of the lifetime (13.8%) and 12-month (7.9%) prevalence rates for SAD (Kessler *et al.*, 1994), as well as rates for SAD found by other more recent community studies (Magee *et al.*, 1996) were higher than the estimates from the (ECA) Study, which was an earlier population study of the prevalence of psychiatric disorders in the US (Robins *et al.*, 1991). One possible reason for the higher estimated prevalence rates is that there were six stem questions used in the NCS interviews as against three employed in the ECA. The high prevalence rates for SAD from more recent community surveys, consistent with the NCS data, suggest that the NCS did not overestimate the prevalence rates of this serious psychiatric disorder.

SOCIAL ANXIETY DISORDER AND PSYCHIATRIC COMORBIDITY

SAD represents a particularly difficult problem in terms of detection since it begins early in life and the affected individuals may not recognize their symptoms of shyness as a treatable psychiatric disorder (Ballenger *et al.*, 1998; Liebowitz *et al.*, 1985; Kasper 1998. Two main subtypes of SAD are currently recognized by the DSM-IV. Approximately 75% of SAD is of the generalized subtype (most or all social situations provoke anxiety and/or avoidance). The remaining one-fourth of individuals with social anxiety endorse one or a few circumscribed social fears which usually involve performance (public speaking or other performance situations). Those individuals with generalized SAD are three times more likely to suffer from comorbid anxiety disorders and twice as likely to suffer from mood disorders as are those with the non-generalized SAD (Mannuzza *et al.*, 1995; Wittchen *et al.*, 1992). SAD appears primarily in the first two decades of life (Davidson *et al.*, 1993; Magee *et al.*, 1996; Schneier *et al.*, 1992); with a median age of onset in the mid-teens. People with SAD are more likely to suffer from major depression, and consequent academic, truancy and other behavioral problems, and alcohol and other substance abuse (Cox *et al.*, 1994; DeWit *et al.*, 1999; Essau *et al.*, 1998; Hovens *et al.*, 1994; Lépine and Pélissolo, 1998; Wittchen *et al.*, 1999). Since feeling awkward and shy are commonly reported by adolescents, it may be difficult or even impossible for those with SAD to describe their symptoms accurately to a peer and be readily understood. Because SAD typically begins early in life, there is a prolonged period of risk for comorbidity and chronicity. At present, there are too few data to evaluate whether comorbidity affects treatment outcome for SAD.

Compared with individuals with uncomplicated SAD, those with comorbid psychiatric disorders are more likely develop alcohol dependence, substance abuse disorders, social and occupational impairment, be higher health care utilizers, and attempt suicide (Lépine and Pélissolo, 1996; Schneier*et al.*, 1992; Wittchen and Beloch, 1996). In primary care samples the prevalence of SAD is high, and comorbidity of SAD is similarly much more common than "pure" SAD (Katzelnick *et al.*, 1999; Stein *et al.*, 1999a) As noted above, the public health implications of comorbidity of SAD are potentially enormous. Based on the model of increased risk suggested by the NCS study, early detection and intervention might prevent the accumulation of multiple comorbid disorders, reduce the tremendous suffering of those affected, and billions of dollars lost to the US economy each year (Greenberg *et al.*, 1999).

Social anxiety disorder and major depression

Major depression (MDD) frequently occurs in those with pre-existing SAD, especially those with generalized SAD. An increased risk for early-onset MDD, apparent persistence or chronicity of mood symptoms associated with SAD is commonly observed (Kessler *et al.*, 1999). Breslau and Peterson (1995) studied a community sample from Detroit, Michigan, and found that primary anxiety disorders (including SAD) were significant risk factors for the development of secondary MDD. Primary anxiety disorders were twice as common in women than in men. Since the presence of an anxiety disorder increases the risk for MDD, Breslau and Peterson suggested this might explain why women are twice as likely as men to develop MDD (i.e. twice as likely to have anxiety, which increases the risk for MDD). Also, individuals with early-onset SAD are more likely to develop MDD during childhood or adolescence (versus adult-onset MDD). These individuals are more likely to develop subsequent alcohol use (Alpert *et al.*, 1999). This suggests that early intervention may prevent the subsequent comorbidity associated with SAD. SAD also commonly co-occurs with bipolar, schizoaffective or psychotic depression, usually with one or more of the other anxiety disorders, and significantly increased rates of stimulant abuse (Cassano *et al.*, 1999). SAD may appear secondary to MDD. Dilsaver and colleagues (1992) assessed SAD in 42 patients with recurrent MDD; of these, 19 of 42 experienced SAD which met DSM-IIIR criteria only while in the context of an episode of MDD. When SAD and MDD co-exist, the clinician is presented with the diagnostic challenge of distinguishing social avoidance/withdrawal due to depression from that associated with SAD.

Social anxiety disorder and panic disorder

SAD commonly co-exists with panic disorder (PD). In clinical samples of patients presenting for treatment of PD with or without agoraphobia, SAD was also detected in up to 45% (Montejo and Liebowitz, 1994). In the majority of cases, SAD appeared prior to the onset of PD. One family study suggested that comorbid SAD and PD may represent a distinct subtype of SAD. Fyer *et al.*, reported the results of a family study comparing treatment-seeking probands with SAD alone, SAD plus PD, and never-ill controls (Fyer *et al.*, 1996). No other comorbid anxiety disorders were present in the probands. They found that the first-degree relatives of individuals with SAD plus PD resembled those with PD alone (i.e. increased levels of PD but not SAD). The families of those with SAD only had increased rates of SAD but not PD. SAD may be non-familial and/or causally related to PD. Stein *et al.* (1989), reported findings from a group of patients with PD only versus those with PD plus SAD. They found that 93% of those with both PD and SAD had experienced a prior MDE compared with 47% of those with PD only. These studies and numerous others suggest that PD and SAD frequently co-exist (Starcevic *et al.*, 1992); whether subtyping according to order of onset will yield clinically significant findings (i.e. with implications for treatment) is still unclear.

Social anxiety disorder and post-traumatic stress disorder

There has been little systematic study of the association of post-traumatic stress disorder (PTSD) and SAD. Evidence exists that a substantial percentage of adult patients with PD or SAD, and in particular women, have experienced higher rates of sexual and/or physical abuse than those without anxiety disorders (Stein *et al.*, 1996a). In one study of women who were victims of completed traumatic rape, there were high levels of SAD, MDD and all the other anxiety disorders; in contrast, women who were robbed or burglarized (i.e. had less serious traumatic events) did not have these additional disorders as frequently (Boudreaux *et al.*, 1998). Whether SAD may be a common sequel of severe traumatic stress (i.e. whether trauma is a risk factor for SAD) has not been studied in detail. Orsillo and colleagues reported the results of a study of psychiatric comorbidity in veterans with combat-related PTSD and compared them with veterans without PTSD. Veterans with PTSD had significantly higher rates of current SAD, MDD, bipolar disorder and PD; higher rates of lifetime MDD, PD, SAD and obsessive-compulsive disorder were also noted (Orsillo *et al.*, 1996a). This same group (Orsillo *et al.*, 1996b) described a group of male Vietnam veterans with PTSD, and, after controlling for relevant variables, found that over 30% had SAD which began after the onset of PTSD. Adversity of homecoming and shame about one's experience in Vietnam were significant predictors of the current level of social anxiety over and above the effects of premilitary anxiety and severity of combat exposure.

In a community study, Davidson *et al.* (1991) reported that PTSD in the general population was associated with a family history of psychiatric illness, poverty, abuse and parental separation prior to age 10. Those with chronic PTSD were more likely to have SAD. David *et al.* (1995) assessed a group of patients with either PD and/or SAD and compared them with a non-clinical sample. Traumatic events in childhood were more commonly reported by the PD and/or SAD patients (63% vs. 35% of comparison subjects). Sexual and/or physical abuse were also significantly increased in the patient group and were most specifically associated with SAD. Engdahl *et al.* (1998) examined 262 men with prior combat exposure and imprisonment by the enemy. They found that both SAD and PD, and other anxiety and mood disorders were more common in individuals with PTSD-related to the war trauma. About half of the SAD and PD diagnoses had arisen after the traumatic event. One recent controlled twin study from Australia indicated that early childhood sexual abuse was associated with a higher rate of adult psychopathology, including (in women only) SAD (Dinwiddie et al., 2000). SAD appears to be a familial disorder, suggesting genetic vulnerability as one etiological variable of importance (Fyer et al., 1993, 1995; Mancini et al., 1996; Rosenbaum et al., 1994; Stein et al., 1998a). However, the association of trauma, either civilian or combat-related, found in community or patient samples raises the question of whether SAD following traumatic stress in childhood, adulthood (or both) is in some way different from SAD which appears in the absence of trauma. Whether treatment outcome varies for SAD arising in these different contexts is not yet clear, but merits further study.

Social anxiety disorder, alcohol and other substance abuse

Individuals with SAD are at substantially increased risk for alcohol abuse and dependence, nicotine dependence and other substance abuse disorders (Degonda and Angst, 1993; Feehan et al., 1994; Hovens et al., 1994; Kessler et al., 1994, 1996b; Lecrubier, 1998; Lépine and Pélissolo, 1998; Lydiard et al., 1992; Mullaney and Trippett, 1979; Myrick and Brady, 1997; Perugi et al., 1990; Schneier et al., 1992; Smail et al., 1984; Tomasson and Vaglum, 1997). Individuals with SAD are more likely to develop dependence on alcohol (Schuckit et al., 1997). Nearly all studies which have examined the relative ages of onset of SAD and problem alcohol use have found that SAD precedes alcohol use, possibly because of the typically early age of onset of SAD (Amies et al., 1982: Clark et al., 1995; Hovens et al., 1994; Kessler et al., 1996b; Kushner et al., 1990; Lépine and Pélissolo 1998; van Ameringen et al., 1991). Individuals who have SAD with comorbid alcohol use disorders are more likely to have additional disorders, such as PD with agoraphobia and MDD (Alpert et al., 1999; Chignon et al., 1991; Otto et al., 1992). Suicide risk is increased in males with SAD and alcohol dependence (Chartier et al., 1998). Although the association of SAD and alcoholism has been established, the effect of alcoholism on the treatment of SAD has received minimal investigation (Thomas et al., 1999; Wesner, 1990). The limited data available indicate that alcohol-related disorders convey a worse prognosis for outcome of SAD following cognitive-behavioral treatment (Martinsen et al., 1998), pharmacological treatment (Versiani et al., 1997), and detoxification from alcohol (Thomas et al., 1999; Tomasson and Vaglum, 1997, 1998). Myrick and Brady (1997) recently reported that 22 of 158 individuals who were admitted for cocaine dependence had SAD; compared to those with cocaine dependence only, the individuals with SAD also had more additional psychiatric disorders, greater symptom severity, and more alcohol and polysubstance abuse.

There are numerous barriers to treatment-seeking for individuals with SAD and alcoholism. Perhaps the greatest barrier is that many individuals with alcohol or

drug-related disorders are unaware that they have a treatable anxiety disorder—
SAD—but rather see their social fears as an enduring part of their constitutional
makeup. Also, SAD sufferers tend to avoid scrutiny, criticism and being the center of
attention. Reluctance to enter highly socially interactive treatment programs for
alcohol and other substance abuse disorders undoubtedly complicates treatment-
seeking behavior in individuals who also have SAD. Such individuals may require
novel treatment approaches, e.g. computer-based (Kobak *et al.*, 1996), and
individualized substance abuse and anxiety treatment in a dual diagnosis treatment
program (Brady and Lydiard, 1993). Given the relatively high rates of SAD in
alcohol-dependent individuals, the cost-effectiveness of more definitive and
comprehensive early intervention seems clear, but further research is required to
confirm this hypothesis.

Social anxiety disorder and other psychiatric disorders

In addition to the disorders noted above, individuals with SAD exhibit high rates of
other psychiatric disorders (Hochstrasser and Angst, 1996; Lépine and Pélissolo, 1996;
Mannuzza *et al.*, 1995; Schneier *et al.*, 1992) such as generalized anxiety disorder
(Borkovec *et al.*, 1995; Goldenberg *et al.*, 1996; Mancuso *et al.*, 1993), bipolar
disorder (Cassano *et al.*, 1999; Kessler *et al.*, 1999; Perugi *et al.*, 1998, 1999; Pini *et al.*,
1997; Savino *et al.*, 1993), obsessive-compulsive disorder (Angst, 1993; Austin *et al.*,
1990; Degonda and Angst, 1993; Perugi *et al.*, 1990), body dysmorphic disorder
(Brawman-Mintzer *et al.*, 1995; Phillips *et al.*, 1998), eating disorders (Brewerton *et
al.*, 1993; Bulik, *et al.*, 1997; Carter *et al.*, 1999; Kendler and Gardner 1998;
Schwalberg *et al.*, 1992) and specific phobias (previously called simple phobias)
(Bienvenu and Eaton, 1998; Kessler *et al.*, 1998; Magee *et al.*, 1996: Merikangas and
Angst, 1995) (see Figure 6.1).

While there has been no systematic study of the treatment of patients with
bipolar disorder and SAD, data from clinical and patient samples noted above
indicate that the two conditions overlap with significant frequency. In such patients,
treatments which might address both bipolar disorder and SAD could be useful.
Gabapentin, an established anticonvulsant with more recent evidence for use as an
anxiolytic, was recently reported to be effective in the treatment of generalized SAD
(Pande *et al.*, 1999). While further research is required, agents like gabapentin, with
therapeutic effects for more than one comorbid disorder, may prove to be useful in
selected patients. The extremely high comorbidity of SAD with specific phobia is of
interest from a research perspective, but currently carries little significance for
clinical practice. In a case series of individuals with either generalized or non-
generalized SAD and obsessive-compulsive disorder, there was evidence of poor
response to treatment with conventional pharmacological treatment with SSRIs,
but a good response to phenelzine (Carrasco *et al.*, 1992). Beyond the minimal
information noted above, the effect of comorbid disorders on treatment outcome
requires further investigation.

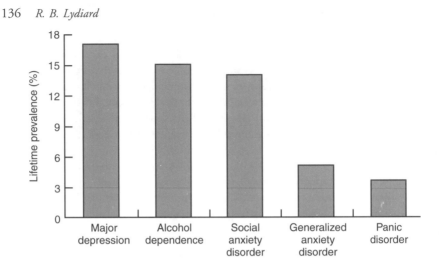

Figure 6.1. Prevalence of social anxiety disorder and other common DSM-III-R disorders. Adapted from Kessler, McGonagle *et al.* (1994), with permission.

SOCIAL ANXIETY DISORDER AND MEDICAL COMORBIDITY

The diagnostic system utilized currently excludes social anxiety due to medical disorders (American Psychiatric Association, 1994). However, social anxiety commonly occurs in the context of several medical disorders, such as benign essential tremor, stuttering and irritable bowel syndrome (George and Lydiard, 1994; Stein, Heuser *et al.*, 1990; Lydiard and Falsetti, 1999). Anecdotally, morbidly obese individuals and burn victims also experience significant social anxiety secondary to their medical conditions. In our experience, social anxiety in these individuals can respond to same the treatments that are used in SAD patients without such medical disorders. The clinical implications of secondary SAD in terms of additional disability/functional impairment have not been investigated. However, based on the limited information available, it seems worthwhile to address SAD specifically even when it appears in the context of a medical (i.e. axis III) disorder.

TREATMENT IMPLICATIONS OF COMORBIDITY IN SOCIAL ANXIETY DISORDER

There is conclusive evidence that in many individuals SAD is accompanied by comorbid psychiatric disorders. These individuals experience more social and occupational impairment and subjective distress, utilize more health care, and have a poorer long-term prognosis than those with SAD only. Given the limited treatment outcome literature on comorbidity in SAD, the clinician is left with little hard evidence on which to base treatment planning. Fortunately, the increased information on the SSRIs, which appear to have relatively broad effects on most of the disorders commonly associated with SAD, suggests that these might be the treatment of choice for generalized SAD (Ballenger *et al.*, 1998). A thorough differential diagnostic assessment, and a systematic trial-and error approach to SAD patients with comorbid psychiatric disorders (Rosenbaum and Pollock, 1994) remain the pillars of optimal treatment.

DIFFERENTIAL DIAGNOSIS OF SOCIAL ANXIETY DISORDER

Discriminating SAD from associated disorders can sometimes present a diagnostic challenge (Moutier and Stein, 1999). Table 6.2 presents several important conditions to be considered in the differential diagnostics, together with comments on the features discriminating SAD from the other disorders. One of the more controversial of these is avoidant personality disorder, which in the vast majority of cases co-exists with generalized SAD. Most experts believe that this "personality disorder" is actually the same as generalized SAD, and note that it has been shown to resolve with treatment for

Table 6.2. Differential diagnoses for social anxiety disorder.

Condition	Diagnostic issues
Post-traumatic stress disorder	Temporally follows traumatic event, cues related to trauma not exclusively to social situations
Panic disorder	Unexpected panic attacks are typical of panic disorder vs. exclusively socially mediated anxiety
Agoraphobia	Fearful avoidance of situations in which panic attacks may occur, not limited to social situations
Major depression or atypical depression	Social withdrawal temporally related to mood disturbance and not to fear of humiliation or embarrassment. Atypical depression with rejection sensitivity is associated with other symptoms (e.g. hypersomnia, hyperphagia, anergy, depressed mood)
Generalized anxiety disorder	Focus of worry not limited to social situations; social discomfort or avoidance is not a key feature
Body dysmorphic disorder	Avoidance of social activity focused on concern over perceived ugliness
Avoidant personality disorder	Often present in generalized social anxiety disorder, may represent more severe end of social anxiety disorder spectrum. Individual desires social activity, but avoids it
Schizotypal/schizoid personality disorders	Avoidance of social situations is preferred by individual and not due to fear of embarrassment or humiliation
Normal shyness	No or minimal interference with social, occupational or family functioning

SAD (Deltito and Stam, 1989; Fahlen, 1995) which raises the question of whether it is a personality disorder or an artifact of the early onset and chronic nature of SAD. Atypical depression is a subtype of MDD characterized by rejection sensitivity. In addition, however, it is also associated with several of the following symptoms: anergy, mood reactivity, hypersomnia and hyperphagia. Atypical depression is more commonly associated with generalized SAD (Mannuzza et al., 1995; Alpert et al., 1999) than the non-generalized subtype.

SELECTIVE SEROTONIN-REUPTAKE INHIBITORS—FIRST LINE TREATMENT FOR SOCIAL ANXIETY DISORDER

Social anxiety disorder is amenable to both cognitive-behavioral and pharmacological treatment, as discussed by Davidson (1998), Jefferson, (1995) and Lydiard (1998). Recently, the International Consensus Group on Depression and Anxiety recommended SSRIs as the therapy of choice for social anxiety disorder (Ballenger et al., 1998).

The initial suggestions of the efficacy of the SSRIs in SAD, initially derived from case reports and open-label studies of SSRIs, have indicated their potential for use in SAD. An acute study utilizing fluvoxamine was the first study to demonstrate the efficacy of an SSRI in a controlled study with a small sample (van Vliet, et al., 1994). This was followed by two crossover studies which included double-blind placebo-controlled treatment with sertraline (Katzelnick et al., 1994) and paroxetine (Stein et al., 1996b) [see Table 6.3]. The latter authors reported that abrupt placebo substitution for paroxetine therapy following successful treatment of generalized SAD led to the relapse of symptoms, while continued paroxetine therapy was of benefit.

Based on the optimistic preliminary data from these smaller studies, three large-scale studies of paroxetine in SAD were undertaken. These studies, which represent the largest combined sample to date ($n = 861$) of patients with SAD treated with SSRIs, were all intentionally similarly structured to allow easy comparison between studies (Baldwin, 2000; Baldwin et al., 1999; Lydiard and Bobes, 2000), and are discussed in some detail below. The studies utilized standardized ratings for social anxiety as well as the other variables usually assessed in anxiety studies. Paroxetine is the first SSRI to receive approval for use in SAD in the UK, other European countries and in the

Table 6.3. Early studies of SSRIs in social anxiety disorder/social phobia.

SSRI	Study design	n	% Responders	Reference
Paroxetine	Open	36	77	Stein et al., 1996
Sertraline	Parallel cross-over	12	42	Katzelnick et al., 1995
Fluvoxamine	Parallel	30	46	van Vliet et al., 1994

United States. It is worth mentioning that the design of subsequent studies assessing the SSRIs in SAD have largely used methods that were employed in these multicenter studies.

Study designs

Flexible-dose studies

Two multicenter, double-blind, placebo-controlled, flexible-dose clinical trials of paroxetine were conducted: one in the US and Canada (Study 382) (Stein *et al.*, 1998b), which included 187 subjects, and one in Europe and South Africa (study 502) (Baldwin *et al.*, 1999), which included 290 subjects. Each study employed a 1-week, single-blind, placebo run-in period followed by a 12-week double-blind treatment phase. The dose of paroxetine was 20 mg/day for the first two weeks. After the initial two weeks, the daily dosage could be increased by 10 mg daily per week to a maximum daily dose of 50 mg paroxetine (or the placebo equivalent).

Fixed-dose study

A still-unpublished 12-week fixed-dose study conducted in the US and Canada was highlighted briefly in a recent review (Lydiard and Bobes, 2000) along with the two flexible-dose studies. A total of 384 patients were randomized to receive a fixed dose of paroxetine 20, 40, or 60 mg/day, or placebo. As with the flexible-dose studies, a 1-week, single-blind, placebo run-in preceded double-blind, random assignment to the treatment groups. Paroxetine was initiated at 20 mg/day one week, increased to 40 mg/day for the 40 or 60 mg/day treatment groups and further increased to 60 mg/day for the 60 mg/day treatment group.

Inclusion and exclusion criteria for all studies

Inclusion and exclusion criteria were similar across all three studies. Subjects were recruited by referral or from advertisements in the media. Outpatients with DSM-IV criteria for SAD were evaluated using the structured interviews for DSM-IV (First *et al.*, 1995; (Sheehan *et al.*, 1994). Men and women aged at least 18 years who fulfilled DSM-IV criteria for SAD, and who had given written informed consent were eligible for the studies. The main exclusion criteria were other axis I disorder(s) which might interfere with assessment of efficacy in the study (e.g. major depression, panic disorder, schizophrenia, bipolar affective disorder, body dysmorphic disorder, recent alcohol or substance abuse or dependence), or a significant risk of suicide. In the two flexible-dose studies, patients with a Hamilton Depression Rating Scale (HAM-D) (Hamilton, 1960) of 15 or more were also excluded, as were patients who required other psychotropic medication (anxiolytics, antidepressants or neuroleptics) or who had a history of paroxetine intolerance. Patients with unstable medical disorders that might interfere with study procedures were also excluded.

Assessment instruments and frequency of assessment

All patients were assessed weekly for the first four weeks of the trial, then at weeks 6, 8, and 12 (endpoint). Two primary efficacy variables were utilized. The first was the proportion of patients with a Clinical Global Impressions (CGI) global improvement (Guy, 1976) score of 1 ("very much improved") or 2 ("much improved") at study endpoint. The second was the mean change from baseline in Liebowitz Social Anxiety Scale (LSAS) (Liebowitz *et al.*, 1988) total score. Secondary measures included changes in anxiety symptoms assessed using the Social Anxiety and Distress Scale (SADS) (Watson and Friend, 1969), and disability assessed using the Sheehan Disability Scale (SDS), a patient self-rated scale which measures impairment of work, social life, and family-life domains.

Results

Patient characteristics

Patient demographic characteristics were similar across the three studies (Table 6.4). The mean age at onset of SAD was 15.8 years and the mean current age of the study population was 36 years (entire patient sample).

Table 6.4. Patient characteristics in three studies of paroxetine treatment vs. placebo for social anxiety disorders.

	Study 382		Study 502		Study 454	
	Paroxetine ($n=94$)	Placebo ($n=93$)	Paroxetine ($n=139$)	Placebo ($n=151$)	Paroxetine ($n=289$*)	Placebo ($n=95$)
Mean age (years)	35.9	36.7	34.7	37.3	37.7	34.7
Age range (years)	18–59	18–76	18–67	18–85	20–70	18–65
Sex (%)						
Male	53	60	46	46	59	58
Female	47	40	54	54	41	42
Race (%)**						
Caucasian	76	86	89	90	81	83
Black	16	9	6	3	9	11
Other	8	5	6	7	10	6

* Combined data from the three active treatment subgroups.
** Some totals greater than 100% due to rounding.

Efficacy results

Paroxetine-treated patients exhibited clinically and statistically significant improvement in both the primary efficacy measures (CGI and LSAS scores), compared with placebo-treated patients.

The proportion of responders on the CGI global improvement scale ("much improved" or "very much improved") in the flexible-dose studies were 55% in the paroxetine group compared with 24% in the placebo group in study 382, and 66% in the paroxetine versus 32% in the placebo group, in study 502. The mean difference in response between the paroxetine and placebo groups was just over 30% in both studies.

In the fixed-dose study, similar percentages of patients in the paroxetine groups were rated as responders on the CGI global improvement assessment (Figure 6.2). However, only the 40 mg/day group was statistically significantly different from the placebo group. Interestingly, the percentages of patients rated as responders in the three active fixed-dose study groups (45%, 47%, and 43% at 20, 40, and 60 mg/day respectively) were lower than in either flexible-dose study (55% and 66%), but the placebo response rates were comparable (20–30% range) across all three studies. The lower response rates may be due to the fixed-dose design, which does not allow for optimizing the balance between efficacy and adverse effects by dose adjustment, and does not really reflect standard clinical practice as well as the flexible-dose studies.

Across all three studies, patients receiving paroxetine experienced greater improvements in their social anxiety symptoms than placebo-treated patients, as

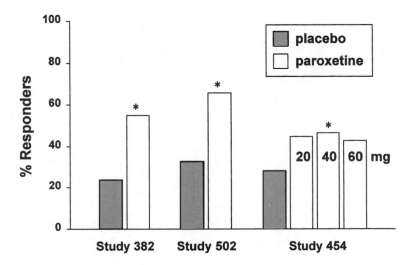

Figure 6.2. Proportion of patients at endpoint with Clinical Global Impressions global improvement scores of 1 or 2 (responders). * < 0.05, paroxetine vs. Placebo.

measured by the average reduction in total LSAS scores from baseline (Figure 6.3). In both flexible-dose studies, the paroxetine-treated patients exhibited significantly more improvement in the total LSAS score ratings than placebo recipients by week 4 (Study 382 was from week 2 onwards) and throughout all of the subsequent assessments to endpoint (week 12). At endpoint, the differences in LSAS score improvement between the paroxetine and placebo groups were statistically significant (paroxetine: study 382, 31 points; study 502, 29 points; placebo: study 382, 15 points; study 502, 16 points). In the fixed dose study, the reduction in LSAS scores in the 20 mg/day dose group (31 points) was statistically significantly greater than in the placebo group (15 points). The two higher-dose groups (paroxetine 40 and 60 mg/day) both exhibited the same degree of improvement (25 points) in LSAS ratings, but this difference was not statistically significantly different from placebo (Figure 6.3).

Secondary efficacy measures

Improvements in all secondary efficacy variables were greater with paroxetine than with placebo. The results from the secondary efficacy measures of the flexible dose studies are shown in Table 6.5. In the fixed-dose study, several of these efficacy variables showed statistical significance for each dose level, but, as might be expected, not all doses showed statistical superiority on all measures. At no time was placebo superior to paroxetine.

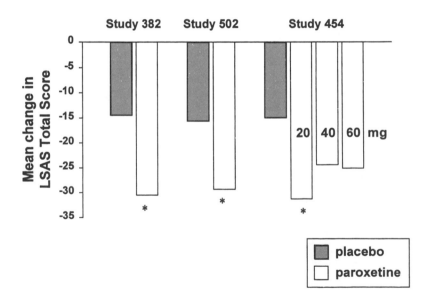

Figure 6.3. Social anxiety symptoms: mean reduction in Liebowitz Social Anxiety Scale (LSAS) total scores at endpoint. * < 0.05, paroxetine vs. Placebo.

Table 6.5. Efficacy of paroxetine in the treatment of social anxiety disorder. Data represent mean change from baseline at endpoint. Adapted from Stein *et al.*, 1998, and Baldwin *et al.*, 1999.

Secondary efficacy measure	Study 382		Study 502	
	Paroxetine	Placebo	Paroxetine	Placebo
CGI, severity of illness	ND	ND	−1.4*	−0.7
LSAS, fear/anxiety	−15.8*	−7.0	ND	ND
LSAS, avoidance	−14.8*	−7.6	ND	ND
SADS, total score	−7.8*	−2.8	−7.2*	−3.9
SDI, work	−1.4*	−0.7	−2.8*	−1.6
SDI, Social life	−2.7*	−1.4	−3.2*	−2.5
SDI, family life	−1.0*	−0.6	−1.8*	−0.8

*Statistically significant improvement with paroxetine compared with placebo, ($p < 0.05$). ND, not described CGI, Clinical Global Impressions; LSAS, Liebowitz Social Anxiety Scale; SADS, Social Anxiety and Distress scale; SDI, Sheehan Disability Index.

Treatment effects on depression

In the European–South African flexible-dose study (502), the change in depression was determined via the HAM-D rating in the two treatment groups. The mean HAM-D total scores at baseline and endpoint, respectively, were 6.2 and 4.2 in for the paroxetine group and 6.7 and 6.5 in the placebo group. The analysis of the treatment effects on depression (HAM-D scores) vs. the effects on SAD symptoms (LSAS and CGI scores) confirmed that treatment outcome with regard to SAD symptoms was independent of effects on depressive symptoms. Similar results were observed in the fixed-dose study.

Paroxetine dosage

The flexible-dose studies allowed a range between 20 and 50 mg/day; the mean dose of paroxetine at study endpoint was 36.6 mg/day in study 382 and 34.7 mg/day in study 502. Not surprisingly, optimal individual patient dosage varied within both flexible-dose studies. In the dose-finding (i.e. fixed-dose) trial, a good response to treatment was observed with 20 or 40 mg/day paroxetine, with no additional efficacy advantage of raising the dose to 60 mg/day (see Figure 6.2).

Tolerability

The most common treatment-emergent adverse experiences in the paroxetine group were abnormal ejaculation, nausea, somnolence, insomnia, headache and asthenia. Headache, insomnia and asthenia, however, were reported at a similar rate in the placebo group (Table 6.6).

Table 6.6. Most common adverse experiences (percentages of patients) reported over 12 weeks of treatment with paroxetine or placebo.

	Paroxetine (%) ($n = 522$)	Placebo (%) ($n = 339$)
Abnormal ejaculation*	32	1
Nausea	25	7
Somnolence	23	5
Insomnia	23	16
Headache	22	22
Asthenia	22	14

* Corrected for gender.

Most adverse experiences in both groups were mild or moderate. The rate of adverse experiences classed as "severe" was similar in the paroxetine (9%) and placebo (6%) groups.

Early termination and dropouts

For all studies combined, lack of efficacy was the most common reason for withdrawal from the placebo group (12%, vs. 2% with paroxetine). However, there were more withdrawals due to adverse experiences from the paroxetine group (16%, vs. 4% with placebo). Patients lost to follow-up amounted to 8% in the paroxetine group and 6% in the placebo group.

Severity of SAD and treatment response

A post-hoc of this large data set by Montgomery (1999) produced evidence that the more severe the SAD, the larger the treatment effect was likely to be. This is somewhat different from the findings seen in depression and some other anxiety disorders. Replication of this important finding awaits future study.

Other selective serotonin-reuptake inhibitors

Recent evidence from larger controlled trials with other SSRIs such as sertraline (van Ameringen et al., 1999a) and fluvoxamine (Stein et al., 1999b) suggest that these agents are approximately equal in efficacy to paroxetine (although no direct comparative studies have been conducted). Other preliminary data for fluoxetine (van Ameringen et al., 1993) and citalopram (Bouwer and Stein, 1998; Lepola et al., 1994) are also encouraging. Finally, preliminary evidence has also been reported that nefazodone (van Ameringen et al., 1999a) and venlafaxine (Altamura et al., 1999; Kelsey, 1995) may also be useful antidepressant agents for the treatment of SAD, but this awaits scientific confirmation. Some of the agents mentioned above are currently being studied in large multicenter trials to establish the efficacy of the individual agents in SAD.

DISCUSSION AND CONCLUSIONS

This article has summarized the current status of the use of SSRIs in the treatment of patients with SAD. As a class, SSRIs show promise for the treatment of SAD and are currently considered first-line medication treatment. The three paroxetine trials described in this review consistently show that paroxetine (20–50 mg/day) is an effective and well-tolerated treatment for SAD. It is likely that similar efficacy will be found for the other SSRIs, as well as for venlafaxine and nefazodone, although this requires confirmation from large, multicenter clinical trials.

The pattern of adverse experiences attributed to paroxetine in these studies is similar to those reported for paroxetine in previous studies in depression; this finding is likely to generalize to the other SSRIs as well.

The process of development of paroxetine as a treatment for SAD described above is the first important step in an ongoing effort to develop effective and safe treatments for SAD. Since approximately 60–70% of patients with social anxiety respond to treatment with SSRIs, there is a clear need for further expansion of the treatment armamentarium. Whether patients who are unresponsive or incompletely responsive to one SSRI may respond to another SSRI or a monoamine oxidase inhibitor remains an open and important clinical question.

It appears that the other SSRIs, some of the newer non-SSRI antidepressant agents, high-potency benzodiazepines and the anticonvulsant gabapentin are also effective treatments for this prevalent and serious disorder (Ballenger *et al.*, 1998; Lydiard, 1998; Pande *et al.*, 1999). Studies comparing these newer agents both with each other and with the other efficacious treatments are needed to provide important clinical information on their relative efficacy and tolerability. (Van Ameringen, Mancini *et al.*, 1993).

REFERENCES

Alpert JE, Fava M *et al.* (1999) Patterns of axis I comorbidity in early-onset versus late-onset major depressive disorder. *Biol Psychiatry*, **46**, 202–211.

Altamura AC, Pioli R *et al.* (1999) Venlafaxine in social phobia: a study in selective serotonin reuptake inhibitor non-responders. *Int Clin Psychopharmacol*, **14**, 239–245.

Amies PL, Gelder MG *et al.* (1983) Social phobia: a comparative clinical study. *Br J Psychiat*, **142**, 174–179.

Angst J. (1993) Comorbidity of anxiety, phobia, compulsion and depression. *Int Clin Psychopharmacol*, **1**, 21–25.

American Psychiatric Association (1994) *Diagnostic and Statistical Manual for Mental Disorders*. Washington, DC: American Psychiatric Association.

Austin LS, Lydiard RB *et al.* (1990) Panic and phobic disorders in patients with obsessive compulsive disorder. *J Clin Psychiat*, **51**, 456–458.

Baldwin DS (2000) Clinical experience with paroxetine in social anxiety disorder. *Int Clin Psychopharmacol*, **15**(suppl 1): S19–S24.

Baldwin D, Bobes J *et al.* (1999) Paroxetine in social phobia/social anxiety disorder. Randomized, double-blind, placebo-controlled study. *Br J Psychiatry*, **175**, 120–126.

Ballenger JC, Davidson JR *et al.* (1998) Consensus statement on social anxiety disorder from the International Consensus Group on Depression and Anxiety. *J Clin Psychiat*, **59**(suppl 17), 54–60.

Bienvenu OJ, Eaton WW (1998) The epidemiology of blood-injection-injury phobia. *Psychol Med*, **28**, 1129–1136.

Borkovec TD, Abel JL *et al.* (1995) Effects of psychotherapy on comorbid conditions in generalized anxiety disorder. *J Consult Clin Psychol*, **63**, 479–483.

Boudreaux E, Kilpatrick DG *et al.* (1998) Criminal victimization, posttraumatic stress disorder, and comorbid psychopathology among a community sample of women. *J Trauma Stress*, **11**, 665–678.

Bouwer C, Stein DJ (1998) Use of the selective serotonin reuptake inhibitor citalopram in the treatment of generalized social phobia. *J Affect Disord*, **49**, 79–82.

Brady KT, Lydiard RB (1993) The association of alcoholism and anxiety. *Psychiat Q*, **64**, 135–149.

Brawman-Mintzer O, Lydiard RB *et al.* (1995) Body dysmorphic disorder in patients with anxiety disorders and major depression: a comorbidity study. *Am J Psychiatry*, **152**, 1665–1667.

Breslau N, Peterson E (1995) Sex differences in depression: a role for preexisting anxiety. *Psychiat Res*. 58: 1–12.

Brewerton TD, Lydiard RB *et al.* (1993) Eating disorders and social phobia. *Arch Gen Psychiat*, **50**(1).

Bulik CM, Sullivan PF *et al.* (1997) Eating disorders and antecedent anxiety disorders: a controlled study. *Acta Psychiat Scand*, **96**, 101–107.

Carrasco JL, Hollander E *et al.* (1992) Treatment outcome of obsessive compulsive disorder with comorbid social phobia. *J Clin Psychiatry*, **53**(11), 387–391.

Carter JD, Joyce PR *et al.* (1999) Gender differences in the rate of comorbid axis I disorders in depressed outpatients. *Depress Anxiety*, **9**, 49–53.

Cassano GB, Pini S *et al.* (1999) Multiple anxiety disorder comorbidity in patients with mood spectrum disorders with psychotic features. *Am J Psychiat*, **156**, 474–476.

Chartier MJ, Hazen AL *et al.* (1998) Lifetime patterns of social phobia: a retrospective study of the course of social phobia in a nonclinical population. *Depress Anxiety*, **7**, 113–121.

Chignon JM, Lépine JP *et al.* (1991) Panic disorder and alcoholism. (In French.) *Encephale*, **17**, 519–523.

Clark DB, Bukstein OG *et al.* (1995) Identifying anxiety disorders in adolescents hospitalized for alcohol abuse or dependence. *Psychiat Serv*, **46**, 618–620.

Cox BJ, Swinson RP *et al.* (1994) Social desirability and self-reports of alcohol abuse in anxiety disorder patients. *Behav Res Ther*, **32**, 175–178.

David D, Giron A *et al.* (1995) Panic-phobic patients and developmental trauma. *J Clin Psychiat*, **56**, 113–117.

Davidson JRT (1998) Pharmacotherapy of social anxiety disorder. *J Clin Psychiat*, **59** (suppl 17), 47–51.

Davidson JR, Hughes D *et al.* (1991) Post-traumatic stress disorder in the community: an epidemiological study. *Psychol Med*, **21**, 713–721.

Davidson JR, Hughes DL *et al.* (1993) The epidemiology of social phobia: findings from the Duke Epidemiological Catchment Area Study. *Psychol Med*, **23**, 709–718.

Degonda M, Angst J (1993) The Zurich study. XX. Social phobia and agoraphobia. *Eur Arch Psychiat Clin Neurosci*, **243**, 95–102.

Deltito JA and Stam M (1989) Psychopharmacological treatment of avoidant personality disorder. *Compr Psychiatry*, 9, 30(6), 498–504.

DeWit DJ, MacDonald K *et al.* (1999) Childhood stress and symptoms of drug dependence in adolescence and early adulthood: social phobia as a mediator. *Am J Orthopsychiat*, **69**, 61–72.

Dilsaver SC, Qamar AB *et al.* (1992) Secondary social phobia in patients with major depression. *Psychiat Res*, **44**, 33–40.

Dinwiddie S, Heath AC *et al.* (2000) Early sexual abuse and lifetime psychopathology: a co-twin-control study. *Psychol Med*, **30**, 41–52.

Engdahl B, Dikel TN *et al.* (1998) Comorbidity and course of psychiatric disorders in a community sample of former prisoners of war. *Am J Psychiat*, **155**, 1740–1175.

Essau CA, Conradt J *et al.* (1998) Frequency and comorbidity of social anxiety and social phobia in adolescents. Results of a Bremen adolescent study. (In German.) *Fortschr Neurol Psychiat*, **66**, 524–530.

Fahlen T (1995) Personality traits in social phobia II: changes during treatment. *J Clin Psychiatry*, **56**(12), 569–573.

Feehan M, McGee R *et al.* (1994) DSM-III-R disorders in New Zealand 18-year-olds. *Aust N Z J Psychiat*, **28**, 87–99.

First M, Spitzer RL *et al.* (1995) Structured clinical interview for DSM-IV—patient edition. Washington, DC: American Psychiatric Press.

Fyer AJ, Mannuzza S *et al.* (1993) A direct interview family study of social phobia. *Arch Gen Psychiat*, **50**, 286–293.

Fyer AJ, Mannuzza S *et al.* (1995) Specificity in familial aggregation of phobic disorders. *Arch Gen Psychiat*, **52**, 564–573.

Fyer AJ, Mannuzza S *et al.* (1996) Panic disorder and social phobia: effects of comorbidity on familial transmission. *Anxiety*, **2**, 173–178.

George MS and Lydiard RB (1994) Social phobia secondary to physical disability. A review of benign essential tremor (BET) and stuttering. *Psychosomatics*, **35**(6), 520–523.

Goldenberg IM, White K *et al.* (1996) The infrequency of "pure culture" diagnoses among the anxiety disorders. *J Clin Psychiat*, **57**, 528–533.

Greenberg PE, Sisitsky T *et al.* (1999) The economic burden of anxiety disorders in the 1990s. *J Clin Psychiat*, **60**, 427–435.

Guy W (1976) *ECDEU Assessment Manual for Psychopharmacology*. Washington, DC: National Institute of Mental Health—US Department of Health, Education, and Welfare.

Hamilton MA (1960) A rating scale for depression. *J Neurol Neurosurg Psychiat*, **23**, 56–62.

Hochstrasser B, Angst J (1996) The Zurich Study: XXII. Epidemiology of gastrointestinal complaints and comorbidity with anxiety and depression. *Eur Arch Psychiat Clin Neurosci*, **246**, 261–272.

Hovens JG, Cantwell DP *et al.* (1994) Psychiatric comorbidity in hospitalized adolescent substance abusers. *J Am Acad Child Adolesc Psychiat*, **33**, 476–483.

Jefferson JW (1995) Social phobia: a pharmacologic treatment overview. *J Clin Psychiat*, **56**(suppl 5), 18–24.

Kasper S (1998) Social phobia: the nature of the disorder. *J Affect Disord*, **50**(suppl 1), S3–S9.

Katzelnick D, Jefferson J *et al.* (1994) Sertraline in social phobia: a double-blind, placebo-controlled crossover pilot study. Presented at the 34th Annual Meeting of NCDEU, May 31–June 3, Marco Island, Fl.

Katzelnick DJ, Kobak KA *et al.* (1999) *The Direct and Indirect Costs of Social Anxiety Disorders in Managed Care Patients I*. Washington, DC: American Psychiatric Association.

Kelsey JE (1995) Venlafaxine in social phobia. *Psychopharmacol Bull*, **31**, 767–771.

Kendler KS and Gardner CO, Jr (1998) Twin studies of adult psychiatric and substance dependence disorders: are they biased by differences in the environmental experiences of monozygotic and dizygotic twins in childhood and adolescence? *Psychol Med*, **28**, 625–633.

Kessler RC, McGonagle KA *et al.* (1994) Lifetime and 12-month prevalence of DSM-III-R psychiatric disorders in the United States. Results from the National Comorbidity Survey. *Arch Gen Psychiat*, **51**, 8–19.

Kessler RC, Nelson CB *et al.* (1996a) Comorbidity of DSM-III-R major depressive disorder in the general population: results from the US National Comorbidity Survey. *Br J Psychiat Suppl*, **30**, 17–30.

Kessler RC, Nelson CB *et al.* (1996b) The epidemiology of co-occurring addictive and mental disorders: implications for prevention and service utilization. *Am J Orthopsychiat*, **66**, 17–31.

Kessler RC, Stang P *et al.* (1999) Lifetime co-morbidities between social phobia and mood disorders in the US National Comorbidity Survey. *Psychol Med*, **29**, 555–567.

Kobak KA, Greist JH *et al.* (1996) Computer-administered clinical rating scales. A review. *Psychopharmacology (Berl)*, **127**, 291–301.

Kushner MG, Sher KJ *et al.* (1990) The relation between alcohol problems and the anxiety disorders. *Am J Psychiat*, **147**, 685–695.

Lecrubier Y (1998) Comorbidity in social anxiety disorder: impact on disease burden and management. *J Clin Psychiat*, **59**(suppl 17), 33–38.

Lecrubier Y, Weiller E (1997) Comorbidities in social phobia. *Int Clin Psychopharmacol*, **12**(suppl 6), S17–S21.

Lépine JP, Pelissolo A (1996) Comorbidity and social phobia: clinical and epidemiological issues. *Int Clin Psychopharmacol*, **11**(suppl 30, 35–41.

Lépine JP, Pelissolo A (1998) Social phobia and alcoholism: a complex relationship. *J Affect Disord*, **50**(suppl 1), S23–S28.

Lepola U, Koponen H *et al.* (1994) Citalopram in the treatment of social phobia: a report of three cases. *Pharmacopsychiatry*, **27**, 186–188.

Liebowitz MR, Gorman JM *et al.* (1985) Social phobia. Review of a neglected anxiety disorder. *Arch Gen Psychiat*, **42**, 729–737.

Liebowitz MR, Gorman JM *et al.* (1988) Pharmacotherapy of social phobia: an interim report of a placebo-controlled comparison of phenelzine and atenolol. *J Clin Psychiat*, **49**, 252–257.

Lydiard RB (1998) The role of drug therapy in social phobia. *J Affect Disord*, **50**(suppl 1), S35–S39.

Lydiard RB, Bobes J (2000) Therapeutic advances: paroxetine for the treatment of social anxiety disorder. *Depress Anxiety*, **11**, 99–104.

Lydiard RB, Brady KT *et al.* (1992) Lifetime prevalence of anxiety and affective disorders in hospitalized alcoholics. *Am J Addictions*, **1**, 321–331.

Lydiard RB, Brawman-Mintzer O *et al.* (1996) Recent developments in the psychopharmacology of anxiety disorders. *J Consult Clin Psychol*, **64**, 660–668.

Lydiard RB and Falsetti SA (1999) Experience with anxiety and depression treatment studies: implications for designing irritable bowel syndrome clinical trials. *Am J Mod*, **107**, 65S–73S.

Magee WJ, Eaton WW *et al.* (1996) Agoraphobia, simple phobia, and social phobia in the National Comorbidity Survey. *Arch Gen Psychiat*, **53**, 159–168.

Mancini C, van Ameringen M *et al.* (1996) A high-risk pilot study of the children of adults with social phobia. *J Am Acad Child Adolesc Psychiat*, **35**, 1511–1517.

Mancuso DM, Townsend MH *et al.* (1993) Long-term follow-up of generalized anxiety disorder. *Compr Psychiat*, **34**, 441–446.

Mannuzza S, Schneier FR *et al.* (1995) Generalized social phobia: reliability and validity. *Arch Gen Psychiat*, **52**, 230–237.

Markowitz JC, Moran ME *et al.* (1992) Prevalence and comorbidity of dysthymic disorder among psychiatric outpatients. *J Affect Disord*, **24**, 63–71.

Martinsen EW, Olsen T *et al.* (1998) Cognitive-behavioral group therapy for panic disorder in the general clinical setting: a naturalistic study with 1-year follow-up. *J Clin Psychi*, **59**, 437–42.

Merikangas KR, Angst J (1995) Comorbidity and social phobia: evidence from clinical, epidemiologic, and genetic studies. *Eur Arch Psychiat Clin Neurosci*, **244**, 297–303.

Merikangas KR, Angst J *et al.* (1996) Comorbidity and boundaries of affective disorders with anxiety disorders and substance misuse: results of an international task force. *Br J Psychiat Suppl*, **30**, 58–67.

Merikangas KR, Stevens DE *et al.* (1998) Co-morbidity and familial aggregation of alcoholism and anxiety disorders. *Psychol Med*, **28**, 773–788.

Montejo J, Liebowitz MR (1994) Social phobia: anxiety disorder comorbidity. *Bull Menninger Clin*, **58**(2 suppl A): A21–A42.

Montgomery SA (1999) Social phobia: diagnosis, severity and implications for treatment. *Eur Arch Psychiat Clin Neurosci*, **249**(suppl 1), S1–S6.

Moutier CY and Stein MB (1999) The history, epidemiology, and differential diagnosis of social anxiety disorder. *J Clin Psychiatry*, **60**(suppl 9), 4–8.

Mullaney JA, Trippett CJ (1979) Alcohol dependence and phobias: clinical description and relevance. *Br J Psychiat*, **135**, 565–573.

Myrick H, Brady KT (1997) Social phobia in cocaine-dependent individuals. *Am J Addict*, **6**, 99–104.

Orsillo SM, Weathers FW *et al.* (1996a) Current and lifetime psychiatric disorders among veterans with war zone-related posttraumatic stress disorder. *J Nerv Ment Dis*, **184**, 307–313.

Orsillo SM, Heimberg RG *et al.* (1996b) Social phobia and PTSD in Vietnam veterans. *J Trauma Stress*, **9**, 235–252.

Otto MW, Pollack MH *et al.* (1992) Alcohol dependence in panic disorder patients. *J Psychiat Res*, **26**, 29–38.

Pande AC, Davidson JR *et al.* (1999) Treatment of social phobia with gabapentin: a placebo-controlled study. *J Clin Psychopharmacol*, **19**(4), 341–348.

Perugi G, Simonini E *et al.* (1990) Primary and secondary social phobia: psychopathologic and familial differentiations. *Compr Psychiat*, **31**, 245–252.

Perugi G, Akiskal HS *et al.* (1998) The high prevalence of "soft" bipolar (II) features in atypical depression. *Compr Psychiat*, **39**, 63–71.

Perugi G, Toni C *et al.* (1999) Anxious-bipolar comorbidity. Diagnostic and treatment challenges. *Psychiat Clin North Am*, **22**, 565–583, viii.

Phillips KA, Gunderson CG *et al.* (1998) A comparison study of body dysmorphic disorder and obsessive-compulsive disorder. *J Clin Psychiat*, **59**, 568–575.

Pini S, Cassano GB *et al.* (1997) Prevalence of anxiety disorders comorbidity in bipolar depression, unipolar depression and dysthymia. *J Affect Disord* 42(2–3): 145–153.

Robins LN, Locke BZ *et al.* (1991) An overview of psychiatric disorders in America. In: LN Robins and DA Reiger, eds. *Psychiatric Disorders in America: The Epidemiologic Catchment Area Study*. New York: Free Press, pp 328–366.

Rosenbaum JF, Biederman J *et al.* (1994) The etiology of social phobia. *J Clin Psychiat*, **55**.

Rosenbaum JF and Pollock MA (1994) The psychopharmacology of social phobia and comorbid disorders. *Bull Menninger Clin*, **58**(suppl), A67–A83.

Savino M, Perugi G *et al.* (1993) Affective comorbidity in panic disorder: is there a bipolar connection? *J Affect Disord*, **28**, 155–163.

Schneier FR, Johnson J *et al.* (1992) Social phobia. Comorbidity and morbidity in an epidemiologic sample. *Arch Gen Psychiat*, **49**, 282–288.

Schuckit MA, Tipp JE *et al.* (1997) The life-time rates of three major mood disorders and four major anxiety disorders in alcoholics and controls. *Addiction*, **92**, 1289–1304.

Schwalberg MD, Barlow DH *et al.* (1992) Comparison of bulimics, obese binge eaters, social phobics, and individuals with panic disorder on comorbidity across DSM-III-R anxiety disorders. *J Abnorm Psychol*, **101**, 675–681.

Sheehan DV, Janavs J *et al.* (1994) MIN.PLUS I. Mini-International Neuropsychiatric Interview, Clinician Rated (version 4.4).

Smail P, Stockwell T *et al.* (1984) Alcohol dependence and phobic anxiety states. A I prevalence study. *Br J Psychiat*, **144**, 53–57.

Starcevic V, Uhlenhuth EH *et al.* (1992) Patterns of comorbidity in panic disorder and agoraphobia. *Psychiat Res,* **42**, 171–183.

Stein MB, Shea CA *et al.* (1989) Social phobic symptoms in patients with panic disorder: practical and theoretical implications. *Am J Psychiaty,* **146**, 235–238.

Stein MB, Heuser IJ *et al.* (1990) Anxiety disorders in patients with Parkinson's disease. *Am J Psychiatry,* **147**(2), 217–220.

Stein MB, Walker JR *et al.* (1996a) Childhood physical and sexual abuse in patients with anxiety disorders and in a community sample. *Am J Psychiat,* **153**, 275–277.

Stein MB, Chartier MJ *et al.* (1996b) Paroxetine in the treatment of generalized social phobia: open-label treatment and double-blind placebo-controlled discontinuation. *J Clin Psychopharmacol,* **16**, 218–222.

Stein MB, Chartier MJ *et al.* (1998a) A direct-interview family study of generalized social phobia. *Am J Psychiat,* **155**, 90–97.

Stein MB, Liebowitz MR *et al.* (1998b) Paroxetine treatment of generalized social phobia (social anxiety disorder): a randomized controlled trial. *JAMA,* **280**, 708–713.

Stein MB, McQuaid JR *et al.* (1999a) Social phobia in the primary care medical setting. *J Fam Pract,* **48**, 514–519.

Stein MB, Fyer AJ *et al.* (1999b) Fluvoxamine treatment of social phobia (social anxiety disorder): a double-blind, placebo-controlled study. *Am J Psychiat,* **156**, 756–760.

Thomas SE, Thevos AK *et al.* (1999) Alcoholics with and without social phobia: a comparison of substance use and psychiatric variables. *J Stud Alcohol,* **60**, 472–479.

Tomasson K, Vaglum P (1997) The 2-year course following detoxification treatment of substance abuse: the possible influence of psychiatric comorbidity. *Eur Arch Psychiat Clin Neurosci,* **247**, 320–327.

Tomasson K, Vaglum P (1998) Social consequences of substance abuse: the impact of comorbid psychiatric disorders. A prospective study of a nation-wide sample of treatment-seeking patients. *Scand J Soc Med,* **26**, 63–70.

van Ameringen, M, Mancini C *et al.* (1991) Relationship of social phobia with other psychiatric illness. *J Affect Disord,* **21**, 93–99.

van Ameringen, M, Mancini C *et al.* (1993) Fluoxetine efficacy in social phobia. *J Clin Psychiat,* **54**, 27–32.

van Ameringen, MA, Swinson RP *et al.* (1999) *A Placebo-Controlled Study of Sertraline in Generalized Social Phobia NR330.* Washington, DC: American Psychiatric Association.

van Ameringen, M, Mancini C *et al.* (1999b) Nefazodone in social phobia. *J Clin Psychiat,* **60**, 96–100.

van Vliet, IM, den Boer JA *et al.* (1994) Psychopharmacological treatment of social phobia; a double-blind placebo controlled study with fluvoxamine. *Psychopharmacology,* **115**, 128–134.

Versiani M, Amrein R *et al.* (1997) Social phobia: long-term treatment outcome and prediction of response—a moclobemide study. *Int Clin Psychopharmacol,* **12**, 239–254.

Watson P, Friend FR (1969) Measurement of social-evaluative anxiety. *J Consult Clin Psychol,* **33**, 448–457.

Wesner RB (1990) Alcohol use and abuse secondary to anxiety. *Psychiatr Clin North Am,* **13**, 699–713.

Wittchen HU, Essau CA *et al.* (1992) Lifetime and six-month prevalence of mental disorders in the Munich Follow-Up Study. *Eur Arch Psychiat Clin Neurosci,* **241**, 247–258.

Wittchen HU, Beloch E (1996) The impact of social phobia on quality of life. *Int Clin Psychopharmacol,* **11**(suppl), 15–23.

Wittchen HU, Stein MB *et al.* (1999) Social fears and social phobia in a community sample of adolescents and young adults: prevalence, risk factors and co-morbidity. *Psychol Med,* **29**, 309–323.

7

SSRIs in obsessive-compulsive disorder

Stuart A. Montgomery

INTRODUCTION

Effective treatment for obsessive-compulsive disorder (OCD) is important as it is a common and frequently disabling illness. Until relatively recently it was thought to affect only 0.05% of the population and was therefore relatively rare. However, these estimates were based on studies of hospitalized patients and undoubtedly under-estimated the true incidence of the disorder. The recognition that effective treatments are available has given rise to considerable research interest in the condition in recent years and large epidemiological studies have been carried out that show OCD to be a common disorder. The Epidemiological Catchment Area survey in the USA reported the lifetime prevalence at 2.5% (Robins and Regier, 1990). This is greater than schizophrenia and similar to panic disorder, making OCD one of the most common psychiatric disorders. OCD has an early age of onset, often starting in childhood or adolescence, and generally runs a chronic, fluctuating course with exacerbations.

OCD is characterized by unwanted thoughts that recur (obsessional ruminations) and unwanted repetitive acts that the patient realizes are foolish but is unable to resist (compulsive rituals). The thoughts and behaviours are not a source of pleasure, although they may serve to reduce discomfort. The obsessions or compulsions, which may be resisted at least initially, cause marked distress, are time consuming and interfere with social functioning; when severe the sufferer may be preoccupied with the obsessional behaviours for much of the day and be unable to pursue his/her normal activities. Comorbid symptoms of other psychiatric disorders are frequent

SSRIs in Depression and Anxiety, Second Edition. Edited by S.A. Montgomery and J.A. den Boer.
© 2001 John Wiley & Sons Ltd.

and half of those with OCD have depressive symptoms that would fulfil criteria for major depression.

RESPONSE OF OCD TO SEROTONERGIC AGENTS

The therapeutic role of the selective serotonin reuptake inhibitors (SSRIs) is of particular interest in OCD, which, from a treatment perspective, appears to be a unique disorder. The results from the body of placebo-controlled studies of the efficacy of pharmacological treatment in OCD show that, for the moment, only drugs that specifically affect the serotonergic system are effective. This contrasts with other psychiatric disorders where the response is not selective, for example depression and panic disorder respond to drugs that affect the noradrenergic system as well as to those that affect the serotonergic system, and schizophrenia responds to drugs with mixed dopaminergic and serotonergic action systems. The specificity of response to serotonergic agents that characterizes the pharmacological treatments for OCD is particularly interesting because of the clues it gives to the biological substrate of the disorder.

The drugs that have been shown to possess antiobsessional efficacy are the SSRIs and clomipramine, which has potent but non-selective effects on serotonin reuptake.

Clomipramine was the first effective pharmacological treatment. Its beneficial effect on obsessional symptoms was observed in the 1960s (Fernandez and Lopez-Ibor, 1967) but it was not until placebo-controlled studies were reported in 1980 that the antiobsessional efficacy of this drug became established. The early studies that demonstrated the superiority of clomipramine compared with placebo in the treatment of OCD were small (Marks *et al.*, 1980; Montgomery, 1980; Thoren *et al.*, 1980) but the antiobsessional efficacy was later confirmed in large placebo-controlled studies (De Veaugh Geiss *et al.*, 1991). Clomipramine has been shown to be effective in the treatment of OCD in children as well as in adults (De Veaugh Geiss *et al.*, 1992; Flament *et al.*, 1985). The consistency of the finding of efficacy with clomipramine, even in small studies, is a measure of the robustness of the effect.

The positive findings with clomipramine were in stark contrast to the results with other tricyclic antidepressants, several of which have been investigated for their therapeutic potential in OCD without success. Imipramine and nortriptyline were not different from placebo in studies that reported a significant therapeutic effect with clomipramine (Thoren *et al.*, 1980; Volavka *et al.*, 1985) and in comparator studies with clomipramine, amitriptyline and desipramine were not associated with an antiobsessional effect (Ananth *et al.*, 1981; Leonard *et al.*, 1988). Desipramine has also been found to be significantly less effective than the SSRI fluvoxamine (Goodman *et al.*, 1990).

Other compounds have been tried in OCD but the results have generally been negative or inconclusive. For example, trazodone was not significantly different from placebo (Pigott *et al.*, 1992b); a preliminary analysis suggests some effect with mianserin, although a definitive study has not been published (Jaskari, 1980). The monoamine oxidase inhibitor phenelzine was reported to be of similar efficacy to clomipramine, although the small study did not include a placebo comparison (Vallejo *et al.*, 1992), and clorgyline was less effective than clomipramine (Insel *et al.*, 1983). The findings with benzodiazepines are inconclusive: a very small study found a difference from placebo and no difference from clomipramine for clonazepam (Hewlett *et al.*, 1992), and buspirone was found to have an effect in one small study (Pato *et al.*, 1991b), in contrast to an earlier report which found no efficacy (Jenike and Baer, 1988).

The lack of response of OCD to non-serotonergic antidepressants that are effective in depression, or to anxiolytic compounds, made it appear likely that the important factor in producing a therapeutic effect in OCD was the potent serotonin reuptake blocking properties of clomipramine. The SSRIs were obvious candidate treatments for OCD. The antiobsessional efficacy demonstrated with the SSRIs is in accord with the view that OCD may be a serotonin-specific illness.

EFFICACY OF SEROTONIN REUPTAKE INHIBITORS IN OCD

The antiobsessional activity of drugs with potent serotonergic reuptake blocking activity was identified in early studies that included small numbers of patients. The studies carried out recently to test the efficacy of new pharmacological treatments are much larger and their size addresses the possibility that the findings in the very small studies may have been due to chance. These studies, which have established the efficacy of these drugs in OCD, have been large, well designed, and have provided evidence of efficacy not only in short-term treatment but in some cases also in long-term treatment.

Fluvoxamine

Fluvoxamine was the earliest of the SSRIs to be investigated in OCD and there have been five placebo-controlled studies, all showing efficacy. Positive results were reported in a series of relatively small studies carried out in the 1980s (Cottraux *et al.*, 1990; Goodman *et al.*, 1989; Perse *et al.*, 1987). A modest but significant advantage compared with placebo was seen after two weeks' treatment in a group parallel comparison that included 42 patients. The effect became highly significant later in the study (Goodman *et al.*, 1989). After 6–8 weeks the advantage was also reflected in the increased number of responders to treatment, defined in the study as "much improved" or "very much improved" on the Clinical Global Improvement (CGI) scale. An even smaller study ($N = 20$) found a significant advantage for fluvoxamine given for 8 weeks in a cross-over design (Perse *et al.*, 1987). In the third early study, 60 patients with OCD were randomized to three groups to receive either fluvoxamine with concomitant exposure therapy, fluvoxamine with concomitant antiexposure with the aim of controlling for the exposure given in the parallel medication group, or placebo plus exposure. The number of patients in each treatment group was consequently small and the likelihood of the study being able to identify significant differences reduced. A difference would in any case be difficult to establish in a study that provided a potentially effective treatment, behaviour therapy, to the placebo control group. In spite of these methodological problems a significant advantage was seen in the fluvoxamine-treated group compared with the placebo plus exposure group in reducing the duration of the rituals.

Two more recent multicentre placebo-controlled studies each included 160 patients. One of these, Goodman et al. (1996), found that in a 10-week study there was a significant advantage for fluvoxamine compared with placebo that could be measured from week 6 onwards on the Yale–Brown Obsessive-Compulsive Scale (Y-BOCS), the most widely used scale for measuring severity and change in OCD studies. The effect was seen both on the total scale score and also on the scales to measure obsessions and compulsions separately. On the National Institute for Mental Health (NIMH)-OC scale, which was also used in this study, a significant difference could also be detected at 4 weeks. The advantage for fluvoxamine was also seen in the number of responders who were much improved or very much improved, an important measure in OCD where mean amelioration scores on rating scores may appear modest.

Similar results were reported in the second multicentre study, with significant differences appearing from 6 weeks on the severity scales, the Y-BOCS and the NIMH-OC scale. On the CGI scale the significant advantage was apparent as early as 4 weeks (Greist et al., 1995c).

Fluoxetine

The antiobsessional efficacy of fluoxetine has been investigated in three multicentre placebo-controlled studies, one 8-week study in Europe and South Africa (Montgomery et al., 1993) and two 13-week studies in the USA (Tollefson et al., 1994b). The data from the two American studies, which followed identical protocols comparing fluoxetine 20, 40 and 60 mg/day with placebo, were pooled for the analysis. In the European study, 217 patients were randomized to fluoxetine 20, 40 or 60 mg/day or placebo. There was a significant advantage for fluoxetine compared with placebo in the overall responder rates defined on the Y-BOCS and much or very much improved on the CGI scale, but the difference as registered by the symptom scales mean scores, although numerically clear, was statistically marginal. A clearer demonstration of the efficacy of fluoxetine was seen in the report of the American studies, which included more patients ($N = 355$) and was therefore better powered and which had a longer treatment duration. Fluoxetine was significantly superior to placebo with the differences beginning at week 5. The greatest difference was seen at the highest dose of 60 mg/day of fluoxetine and this dose–response relationship was significant. A recent report of results in a group of Austrian patients also commented on the better effects of doses of 40 and 60 mg/day of fluoxetine (Zitterl et al., 1999).

The same protocol was used in the European and American studies, except for the extended study duration in the latter, and the data were subsequently pooled for analysis with the American data truncated to 9 weeks for comparability. The analysis of these data showed that there was a significant advantage for all doses of fluoxetine compared with placebo, measured on the Y-BOCS total score and on the obsessions subscale, and for the highest dose there was also a significant advantage on the compulsions subscale (Wood *et al.*, 1993).

Paroxetine

Preliminary reports from a large, placebo-controlled comparison of three doses of paroxetine, 20, 40 and 60 mg/day, have shown the clear efficacy of the two higher doses of paroxetine compared with placebo. In this study, 348 patients with OCD with a history of at least 6 months' duration were treated for a 12-week period. A significant difference from placebo was demonstrated in the 40 and 60 mg/day groups on both the Y-BOCS scale and the NIMH-OC scale. At week 12, both the 40 mg/day dose and the 60 mg/day dose showed a significant advantage over the 20 mg/day dose of paroxetine (Wheadon *et al.*, 1993). These differences were registered on both the scales used in the study, the Y-BOCS and the NIMH-OC scale. This was a large study including 348 patients treated for 12 weeks.

An important placebo-controlled multicentre study compared paroxetine given in a flexible dose of 10–60 mg/day (mean 37.5 mg/day) with clomipramine given in a dose of 25–250 mg/day (mean 113.1 mg/day). This too was a large study, with 399 patients entering the 12-week study (Zohar and Judge, 1996). Paroxetine was significantly superior to placebo at week 12 on all the primary efficacy measures: the number of patients achieving 25% or greater reduction in the Y-BOCS, the change in Y-BOCS total score, and the change in NIMH-OC scale total score. The significant difference from placebo was already present at week 6. Secondary analyses included the obsession and compulsion subscales of the Y-BOCS, and paroxetine was significantly better than placebo on both, demonstrating that it exerts a therapeutic effect on both aspects of OCD.

The inclusion of clomipramine as a reference comparator in this study is valuable for the added weight it lends to the demonstration of the efficacy of paroxetine. A large body of placebo-controlled studies supports the efficacy of clomipramine, which was the first antiobsessional drug to be identified, and its efficacy in this study serves to validate the patient population. Both paroxetine and clomipramine were better than placebo and there was no significant difference between the two active drugs in their efficacy measured on the CGI scales or the obsessional symptom scales. There were some advantages for paroxetine, however, in the effect on depressive symptoms and in terms of better tolerability, as discussed below.

Sertraline

Sertraline has been investigated in a number of placebo-controlled trials including studies that used a flexible-dose regime and fixed-dose studies. Sertraline was used in doses 50–200 mg/day in the first flexible-dose study, which was small (87 patients), with a duration of 8 weeks (Chouinard et al., 1990). The second flexible-dose study, which used the same dose range, was larger (167 patients) and had a longer duration of 12 weeks (Kronig et al., 1999). Both studies found a significant advantage for sertraline compared with placebo ($p < 0.05$). In the 12-week fixed dose study of sertraline, which compared doses of 50, 100 and 200 mg/day and placebo with approximately 80 patients per group, improvement was significantly greater than placebo in the 50 mg/day dose group and the 200 mg/day dose group measured on the Y-BOCS, the NIMH-OC, and the CGI scales. The advantage was less clear cut in the 100 mg/day dose group, where a statistically significant difference was registered only on the NIMH-OC scale. The difference in response between the doses of sertraline was not significant and when the data from all groups were pooled, a significant advantage for sertraline was observed compared with placebo.

Citalopram

Open treatment studies suggested that citalopram might be effective in treating OCD and the efficacy of this SSRI has been confirmed in a recent placebo-controlled study.

All the tested doses of citalopram (20 mg, 40 mg and 60 mg) were shown to be better than placebo in a large 12-week fixed dose study (Montgomery et al., 2000). The discontinuation rate in the study was low at 15–17% in all groups. As with other SSRIs, the higher doses tended to be associated with the best and the earliest response. The presence of low levels of comorbid depressive symptoms appeared to weaken the response compared with that in pure OCD, although citalopram was better than placebo in both groups of patients. This observation reinforces the view that these depressive symptoms are part of OCD rather than reflecting major depression. The long-term efficacy of citalopram has not yet been tested.

Case reports of efficacy from other serotonin reuptake inhibitors

The consistency of the results from placebo-controlled studies showing antiobsessional efficacy with SSRIs provides clear support for the view that this a pharmacological effect of this class of compounds. It can be expected that other members of this class will also have antiobsessional efficacy. Adequate placebo-controlled studies have not been published for other drugs having an important effect in inhibiting the reuptake of serotonin. However, open case reports with venlafaxine, which has serotonergic reuptake blocking properties but which also has an effect on noradrenergic receptors, have been positive in OCD (Rauch et al., 1998), and the preliminary report of a very small placebo-controlled study indicated antiobsessional activity (Yaryura-Tobias and Neziroglu, 1996).

SSRIs or clomipramine

Since the antiobsessional activity of clomipramine was first identified (Fernandez and Lopez-Ibor, 1967) an impressive body of placebo-controlled studies has produced remarkably consistent evidence of the efficacy of this drug in treating OCD (Montgomery, 1980; Thoren *et al.*, 1980; Marks *et al.*, 1980; Insel *et al.*, 1983; Flament *et al.*, 1985; Marks *et al.*, 1988; De Veaugh Geiss *et al.*, 1991, 1992).

The relative efficacy of clomipramine and the SSRIs in treating OCD has been the subject of considerable discussion, and a number of reviews and meta-analyses of published studies of the efficacy of clomipramine and of the SSRIs have appeared (Cox and Swinson, 1993; Greist *et al.*, 1995b; Piccinelli *et al.*, 1995; Stein *et al.*, 1995). Two of these have suggested that a greater effect is seen with clomipramine than the SSRIs (Greist *et al.*, 1995b; Stein *et al.*, 1995) but the study of Cox *et al.* (1993) found no significant difference between the SSRIs examined and clomipramine, and Piccinelli *et al.* (1995), whilst noting an apparently larger decrease in the Y-BOCS with clomipramine, pointed out a lack of significant difference where direct comparison was available.

Meta-analyses can be a useful method of investigating and quantifying possible trends which in individual studies may be too small to identify. This approach is, however, beset by methodological difficulties and the results must be interpreted with great caution. The heterogeneity of the studies included is a substantial problem, which limits the conclusions that can be drawn from meta-analyses. This is a particularly important factor in assessing the results of the meta-analyses of the treatment studies in OCD. These meta-analyses, which compare recent studies of SSRIs with studies conducted many years ago with clomipramine, may be misleading.

Over the years since the early studies of clomipramine were carried out there appears to have been a change in the response rates observed, which renders the comparison of early and recent studies of questionable validity. In the early studies the response to placebo was low, typically 10% or less. In more recent studies much higher placebo response rates have been reported and rates of 15–20% or more are not unusual. At the same time, the recorded size of the response to active treatment appears to have decreased in recent studies. The reasons for this are not entirely clear, although it is thought likely that the clinical characteristics of the study populations have changed. It is conceivable that only patients with very severe, persistent OCD were included in the early studies, and in this group a low response to placebo and a clear response to an effective drug could be expected. Since the efficacy of pharmacological treatment for OCD has become more widely recognized, the range of patients being treated has broadened to include those with a more intermittent course, or those with milder disorder. This may well result in apparently higher responses to placebo and a less dramatic drug effect would be expected in those with mild OCD. The proportion of those who are resistant or partially resistant to pharmacotherapy has increased as the antiobsessional treatments have become more widely available, and a lower response to treatment in recent placebo-controlled studies can be expected when compared with earlier studies carried out in a drug-naïve population.

Whatever the reason for the changes in the response to pharmacological intervention, such differences invalidate the comparison of effect sizes seen in recent studies with those seen in early studies and underline the risk involved in the use of historical controls. A safer and more scientific method of comparison is the head-to-head, double-blind comparison of clomipramine and SSRIs, and an increasing number of these studies are being reported. Some of the studies have been very small and could not therefore avoid the risk of a Type II error. However, larger studies have also been carried out and the results are in accord.

Direct comparisons have been carried out of fluoxetine in one small study (Pigott *et al.*, 1990) and one 55-patient study (Lopez-Ibor *et al.*, 1996), with fluvoxamine in five studies (Freeman *et al.*, 1994; Koran *et al.*, 1996; Milanfranchi *et al.*, 1997; Smeraldi *et al.*, 1992; Mundo *et al.*, 2000), with paroxetine (Zohar and Judge, 1996) and with sertraline (Bisserbe *et al.*, 1997). The SSRIs were of a similar level of efficacy to clomipramine in all of these studies, with the exception of the study of sertraline, which was significantly better than clomipramine. The study of sertraline was relatively large (168 patients) and compared sertraline and clomipramine in a flexible dose of 50–200 mg/day over 16 weeks.

The comparison with paroxetine is of particular note since it included a placebo arm. Both paroxetine and clomipramine were effective in this study compared to placebo. There was no difference in antiobsessional effect of the two active drugs but there was an advantage for paroxetine in treating the depressive symptoms. This is an important finding because depressive symptoms occur frequently in OCD and 30%

Table 7.1. Comparisons of serotonin reuptake inhibitors with clomipramine.

Study	N	SSRI (mg/day)	Comparator (mg/day)	Result
Pigott *et al.*, 1990	11	Fluoxetine ≤ 80	Clomipramine ≤ 250	No difference
Lopez-Ibor *et al.*, 1996	55	Fluoxetine 40	Clomipramine ≤ 150	No difference
Smeraldi *et al.*, 1992	10	Fluvoxamine ≤ 200	Clomipramine ≤ 200	No difference
Freeman *et al.*, 1994	64	Fluvoxamine ≤ 200	Clomipramine ≤ 250	No difference
Koran *et al.*, 1995	79	Fluvoxamine 100–300	Clomipramine 100–250	No difference
Milanfranchi *et al.*, 1997	26	Fluvoxamine ≤ 300	Clomipramine ≤ 300	No difference
Mundo *et al.*, 2000	133	Fluvoxamine ≤ 300	Clomipramine ≤ 300	No difference
Zohar and Judge, 1996	300	Paroxetine ≤ 60	Clomipramine ≤ 250	No difference for OCD Paroxetine better for depression
Bisserbe *et al.*, 1997	168	Sertraline ≤ 200	Clomipramine ≤ 200	Sertraline better on some measures

or more of patients would fulfil criteria for major depression (Rasmussen & Eisen, 1992).

Some of these head-to-head comparisons were rather small studies and others used doses which were possibly less than optimal, but overall the studies support the conclusion that the SSRIs and clomipramine have similar levels of antiobsessional efficacy (see Table 7.1).

DOSE OF SSRI IN OCD

It is important to establish the minimum effective dose of any medication in order to avoid exposing patients unnecessarily to the increased risk of side effects associated with higher doses. It has been a widely held clinical opinion that high doses are required for efficacy in OCD, certainly higher than the standard doses used in depression. There is, however, a bias towards using high doses inherent in the way drugs are developed. In the absence of clear indicators on the choice of optimum dose, flexible dosage regimes are often used, the dose being raised until a response is seen or side effects appear. This approach causes difficulty with depression, where the characteristic delay in response may lead to the response being attributed to a higher dose although it may have been the lower dose that initiated the response. The approach causes even greater difficulty with OCD, where the response tends to be slow and incremental over long periods.

There has been some evidence that low doses of antiobsessional drugs may be effective, for example clomipramine 75 and 150 mg/day (Montgomery, 1980; Thoren *et al.*, 1980). However, a better design is to compare the efficacy of three doses and placebo at the same time. The results from the large fixed-dose studies that have now been carried out confirm the clinical view that for many patients higher doses are needed.

The fixed-dose study of sertraline reported that both the high dose of 200 mg/day and the low dose of 50 mg/day were effective in the treatment of OCD, but not the 100 mg/day dose (Greist *et al.*, 1995a). There was a numerically greater improvement associated with the 200 mg/day group but this was not significant and it is not possible to predict whether in a larger study this potentially greater effect would be reflected in a dose–response relationship. The benefit of higher doses has been demonstrated with two other SSRIs, fluoxetine and paroxetine.

Fluoxetine has been investigated in studies in Europe and in the USA. In the European study, which was of shorter duration (8 weeks), pairwise comparison against placebo showed a significantly higher response rate in the groups receiving 40 or 60 mg/day fluoxetine. This difference was not observed in the group treated with 20 mg/day (Montgomery *et al.*, 1993). In the two studies carried out in the USA, which continued for 13 weeks and included a total of 355 patients, all three dosages of fluoxetine were significantly better than placebo but there was a trend towards a dose–response relationship, with better effect seen in the 60 mg/day dose (Tollefson *et al.*, 1994b). The lack of a significant difference between fluoxetine 20 mg/day and placebo in the study of Montgomery *et al.* (1993) may therefore have reflected a Type II error. On the other hand, in view of the dose–response relationship seen in the US study, it suggests that in some patients higher doses may be advantageous.

A dose–response relationship was seen in the 12-week study of fixed doses of 20, 40 and 60 mg/day of paroxetine compared with placebo, with patients treated with 40 or 60 mg/day having a better response (Wheadon *et al.*, 1993). There was no significant difference between the 20 mg/day dose and placebo and the advantage for both of the higher doses was statistically significant compared with the 20 mg/day dose. The large study which investigated 399 patients treated with either paroxetine, clomipramine or placebo used a flexible-dose regime, so that the advantage of high vs. low doses cannot be directly assessed in this study. However, treatment was initiated at 10 mg/day for the first 3 days and titrated in all patients to 20 mg on day 4. After 1 week the dose was titrated according to efficacy and/or side effects between 10 and 60 mg/day. The average dose of paroxetine in the study was 37.5 mg/day indicating that, at least for some patients, higher doses were needed than the standard dose of 20 mg/day recommended for depression (Zohar and Judge, 1996).

Overall, the balance of the results supports the clinical view that for the most part higher doses of SSRIs than those used in depression are more likely to produce a better therapeutic effect. If treatment is initiated at a lower dose, the evidence from the studies makes it clear that patients should be reviewed and the dose raised if response is unsatisfactory.

SIDE EFFECTS AND TOLERABILITY

The need for higher doses complicates the treatment of OCD since the level of side effects undoubtedly rises with the increased doses. This is well known from the efficacy trials in depression and is also reported in the trials of OCD. For example, the fixed-dose study of fluoxetine carried out in the USA noted a tendency for the incidence of side effects to increase in the higher dosages, although this rise was not reflected in an increase in dropouts due to side effects (Tollefson *et al.*, 1994b).

The issue of side effects is an important one since poorly tolerated drugs are likely to have considerable impact on compliance with treatment and therefore on clinical outcome. It is a particular issue in OCD, where patients often find it difficult to tolerate any side effects, which worry them and exacerbate their obsessional thoughts. It is therefore difficult to persuade them to persist with a medication that produces a high level of unwanted side effects. The tolerability of medication is also important in long-term conditions, such as OCD, where patients will be required to take medication over very long periods of time.

The usefulness of clomipramine is restricted because of its unwanted side effects. In common with other older tricyclic antidepressants, clomipramine is associated with important anticholinergic action which gives rise to dry mouth, blurred vision, constipation, etc. The anticholinergic side effects are frequently so unpleasant that patients are unable to continue taking medication. Clomipramine is not selective in its pharmacological action; its effects on systems other than serotonin account for its heavy side-effects burden. The SSRIs, which lack important pharmacological activity on other systems, offer an effective treatment for OCD that is better tolerated and more acceptable to patients.

The SSRIs have characteristic serotonergic side effects, in particular nausea and transient increases in anxiety. However, in general the side effects are relatively mild and well tolerated by patients. This is important in the treatment of any disorder, but may be critical in OCD. Analysis of large databases from studies in depressed patients have shown that significantly more patients withdraw prematurely from treatment with tricyclic antidepressants, compared with SSRIs (Montgomery *et al.*, 1994; Montgomery and Kasper, 1995; Anderson and Tomenson, 1995). OCD patients, who are more sensitive to side effects, or who may be more obsessional about them, will stand a better chance of continuing treatment with SSRIs. This effect was seen in a comparison of sertraline with clomipramine (Bisserbe *et al.*, 1997) in which the withdrawals due to adverse events were 26% in the clomipramine-treated patients, mostly occurring within the first month, compared with 11% in the sertraline-treated group.

SAFETY

As well as being associated with fewer withdrawals due to side effects, particularly anticholinergic side effects, the SSRIs have a much improved safety profile compared with clomipramine. Clomipramine is associated with a substantially elevated level of convulsions, reported at 1.5–2% in the higher doses often used in OCD, compared with 0.1–0.5% in higher doses of different SSRIs. This high rate of convulsions with clomipramine has led to a recommendation that the dose should not exceed 250 mg/day. Moreover, clomipramine is associated with a higher level of cardiotoxicity. This is reflected in the rate of deaths from overdose which, although lower than with some other older tricyclic antidepressants, is higher than with the SSRIs, which are clearly the safer alternative.

DIFFERENCES BETWEEN SSRIs

On the basis of a risk–benefit assessment, SSRIs should be the first-choice treatment. There appears to be little to choose between them and although each clinician may have a particular favourite, there are few comparator data to provide a rational, data-driven basis for choice. Selection of an SSRI may need to be made on the basis of other drugs the patient might need to take and the possibility of drug–drug interactions. Fluoxetine and paroxetine, and to a lesser extent sertraline, are potent inhibitors of P-450 isoenzyme CYP 2D6, which metabolizes commonly-used drugs such as tricyclic antidepressants, antipsychotics and β-blockers. Fluvoxamine inhibits CYP 1A2, which metabolizes warfarin and the hydroxylation of tricyclic antidepressants, and CYP 3A4, which metabolizes benzodiazepines and some antiarrhythmics.

The very long half-life of fluoxetine and its active metabolite make it difficult to make a change in the drugs a patient is taking, since 5–6 weeks are needed to wash the drug out, although a variable combination of new and old drug may sometimes be envisaged. The long half-life of fluoxetine may, however, be an advantage for patients who might discontinue high-dose treatment abruptly. Some discontinuation side effects can be expected with all antidepressants if treatment is withdrawn suddenly, and the longer half-life of fluoxetine, which ensures a slower withdrawal, may reduce this risk. In all cases, as with other antidepressants, it is good clinical practice to discontinue treatment slowly.

LONG-TERM TREATMENT

Antiobsessional drugs appear to be effective in short-term treatment in 60–80% of patients (Goodman et al., 1992; Perse, 1988) but the response is mostly partial. Some residual symptoms persist, although function is improved. The chronic nature of the disorder and the quality of response suggests the need for long-term treatment strategies. The characteristic response of OCD is a steady incremental improvement that continues over many weeks. OCD may require treatment measured in months, and there is evidence that further improvement is seen between the end of the acute treatment period and the end of a subsequent 6-month treatment period. Although some patients may respond within the first few weeks of treatment, many respond much later. It is therefore important that courses of treatment should be of adequate length.

The ability of a treatment to maintain or improve response is normally tested by the placebo-substitution or relapse-prevention design, rather than by extension-treatment designs where the individual remains on the same treatment. Recommendations for long-term treatment depend on formal long-term studies rather than on open reports which are prone to bias.

Early open retrospective follow-up of patients who had responded to pharmacological treatment indicated that the improvement in symptoms was only maintained as long as medication was continued, and that relapse would occur rapidly if it was discontinued (Thoren et al., 1980). Even patients who have remained well during treatment for periods of up to 2 years may apparently relapse when the medication is withdrawn. A small placebo-controlled study of clomipramine found that 90% of patients whose OCD had been successfully controlled on clomipramine for up to 27 months suffered significant deterioration of their symptoms following discontinuation to placebo (Pato et al., 1988). The worsening could not be explained as a drug discontinuation reaction, as there was a steady increasing deterioration through the 7-week discontinuation period. When the drug was restarted the patients again improved. This deterioration when effective antiobsessional treatment is withdrawn is also seen with SSRIs, as a small study with fluoxetine showed (Pato et al., 1991a). The study was too small for definitive conclusions, but four of five patients withdrawn from fluoxetine suffered a deterioration of their OCD. The time frame of the worsening of symptoms was slower than the earlier study of clomipramine, an effect possibly related to the longer elimination half-life of fluoxetine, which should have maintained therapeutic levels in the blood for some time after discontinuation.

The benefit obtained by maintaining treatment with clomipramine for a year was reported by Katz *et al.* (1990). This finding is limited by the methodology of the study, which was a double-blind follow-up of responders in a large 10-week study (De Veaugh Geiss *et al.*, 1989). Because most of the responders in this study had been treated with clomipramine, the comparison groups in the follow-up were unbalanced, but nevertheless this must be taken as evidence of long-term efficacy.

SSRIs IN LONG-TERM TREATMENT OF OCD

A number of long-term studies, some for periods of longer than a year, have shown that response to SSRIs is sustained if medication is continued (See Table 7.2). The most thorough investigation has concerned paroxetine, whose efficacy has been tested in a double-blind placebo-controlled relapse-prevention design and for which double-blind extension data following a placebo-controlled acute treatment study are also available. Assessment of the long-term efficacy of other SSRIs includes: 1-year double-blind extension data from the placebo-controlled study of sertraline (Greist *et al.*, 1995b), with open follow-up for a further year (Rasmussen *et al.*, 1997); a comparison of fluvoxamine and behaviour therapy (Cottraux *et al.*, 1990); and open extension data of treatment responders to fluoxetine continued for 24 weeks (Tollefson *et al.*, 1994a).

The efficacy of paroxetine in long-term treatment was demonstrated in a placebo-substitution relapse-prevention design. Patients who responded to treatment and completed a 12-week double-blind comparison of paroxetine, clomipramine and placebo (Zohar and Judge, 1996) were continued on open treatment with paroxetine, given in a flexible dose of 20–60 mg/day for 6 months. Those patients who were defined as responders at the end of this phase of treatment were then randomized double-blind to placebo or to continue to receive paroxetine for 6 months. The results from two studies with identical protocols were pooled for this analysis, which included 397 patients (Dunbar *et al.*, 1995).

A significant advantage for paroxetine compared with placebo was demonstrated in the double-blind placebo substitution study with fewer relapses in the paroxetine-treated group (38.9% vs. 60.3%, $p < 0.05$). The significant advantage was also seen in the analysis of time to relapse and in the analysis of the risk ratio, which indicates that patients treated with placebo were 2.4 times more likely to relapse than those treated with paroxetine ($p = 0.003$). Small gains continued to be made in the paroxetine group during the double-blind study and the improvement in Y-BOCS scores was significantly greater than placebo throughout the study and the improvement in CGI scale scores at several visit points.

Table 7.2. Double-blind long-term treatment studies with selective serotonin reuptake inhibitors in OCD.

Study	Design	Duration	N	Result
Clomipramine				
Katz et al., 1990	Placebo. Double-blind extension data	10 Weeks acute + 52 weeks	124	Efficacy maintained
Fluoxetine				
Tollefson et al., 1994	Placebo. Double-blind extension data	13 Weeks acute + 24 weeks	76	Fluoxetine better than placebo
Sertraline				
Greist et al., 1995	Placebo. Double-blind extension data	12 Weeks acute + 40 weeks	118	Sertraline better than placebo
Fluvoxamine				
Cottraux et al., 1990	Placebo + exposure vs. fluvoxamine + exposure vs. fluvoxamine + antiexposure	24 Weeks	60	Fluvoxamine better than placebo
Paroxetine				
Dunbar et al., 1995	Placebo double-blind relapse prevention	12 Weeks acute; 26 weeks maintenance; 26 weeks relapse prevention	145	Paroxetine better than placebo

The second long-term study of paroxetine was a double-blind extension of a 12-week acute comparison of paroxetine, clomipramine and placebo, in which responders to treatment in the acute study continued the same medication for 8 months. This study showed that the therapeutic benefit obtained during the acute treatment period was maintained in the subsequent 8-month extension period. Continued improvement was observed in both the paroxetine- and clomipramine-treated patients, but there was a worsening in the placebo group.

The advantage of continuing medication is also apparent in a 40-week double-blind extension study comparing sertraline and placebo in 118 patients who had responded to treatment in a 12-week acute treatment study (Greist *et al.*, 1995a). Response in the sertraline-treated group was maintained during the 1-year study and indeed, further small gains were made, measured on the Y-BOCS, the NIMH-OC scales, and the CGI scale (Greist *et al.*, 1995b). The difference in response at the end of the study showed that the significant advantage for sertraline compared with placebo was maintained. Some insight is gained into the need for treatment over still longer periods from the finding of a subsequent open extension study, which followed up those patients who remained well at 1 year for a further 52 weeks (Rasmussen *et al.*, 1997). Direct comparison of the two treatment groups in this period is difficult to interpret, since only a small number of patients who had responded to placebo initially maintained their response during the whole 1-year double-blind study. It is, however, important to note that those patients who remained on treatment with sertraline for the whole 2 years continued to improve throughout the study.

Long-term treatment with fluvoxamine has been tested over 6 months (Cottraux *et al.*, 1990) using a study design that should have made it difficult to demonstrate efficacy. Despite behaviour therapy being given to all patients, the addition of fluvoxamine was significantly more effective than placebo, suggesting that the behavioural treatment was having at best only a weak effect that was not enough to obscure the clear-cut efficacy of the SSRI. Further evidence of efficacy was seen in persistent continued therapeutic gains in responders to acute treatment, who continued on an open basis on long-term treatment.

The overall message from the long-term treatment studies is that antiobsessional drugs are effective in the long term as well as in acute treatment and that they continue to be effective for considerable periods. If pharmacological treatment is discontinued a considerable number of patients can be expected to relapse, and medication therefore needs to be continued for very long periods. Persuading patients to continue with medication is made easier by the finding that persistence with treatment appears to be rewarded with gains in improvement of the OCD.

OCD AND DEPRESSION

It was initially suggested that the antiobsessional effect of clomipramine was a reflection of the antidepressant effect of this drug. This was a reasonable proposition, since OCD treatments are all antidepressants and quite profound depressive symptomatology is often associated with the disorder. The question requires an answer regardless of whether the antiobsessional effect is mediated by an effect on the serotonin system or not. The proposition has been specifically tested in a study that excluded patients with depression, which showed clomipramine to be effective (Montgomery, 1980), a finding that was supported by a later small study (Marks *et al.*, 1988) and confirmed in a large multicentre centre (De Veaugh Geiss *et al.*, 1991). Retrospective analysis of studies that included patients with marked depressive symptoms has also shown that the response of the OCD was independent of the level of depression at the start of the study (Thoren *et al.*, 1980).

OCD differs from depression in a number of important ways. The most important is clearly the specificity of response of OCD to serotonin reuptake inhibitors, but the quality of the response is also different. In OCD, although a response may be seen early in treatment (De Veaugh Geiss *et al.*, 1991; Goodman *et al.*, 1989; Montgomery, 1980) the characteristic response pattern is a slow incremental improvement over many weeks or months. The placebo response has also tended to be low in OCD in contrast to depression, where placebo response rates of around 40% are expected and 50% is not uncommon. In the early OCD studies placebo response rates of 5–15% were reported. The reported rates have increased in more recent studies, possibly as a result of patients with milder or fluctuating disorder coming for treatment as the efficacy and availability of treatment has become more widely known. Nevertheless, the response to placebo is characteristically lower than in depression.

A substantial proportion of individuals with OCD, estimated as at least 30% (Rasmussen and Eisen, 1992), have marked depressive symptoms and these patients risk receiving a diagnosis of depression from the unwary practitioner who overlooks the importance of the OCD symptoms. From the treatment point of view, it is particularly important to note that the depressive symptoms associated with OCD share the same specificity of response as the OCD. The depressive symptoms do not respond to antidepressants that lack potent serotonergic activity but only improve in parallel to the obsessional symptoms and only to antiobsessional medication. This is seen in comparisons of desipramine and fluvoxamine (Goodman *et al.*, 1990; Zohar and Insel, 1987). Desipramine, in spite of being an effective antidepressant, did not improve the depressive symptoms suffered by the OCD patients, whereas fluvoxamine improved both the OCD and the depression. Preliminary results from a comparison of sertraline and desipramine reached similar conclusions (Hoehn-Saric *et al.*, 1997). Comparison of the response to treatment with clomipramine or nortriptyline and amitriptyline in patients with OCD with varying levels of depression found significantly greater efficacy with clomipramine (Ananth *et al.*, 1981; Thoren *et al.*, 1980). It does not appear to be possible to treat the depressive symptoms with an antidepressant independently of the OCD; the primary target has to be the vigorous treatment of the OCD symptoms. Similarly, if effective antiobsessional treatment is withdrawn, as for example in the study of Pato *et al.* (1988), a rapid resurgence of depressive symptoms as well as OCD symptoms is seen. It is appropriate, therefore, to think of the depressive symptoms as being integral to the OCD, rather than as a separate or secondary illness. Clinicians would do well to recognize that so-called comorbidity of OCD and major depression is spurious and that the depressive symptoms seen in the presence of OCD are part of OCD and not of major depression.

AGE AND OCD

OCD is a disorder with an early age of onset and treatment of children and adolescents with OCD has to be considered. Few clinical efficacy studies have been conducted specifically in children, but the results of those that have been carried out indicate that the same treatments that are effective in adults may also be expected to produce a response in adolescent or childhood OCD. The important study of Flament *et al.* (1985) demonstrated the efficacy of clomipramine in treating adolescents with OCD, and the finding has been confirmed in studies by Leonard *et al.* (1988) and in the large study of DeVeaugh Geiss *et al.* (1992). As might be expected, the SSRIs also appear to be effective in childhood OCD (Riddle *et al.*, 1992; March *et al.*, 1998, Rosenberg *et al.*, 1999). A large study in 107 children and 80 adolescents with OCD found that sertraline in doses up to 200 mg daily was effective compared with placebo (March *et al.*, 1998). Neither age nor sex predicted response. Adverse events associated with sertraline in children and adolescents appear to be similar to those seen in adults. An open study of paroxetine in doses of 10–60 mg daily indicates that this drug may provide a relatively safe and effective therapy for short-term treatment of OCD in paediatric patients (Rosenberg *et al.*, 1999). Symptomatology was assessed using the Y-BOCS children's version and a significant reduction was seen during treatment with paroxetine. The dose had to be reduced in some patients because of the appearance of side effects, but the unwanted effects did not cause withdrawal from treatment. Age does not appear to be a factor that alters the response to pharmacological treatment, and neither youth nor advanced age should restrict access to effective treatment. However, the pharmacokinetics need to be addressed the safety issues related to treatment weighed with greater care.

COMBINATION TREATMENTS

Although the antiobsessional efficacy of the SSRIs and clomipramine is now well established, a substantial proportion of patients, around 30–40%, respond poorly or do not respond at all to treatment. The problem of treatment resistance and its management is complicated by our lack of understanding of the underlying pathophysiology of OCD. A number of strategies are proposed but the evidence from controlled studies to support a recommendation for these approaches is meagre. Pharmacological treatment for the treatment-resistant OCD patient may substitute another conventional antiobsessional agent if pharmacological treatment is unsuccessful, or alternatively may use augmentation strategies.

The initial pharmacological treatment with one of the first-line SSRI therapies should have been continued for sufficient time at an adequate dose before assuming that a patient is not responding to treatment. If patients do not respond to an adequate dose maintained for at least 8–10 weeks, an alternative SSRI or, if this approach has failed, clomipramine, is recommended. Caution is needed if clomipramine is administered immediately following fluoxetine, because the long half-life of fluoxetine and its inhibition of cytochrome P-450 2D6 isoenzymes would increase the plasma levels of clomipramine. Caution dictates the use of lower initial doses of clomipramine. Alternatively, if the patient has not responded to clomipramine, a move to SSRIs can be tried as an alternative, although there are few data regarding the efficacy of SSRIs in OCD patients who are non-responders to clomipramine.

A combination of serotonergic therapies has been proposed as an approach to treating resistant OCD with the rationale of attempting to increase the serotonergic activity. For example, the combination of clomipramine with an SSRI has been suggested. One small open study compared citalopram plus clomipramine with citalopram alone in patients who had not responded to treatment with clomipramine or fluoxetine (Pallanti et al., 1999). Patients treated with the combination were reported to experience a significantly greater decrease in OCD symptoms than those treated with citalopram alone. Other approaches have been to add to clomipramine or SSRI either a neuroleptic, fenfluramine, lithium, tryptophan or buspirone. It is, however, very important to bear in mind the possible interaction between drugs when they are combined. For example, an increase in the blood levels of tricyclic antidepressants is reported when they are combined with SSRIs, as well as increased cardiotoxicity and risk of convulsions (Preskorn et al., 1994).

Neuroleptics on their own have not been found to be effective antiobsessional agents, but controlled trials of their use as augmenting agents have shown them to be effective in some OCD patients. Some patients who do not respond to treatment have been found to be suffering from Gilles de la Tourette's syndrome, a tic disorder. This group of patients are thought by many to be a distinct subtype of OCD. The study of McDougle et al. (1990) found that the addition of a dopamine blocker given in low doses in addition to an SSRI had a significant therapeutic benefit in SSRI-resistant OCD patients with associated tic disorder but not in SSRI-resistant OCD without tic disorder.

Fenfluramine, a serotonin releaser and reuptake inhibitor, has been reported to be associated with further decrease in OCD symptoms when combined with SSRIs in several open case reports (Hollander and Liebowitz, 1988; Judd et al., 1991) but there are no double-blind controlled studies and therefore this approach cannot be recommended.

Other combination therapies have proved even less successful. In spite of optimistic open reports augmentation with lithium was not effective in the only double-blind placebo-controlled study of this combination (McDougle et al., 1991). Buspirone, a partial 5-HT$_{1A}$ agonist, has been investigated in OCD both alone, where no difference from clomipramine was reported in a short study (Pato et al., 1991b), and as an augmenting agent. Open studies suggested that some improvement is seen when buspirone is added to an SSRI (Markovitz *et al.*, 1990). However, in controlled studies the result is negative and significant advantages are not reported for the combination (Grady *et al.*, 1993; Pigott *et al.*, 1992a)

PHARMACOTHERAPY AND BEHAVIOUR THERAPY

Psychological treatments provide the second major approach to the management of OCD but evidence of efficacy from rigorously controlled studies has been relatively limited. The early literature that reported the efficacy of behaviour therapy is based on a small number of studies conducted a long time ago and these were flawed by methodological shortcomings. The early studies reported on a series of patients that was increased in size by the addition of extra patients in subsequent publications, rather than drawing on separate samples (Rachman *et al.*, 1973; Hodgson and Marks, 1972; Marks *et al.*, 1975). There is doubt about the blinding of the study and whether patients were sometimes added without either random assignment or the blind being maintained.

Relaxation therapy was used as a control in the early studies, all of which were of too short a duration for adequate testing of efficacy (Marks *et al.*, 1975; Marks *et al.*, 1980; Roper *et al.*, 1975). Later studies by Marks *et al.* (1988) and Cottraux *et al.* (1990) used antiexposure therapy as a control. There are some doubts as to whether this provides a neutral control group, as it may be argued that antiexposure could make the OCD worse. The significant advantage for behaviour therapy compared with antiexposure reported by Marks *et al.* (1988) has to be considered in this context. The study of Cottraux *et al.* (1990), which compared exposure plus fluvoxamine with antiexposure plus fluvoxamine, failed to replicate the finding of a significant advantage for exposure treatment.

A recent study (Lindsay *et al.*, 1997) has, however, carried out a careful controlled study of behaviour therapy using a credible neutral control treatment group. Exposure and response prevention, considered by the investigators to be the psychological treatment of choice, was compared in this small ($N = 18$) study with a control group who received a general anxiety management intervention. Both treatment groups received the same amount of therapist contact time. The study found that the OCD was improved in the behaviour therapy group and the symptom reductions could be attributed to the specific techniques of exposure and response prevention. The finding confirms the efficacy of behaviour therapy in patients with relatively severe OCD.

There have been few controlled studies of behaviour therapy in long-term treatment. The reports of open treatment have been optimistic: a review of 273 patients treated with behaviour therapy in open trials (Foa and Kozak, 1995) reported that 51% of patients were much improved, and at follow-up 76% of all patients had maintained a symptom reduction of at least 60%. However, open reports may have overestimated the benefits by reporting those with a good response who continued on treatment rather than carrying out an intention to treat analysis of all patients. The only controlled study used deep muscle relaxation treatment as a control and discontinued behaviour therapy for a period of 6 months (Hiss *et al.*, 1994). This study showed a significantly higher relapse in the group discontinued on to relaxation treatment compared with those continued on behavioural treatment. The results suggest that behavioural treatments should not be lightly discontinued. This result is very important because it shows that behaviour therapy has less enduring effects than is claimed on the basis of open treatment. The relapse rate seen on discontinuation of behaviour therapy is high and of the same order as seen in discontinuation in drug treatment studies. The results of the study provide strong support for the claim that, for a large proportion of patients treated for OCD, discontinuation of treatment, whether behaviour therapy or drugs, will lead to relapse. Clinicians and patients would do well to take account of these results and avoid premature discontinuation of treatment.

Some of the studies included behaviour therapy and concomitant drug treatment (Flament *et al.*, 1985; Marks *et al.*, 1988; Thoren *et al.*, 1980). The presence of the behaviour therapy did not appear to diminish the significant difference observed between the antiobsessional drug and placebo. Indeed, a positive interreaction between behaviour of therapy and pharmacotherapy, with best response achieved with the combined therapy, is seen in the studies of Marks *et al.* (1980) and Cottraux *et al.* (1990). This supports the generally held clinical opinion that the best response is seen when both modalities of treatment are used to the optimum.

Most clinicians who specialize in the treatment of OCD are of the opinion that for optimum treatment results it is appropriate to use both antiobsessional drugs and antiobsessional psychological treatments. Antiobsessional drugs appear to work well even if the disorder is severe, whereas behaviour therapy with or without cognitive restructuring appears to have its best effect in those with mild to moderate severity of illness. Many clinicians begin treatment with drugs and move in with a cognitive-behavioural programme at the point at which the response to treatment with drugs is beginning to have an effect on function. The rehabilitative advantages of the psychological treatment can then help to maintain and improve the response and provide supportive coping strategies. In those with mild or fluctuating OCD, who represent up to 30% of those attending for treatment, we cannot be sure of the optimum length of long-term treatment. It may well be that this group may discontinue treatment cautiously after a year without deleterious effects. For the more severe group, although there are no controlled trials beyond a year, all the evidence points to the need to continue treatment indefinitely in this severe, chronic and disabling disorder.

REFERENCES

Ananth JV, Pecknold JC, van den Steen N, Engelsmann F (1981) Double-blind comparative study of clomipramine and amitriptyline in obsessive neurosis. *Prog Neuropsychopharm Biol Psychiat*, **5**, 257–262.

Anderson IM, Tomenson BM (1995) Treatment discontinuation with selective serotonin reuptake inhibitors compared with tricyclic antidepressants: a meta-analysis. *Br Med J*, **310**, 1433–1438.

Bisserbe JC, Lane RM, Flament MF (1997) A double-blind comparison of sertraline and clomipramine in outpatients with obsessive-compulsive disorder. *Eur Psychiat*, **12**, 82–93.

Chouinard G, Goodman WK, Greist JH, Jenike MA, Rasmussen SA, White K (1990) Results of a double-blind serotonin uptake inhibitor sertraline in the treatment of obsessive-compulsive disorder. *Psychopharm Bull*, **26**(3), 279–284.

Cottraux J, Mollard E, Bouvard M, Marks IM, Sluys M, Nury AM, Bouge R, Cialdella P (1990) A controlled study of fluvoxamine and exposure in obsessive-compulsive disorders. *Int Clin Psychopharmacol*, **5**, 17–30.

Cox BJ, Swinson RP (1993) Clomipramine, fluoxetine, and behavior therapy in the treatment of obsessive-compulsive disorder: a meta-analysis. *J Behav Therap Exp Psychiat*, **24**, 149–153.

De Veaugh Geiss J, Landau P, Katz RJ (1989) Treatment of obsessive-compulsive disorder with clomipramine. *Psychiat Ann*, **19**, 97–101.

De Veaugh Geiss J, Katz RJ, Landau P et al. (1991) Clomipramine in the treatment of patients with obsessive-compulsive disorder. *Arch Gen Psychiat*, **48**, 730–738.

De Veaugh Geiss J, Moroz G, Biederman J et al. (1992) Clomipramine hydrochloride in childhood and adolescent obsessive-compulsive disorder: a multicentre trial. *J Am Acad Child Adolesc Psychiatr*, **31**, 45–49.

Dunbar GC, Steiner M, Bushnell WD (1995) Long-term treatment and prevention of relapse of obsessive compulsive disorder with paroxetine. *Eur Neuropsychopharmacol*, **5**, 372(abstr).

Fernandez CE, Lopez-Ibor JJ (1967) Monochlorimipramine in the treatment of psychiatric patients resistant to other therapies. *Actas Luso Esp Neurol Psiquiatr Cienc*, **26**, 119–147.

Flament MF, Rapoport JL, Berg CJ (1985) Clomipramine treatment of childhood OCD: a double-blind controlled study. *Arch Gen Psychiat*, **42**, 977–983.

Foa E, Kozak M (1995) Obsessive-compulsive disorder: long-term outcome of psychological treatment. In: M Mavissakalian, RF Prien (eds) *Long-term Treatments of Anxiety Disorders*. Washington, DC: American Psychiatric Press.

Freeman CP, Trimble MR, Deakin JFW et al. (1994) Fluvoxamine or clomipramine in the treatment of obsessive-compulsive disorder? A multicenter, randomized, double-blind, parallel group comparison. *J Clin Psychiat*, **55**, 301–305.

Goodman WK, Price LH, Rasmussen SA, Delgado PL, Heninger GR, Charney DS (1989) Efficacy of fluvoxamine in obsessive-compulsive disorder. *Arch Gen Psychiat*, **46**, 36–44.

Goodman WK, Price LH, Delgado PL, Palumbo J, Krystal JH, Nagy LM, Rasmussen SA, Heninger GR, Charney DS (1990) Specificity of serotonin reuptake inhibitors in the treatment of obsessive-compulsive disorder: comparison of fluvoxamine and desipramine. *Arch Gen Psychiat*, **47**, 577–585.

Goodman WK, McDougle CJ, Price LH (1992) Pharmacotherapy of obsessive-compulsive disorder. *J Clin Psychiat*, **53**, 29–37.

Goodman WK, Kozak MJ, Liebowitz M, White KL (1996) Treatment of obsessive-compulsive disorder with fluvoxamine: a multicentre, double-blind, placebo-controlled trial. *Int Clin Psychopharmacol*, **11**, 21–30.

Grady TA, Pigott TA, L'Heureux F, Hill JL, Bernstein SE, Murphy DL (1993) Double-blind study of adjuvant buspirone for fluoxetine-treated patients with obsessive-compulsive disorder. *Am J Psychiat*, **150**, 819–821.

Greist JH, Chouinard G, DuBoff E, Halaris A, Suck Won Kim, Koran LM, Liebowitz MR, Lydiard RB, Rasmussen S (1995a) Double-blind parallel comparison of three dosages of sertraline and placebo in outpatients with obsessive-compulsive disorder. *Arch Gen Psychiat*, **52**, 289–295.

Greist JH, Jefferson JW, Kobak KA, Chouinard G, DuBoff E, Halaris A, Kim SW, Koran LM, Liebowitz MR, Lydiard RB, McElroy SL, Mendels J, Rasmussen S, White K, Flicker C

172   S.A. Montgomery

(1995b) A 1-year double-blind placebo-controlled fixed dose study of sertraline in the treatment of obsessive-compulsive disorder. *Int Clin Psychopharmacol*, **10**, 57–65.

Greist JH, Jenike MA, Robinson DS, Rasmussen SA (1995c) Efficacy of fluvoxamine in obsessive-compulsive disorder: results of a multicentre, double-blind, placebo-controlled trial. *Eur J Clin Res*, **7**, 195–204.

Hewlett WA, Vinogradov S, Agras WS (1992) Clomipramine, clonazepam, and clonidine treatment of obsessive-compulsive disorder. *J Clin Psychopharmacol*, **12**, 420–430.

Hiss H, Foa E, Kozak MJ (1994) Relapse prevention program for treatment of obsessive-compulsive disorder. *J Consult Clin Psychol*, **62**, 801–808.

Hodgson R, Marks IM (1972) The treatment of obsessive-compulsive neurosis: follow-up and further findings. *Behav Res Ther*, **10**, 181–189.

Hoehn-Saric R, Harrison W, Clary C (1997) Obsessive-compulsive disorder with comorbid major depression: a comparison of sertraline and desipramine treatment. *Eur Neuropsychopharmacol*, **7**, 180–181 (abstr).

Hollander E, Liebowitz M (1988) Augmentation of antiobsessional treatment with fenfluramine. *Am J Psychiat*, **145**, 1314–1315.

Insel TR, Murphy DL, Cohen RM, Alterman I, Kilts C, Linnoila M (1983) Obsessive-compulsive disorder—a double blind trial of clomipramine and clorgyline. *Arch Gen Psychiat*, **40**, 605–612.

Jaskari MO (1980) Observations on mianserin in the treatment of obsessive neuroses. *Curr Med Res Opin*, **6**, 128–131.

Jenike MA, Baer L (1988) An open trial of buspirone in obsessive-compulsive disorder. *Am J Psychiat*, **145**, 1285–1286.

Judd FK, Chua P, Lynch C *et al.* (1991) Fenfluramine augmentation of clomipramine treatment of obsessive-compulsive disorder. *Aust J Psychiat*, **25**, 412–414.

Katz RJ, De Veaugh Geiss J, Landau P (1990) Clomipramine in obsessive-compulsive disorder. *Biol Psychiat*, **28**, 401–404.

Koran LM, McElroy SL, Davidson JRT, Rasmussen SA, Hollander E, Jenike MA (1996) Fluvoxamine vs. clomipramine for obsessive-compulsive disorder: a double-blind comparison. *J Clin Psychiat*, **16**, 121–129.

Kronig MH, Apter J, Asnis G, Bystritsky A *et al.* (1999) Placebo-controlled, multicentre study of sertraline treatment for obsessive-compulsive disorder. *J Clin Psychopharmacol*, **19**, 172–176.

Leonard HL, Swedo SE, Rapoport JL, Coffey M, Cheslow DL (1988) Treatment of childhood obsessive-compulsive disorder with clomipramine and desmethylimipramine: a double-blind crossover comparison. *Psychopharm Bull*, **24**, 93–95.

Lindsay M, Crino R, Andrews G (1997) Controlled trial of exposure and response prevention in obsessive-compulsive disorder. *Br J Psychiat*, **171**, 135–139.

Lopez-Ibor JJ, Saiz J, Cottraux J, Note I, Viñas R, Bourgeois M, Hernandez M, Gomez-Perez JC (1996) Double-blind comparison of fluoxetine vs. clomipramine in the treatment of obsessive-compulsive disorder. *Eur Neuropsychopharmacol*, **6**, 111–118.

March JS, Biederman J, Wolkow R, Safferman A *et al.* (1998) Sertraline in children and adolescents with obsessive-compulsive disorder: a multicentre randomised controlled trial. *JAMA*, **280**, 1752–1756

Markovitz PJ, Stagno SJ, Calabrese JR (1990) Buspirone augmentation of fluoxetine on obsessive-compulsive disorder. *Am J Psychiat*, **147**, 798–800.

Marks IM, Hodgson R, Rachman S (1975) Treatment of chronic obsessive-compulsive neurosis by *in vivo* exposure. *Br J Psychiat*, **127**, 349–364.

Marks IM, Stern RS, Mawson D, Cobb J, McDonald R (1980) Clomipramine and exposure for obsessive-compulsive rituals. *Br J Psychiat*, **136**, 1–25.

Marks IM, Lelliott P, Basoglu M, Noshirvani H, Monteiro W, Cohen D, Kasvikis Y (1988)

Clomipramine, self-exposure and therapist-aided exposure for obsessive-compulsive rituals. *Br J Psychiat*, **152**, 522–534.

McDougle CJ, Goodman WK, Price LH, Delgado PL, Krystal JH, Charney DS, Heninger GR (1990) Neuroleptic addition in fluvoxamine-refractory obsessive-compulsive disorder. *Am J Psychiat*, **147**, 652–654.

McDougle CJ, Price LH, Goodman WK, Charney DS, Heninger GR (1991) A controlled trial of lithium augmentation in fluvoxamine refractory obsessive-compulsive disorders lack of efficacy. *J Clin Psychopharmacol*, **11**, 175–184.

Milanfranchi A, Ravagli S, Lensi P, Marazziti D, Cassano GB (1997) A double-blind study of fluvoxamine and clomipramine in the treatment of obsessive-compulsive disorder. *Int Clin Psychopharmacol*, **12**, 131–136.

Montgomery SA (1980) Clomipramine in obsessional neurosis: a placebo-controlled trial. *Pharmaceut Med*, **1**, 189–192.

Montgomery SA, McIntyre A, Osterheider M, Sarteschi P, Zitterl W, Zohar J, Birkett M, Wood AJ and The Lilly European OCD Study Group (1993) A double-blind, placebo-controlled study of fluoxetine in patients with DSM-III-R obsessive-compulsive disorder. *Eur Neuropsychopharmacol*, **3**, 143–152.

Montgomery SA, Henry J, McDonald G, Dinan T, Lader M, Hindmarch I, Clare A, Nutt D (1994) Selective serotonin reuptake inhibitors: meta-analysis of discontinuation rates. *Int Clin Psychopharmacol*, **9**, 47–53.

Montgomery SA, Kasper S (1995) Comparison of compliance between serotonin reuptake inhibitors and tricyclic antidepressants: a meta-analysis. *Int Clin Psychopharmacol*, **9 S4**, 33–40.

Montgomery SA, Kasper S, Stein D *et al.* (2000, in press) Citalopram 20 mg, 40 mg and 60 mg are all effective and well tolerated compared with placebo in obsessive compulsive disorder. *Int Clin Psychopharmacol*, **16**.

Mundo E, Mainia G, Uslenghi C (2000) Multicentre, double-blind comparison of fluvoxamine and clomipramine in the treatment of obsessive-compulsive disorder. *Int Clin Psychopharmacol*, **15**, 69–76.

Pallanti S, Quercioli L, Paiva RS, Koran LM (1999) Citalopram for treatment-resistant obsessive-compulsive disorder. *Eur Psychiat*, **14**, 101–106.

Pato M, Zohar-Kadouch R, Zohar J, Murphy DL (1988) Return of symptoms after discontinuation of clomipramine in patients with obsessive-compulsive disorder. *Am J Psychiat*, **145**, 1543–1548.

Pato M, Murphy DL, De Vane CL (1991a) Sustained plasma concentrations of fluoxetine and/or norfluoxetine four and eight weeks after fluoxetine discontinuation. *J Clin Psychopharmacol*, **11**, 224–225.

Pato M, Pigott TA, Hill JL, Grover GN, Bernstein SE, Murphy DL (1991b) Controlled comparison of buspirone and clomipramine in obsessive-compulsive disorder. *Am J Psychiat*, **148**, 127–129.

Perse TL (1988) Obsessive-compulsive disorder: a treatment review. *J Clin Psychiat*, **49**, 48–55.

Perse TL, Greist JH, Jefferson JW, Rosenfeld JW, Dar R (1987) Fluvoxamine treatment of obsessive-compulsive disorder. *Am J Psychiat*, **144**, 1543–1548.

Piccinelli M, Pini S, Bellantuono C, Wilkinson G (1995) Efficacy of drug treatment in obsessive-compulsive disorder. *Br J Psychiat*, **166**, 421–443.

Pigott TA, Pato M, Bernstein SE *et al.* (1990) Controlled comparison of clomipramine and fluoxetine in the treatment of obsessive-compulsive disorder. *Arch Gen Psychiat*, **47**, 926–932.

Pigott TA, L'Heureux F, Hill JL (1992a) A double-blind study of adjuvant buspirone hydrochloride in clomipramine-treated OCD patients. *J Clin Psychopharmacol*, **12**, 11–18.

Pigott TA, L'Heureux F, Rubenstein CS, Bernstein SE, Hill JL, Murphy DL (1992b) A double-blind placebo controlled study of trazodone in patients with obsessive-compulsive disorder. *J Clin Psychopharmacol*, **12**, 156–162.

Preskorn SH, Alderman J, Chung M, Harrison W, Messig M, Harris S (1994) Pharmacokinetics of desipramine coadministered with sertraline or fluoxetine. *J Clin Psychopharmacol*, **14**, 90–98.

Rachman S, Marks IM, Hodgson R (1973) The treatment of obsessive compulsive neurotics by modelling and flooding in vivo. *Behav Res Ther*, **11**, 463–471.

Rasmussen S, Eisen J (1992) The epidemiology and clinical features of obsessive-compulsive disorder. *Psychiatr Clin N Am*, **14**, 743–758.

Rasmussen S, Hacket E, DuBoff E, Greist JH, Halaris A, Koran LM, Liebowitz M, Lydiard RB, McElroy SL, Mendels J, O'Connor K (1997) A 2-year study of sertraline in the treatment of obsessive-compulsive disorder. *Int Clin Psychopharmacol*, **12**, 309–316.

Rauch SL, O'Sullivan RL, Jenike MA (1998) Open treatment of obsessive-compulsive disorder with venlafaxine: a series of ten cases. *J Clin Psychopharmacol*, **16**, 81–83.

Riddle MA, Scahill L, King RA et al. (1992) Double-blind, crossover trial of fluoxetine and placebo in children and adolescents with obsessive-compulsive disorder. *J Am Acad Child Adolesc Psychiatr*, **31**, 1062–1069.

Robins LN, Regier DA (1990) *Psychiatric Disorders in America: The Epidemiological Catchment Area Study*. New York, Free Press.

Roper G, Rachman S, Marks IM (1975) Passive and participant modelling in exposure treatment of obsessive-compulsive neurotics. *Behav Res Ther*, **13**, 271–279.

Rosenberg, DR, Stewart CM, Fitzgerald KD, Tawile V et al. (1999) Paroxetine open-label treatment of pediatric outpatients with obsessive-compulsive disorder. *J Am Acad Child Adolesc Psychiat*, **38**, 1180–1185.

Smeraldi E, Erzegovesi S, Bianchi I et al. (1992) Fluvoxamine vs. clomipramine treatment in obsessive-compulsive disorder: a preliminary study. *New Trends Exp Clin Psych*, **8**, 63–65.

Stein DJ, Spadaccini E, Hollander E (1995) Meta-analysis of pharmacotherapy trials for obsessive-compulsive disorder. *Int Clin Psychopharmacol*, **10**, 11–18.

Thoren P, Asberg M, Cronholm B, Jornestedt L, Traskman L (1980) Clomipramine treatment in obsessive compulsive disorder. I. A controlled clinical trial. *Arch Gen Psychiat*, **37**, 1281–1285.

Tollefson GD, Birkett M, Koran LM et al. (1994a) Continuation treatment of OCD: a double-blind and open-label experience with fluoxetine. *J Clin Psychiat*, **55**, 69–76.

Tollefson GD, Rampey AH, Potvin JH, Jenike MA, Rush AJ, Dominguez RA, Koran LM, Shear MK, Goodman WK, Genduso LA (1994b) A multicenter investigation of fixed-dose fluoxetine in the treatment of obsessive-compulsive disorder. *Arch Gen Psychiat*, **51**, 559–567.

Vallejo J, Olivares J, Marcos T, Bulbena A, Menchon JM (1992) Clomipramine vs. phenelzine in obsessive-compulsive disorder. A controlled clinical trial. *Br J Psychiat*, **161**, 665–670.

Volavka J, Neziroglu F, Yaryura-Tobias JA (1985) Clomipramine and imipramine in obsessive-compulsive disorders. *Psychiatr Res*, **14**, 85–93.

Wheadon D, Bushnell WD, Steiner M (1993) A fixed dose comparison of 20, 40 or 60 mg of paroxetine to placebo in the treatment of obsessive-compulsive disorder. Presented at the American College of Neuropsychopharmacology Annual Meeting, Puerto Rico, December.

Wood A, Tollefson GD, Birkett M (1993) Pharmacotherapy of obsessive-compulsive disorder—experience with fluoxetine. *Int Clin Psychopharmacol*, **8**, 301–306.

Yaryura-Tobias JA, Neziroglu F (1996) Venlafaxine in obsessive-compulsive disorder. *Arch Gen Psychiat*, **53**, 653–654.

Zitterl W, Meszaros K, Hornik K, Twaroch T et al. (1999) Efficacy of fluoxetine in Austrian patients with obsessive-compulsive disorder. *Wien Klin Wochenschr*, **111**, 439–442.

Zohar J, Insel TR (1987) Obsessive-compulsive disorder: psychobiological approaches to diagnosis, treatment and pathophysiology. *Biol Psychiat*, **22**, 667–687.

Zohar J, Judge R (1996) Paroxetine vs. clomipramine in the treatment of obsessive-compulsive disorder. *Br J Psychiat*, **169**, 468–474.

8

Serotonin and serotonergic drugs in post-traumatic stress disorder

Jonathan R.T. Davidson and Kathryn M. Connor

INTRODUCTION

In this chapter the concept of post-traumatic stress will be reviewed, along with clinical features of post-traumatic stress disorder (PTSD), its course and outcome. Recent information on economic and health costs of the disorder will also be addressed. Indications for treatment will be covered, with a review of the neurobiology of PTSD, as it bears on serotonergic systems. Finally, the place of serotonergically active drugs in PTSD will be addressed, based on the current limited knowledge base.

DEFINITION, COURSE, IMPAIRMENT

Post-traumatic stress disorder has been described throughout medical history, under a wide range of diagnostic labels. At least 28 different terms have been used to describe this syndrome (Resnick, 1995), many of which emphasize its somatic aspects, others the psychological, depressive and phobic avoidance components. The term post-traumatic stress disorder first originated in 1980 in the American Psychiatric Association's *Diagnostic and Statistical Manual of Mental Disorders*, 3rd edn. A number of changes took place when the revised edition of this, DSM-III-R, came out (American Psychiatric Association, 1987), with further refinements in DSM-IV

SSRIs in Depression and Anxiety, Second Edition. Edited by S.A. Montgomery and J.A. den Boer.
© 2001 John Wiley & Sons Ltd.

(American Psychiatric Association, 1994). In DSM-IV, the principal changes had to do with the redefinition of what constituted a trauma, along with the reclassification of one symptom, physiological hyperarousal in response to trauma cues. This had previously been a hyperarousal symptom and was repositioned as a recurrent intrusive recollection symptom. A third important change was the requirement of both phobic avoidance *and* withdrawal/numbing symptomatology, in contrast to the DSM-III-R requirement that one or other would be sufficient. This effectively turned PTSD into a quadripartite disorder, in comparison to the tripartite symptom clusters of DSM-III-R. Other comparatively minor changes in wording were introduced and the acute vs. chronic dichotomy was also brought back, having been dropped in DSM-III-R.

The symptoms of PTSD are summarized in Table 8.1, and reflect the two-part definition of a trauma, as well as the three sets of symptom groupings: recurrent intrusive recollections (criterion B), avoidance and numbing/withdrawal (criterion C) and hyperarousal (criterion D). In addition, functional limitations or clinically significant distress are required, and there must also be a minimum duration of symptoms. As pointed out, C criteria really constitute two separate symptom domains and in the future it is envisioned that these would occupy separate categories in any diagnostic definition.

In his review on the course of PTSD, Blank (1993) notes that sometimes the disorder fades in a short time, especially if there are subclinical manifestations falling short of the diagnostic threshold. Intrusive symptoms tend to be more prominent at some points, especially at first, with avoidance and numbing symptoms tending to become more prominent later. However, this is by no means an invariable pattern, and it is generally the case the hyperarousal and startle symptoms initiate the illness process and may well drive much of the other symptomatology, which can be seen as adaptive to tolerable and unremitting levels of high arousal and vigilance. There is compelling evidence for acute, chronic, delayed and intermittent forms of PTSD. While sometimes symptoms get worse with age, some improvement generally takes place. In the National Comorbidity Survey (Kessler *et al.*, 1995), approximately 40% of all cases identified with PTSD continued to exhibit the diagnosis after a period of 10 years. The authors did note, however, that the provision of unspecified treatments for PTSD was associated with a considerably shorter duration of illness, although the chronicity rate of 40% remained the same in both groups. It is possible that a selection bias operated in the sample who sought out treatment. It is also worth noting that with well-targeted somatic or behavioral treatments, the prognosis might be better. Rothbaum *et al.* (1992) have noted that following rape approximately 90–95% of women develop an acute PTSD, dropping down to approximately 50% at 3 months. It is in the latter group that the disorder tended to be more persistent at 1 year.

Solomon and Davidson (1997) have noted a high prevalence rate (approximately 8–9%) of PTSD in the US population. Rates of exposure to trauma are considerably higher, in the range of 40–50%, which means that by no means all individuals exposed to trauma develop PTSD. Risk factors include: family history of anxiety, depression, sociopathy, previous history of depression or anxiety; gender; extent and toxicity of the

Table 8.1. Diagnostic criteria for post-traumatic stress disorder.

A. The person has been exposed to a traumatic event in which both of the following were present:
    (1) The person experienced, witnessed or was confronted with an event or events that involved actual or threatened death or serious injury, or a threat to the physical integrity of self or others
    (2) The person's response involved intense fear, helplessness or horror. Note: In children, this may be expressed instead by disorganized or agitated behavior

B. The traumatic event is persistently re-experienced in one (or more) of the following ways:
    (1) Recurrent and intrusive distressing recollections of the event, including images, thoughts or perceptions
    (2) Recurrent distressing dreams of the event
    (3) Acting or feeling as if the traumatic event were recurring (includes a sense of reliving the experience, illusions, hallucinations and dissociative flashback episodes, including those that occur on awakening or when intoxicated)
    (4) Intense psychological distress at exposure to internal or external cues that symbolize or resemble an aspect of the traumatic event
    (5) Physiological reactivity on exposure to internal or external cues that symbolize or resemble an aspect of the traumatic event

C. Persistent avoidance of stimuli associated with the trauma and numbing of general responsiveness (not present before the trauma), as indicated by three (or more) of the following:
    (1) Efforts to avoid thoughts, feelings or conversations associated with the trauma
    (2) Efforts to avoid activities, places or people that arouse recollections of the trauma
    (3) Inability to recall an important aspect of the trauma
    (4) Markedly diminished interest or participation in significant activities
    (5) Feeling of detachment or estrangement from others
    (6) Restricted range of affect (e.g. unable to have loving feelings)
    (7) Sense of a foreshortened future (e.g. does not expect to have a career, marriage, children or a normal lifespan)

D. Persistent symptoms of increased arousal (not present before the trauma), as indicated by two (or more) of the following:
    (1) Difficulty falling or staying asleep
    (2) Irritability or outbursts of anger
    (3) Difficulty concentrating
    (4) Hypervigilance
    (5) Exaggerated startle response

E. Duration of the disturbance (symptoms in criteria B, C and D) is more than 1 month

F. The disturbance causes clinically significant distress or impairment in social, occupational or other important areas of functioning

Specify if:
    Acute: if duration of symptoms is less than 3 months
    Chronic: if duration of symptoms is 3 months or more
Specify if:
    With delayed onset: if onset of symptoms is at least 6 months after the stressor

trauma; personality disorder; lack of available supports. With the passage of time, risk factors associated with chronic PTSD are related more to the individual and his/her environment, rather than to the trauma itself.

In their review, Solomon and Davidson (1997) note that PTSD in the community is associated with increased rates of physical morbidity, especially hypertension, bronchial asthma and peptic ulcer disease. Increased rates of psychiatric comorbidity are evident, and cover a wide range of mental illness. People with PTSD are at least two to four times more likely than those without PTSD to have depression, other anxiety disorders, substance abuse and, most especially, somatization disorder, for which the odds ratio indicated a 90-fold increased likelihood of the co-association between PTSD and somatization disorder. This speaks both to the dissociative and/or conversion processes inherent to PTSD, as well as the highly colored somatic presentation of the illness, as has been highlighted in the many alternative names for the disorder. Breslau *et al.* (1991) found that 83% of people with PTSD also had another psychiatric disorder, and similar findings were noted by Kessler *et al.* (1995), who observed that 88% of men and 79% of women with PTSD had a history of at least one other psychiatric disorder.

Functional impairment was considerable. For instance, victimized women enrolled in a Health Maintenance Organization (HMO) had increased rates of chronic pelvic pain, gastrointestinal disorders, headaches and psychogenic seizures (Koss *et al.*, 1990; Kimerling and Calhoun, 1994). Sexually assaulted women are at risk for poorer physical health (Kimerling and Calhoun, 1994; Golding, 1994). The view has been advanced (Friedman and Schnurr 1995; Wolfe *et al.*, 1994) that PTSD mediates the effects of trauma and impaired physical health, rather than exposure to the trauma *per se*. While PTSD is associated with a higher use of medical health care services, there is marked reluctance for such people to avail themselves of mental health resources (Solomon and Davidson, 1997). As few as 2–8% of crime victims received professional mental health services, although rates are slightly higher for those who are victims of sexual assault. Nevertheless, victims with criminal or sexual assault-induced PTSD seek mental health treatment at a very low rate.

In terms of costs, there are relatively few data available. This is one of the urgent and unanswered aspects of PTSD. Koss *et al.* (1990) noted that severely victimized women had outpatient medical expenses at least twice greater than those of non-victimized controls in the same HMO. Miller *et al.* (1996) have noted that the direct costs of personal crime in the USA amounted to $105 billion, including medical costs, loss of earnings and public assistance programs. When taking into account intangible costs such as pain, suffering, willingness to pay out-of-pocket and jury-awarded compensation, the cost of crime to its victims increased to an estimated $450 billion. Miller *et al.* also estimated that mental health costs accounted for 37% of the total costs from criminal victimization in 1989 (Miller *et al.*, 1993). If this assumption is correct, then the mental health costs of crime are approximately $166 billion annually, and this is no more than a fraction of the total mental health costs attributable to all PTSD. Only a small proportion of these costs are actually related to the delivery of professional mental health treatment.

It is quite clear, then, from even the limited data available that PTSD is an immensely costly health problem.

PSYCHOBIOLOGY OF PTSD: THE PLACE OF SEROTONIN

Lines of evidence from animal models of the traumatic stress syndrome, serotonergic probe studies in patients with PTSD and clinical pharmacology trials all provide strong evidence that serotonergic pathways are integrally involved with PTSD.

The animal model data will be reviewed. As early as 1972, Weissman and Harbert (1972) noted that treatment of animals with PCPA, a serotonin-depleting agent, resulted in sustained wakefulness and generalized hyper-responsivity. Taken as a whole, the authors commented that these behavioral data may be interpreted as suggesting that a well-modulated serotonergic system underlies behavioral inhibition, and that a relative absence of serotonin produces hypersensitivity to environmental cues. Although at the time PTSD was not well recognized, the relevance of their findings to this syndrome are quite clear. Further studies have indicated that conditioned fear stimuli activate 5-HT neurones in the dorsal raphe nucleus, projecting to 5-HT$_2$ or 5-HT$_{1C}$ receptors in the amygdala and other forebrain structures (Hensman *et al.*, 1991; Deakin, 1988). Joseph and Kennett (1983) have observed that the stress-induced corticosteroid response depends upon increased availability of tryptophan, and that competing amino acids, such as valine, prevent restraint stress-induced increases in brain trytephan and serotonin turnover. Administration of valine also attenuates the corticosteroid response to this stress, an effect which is reversed by co-administration of tryptophan. It is clear, then, that an intact serotonergic system is necessary for the adequacy of stress-induced corticosteroid responses. Kennett *et al.* (1985) suggest that enhanced 5-HT-dependent behaviors following stress are reflective of adaptive processes.

A number of studies in patients with PTSD lend support to the serotonin story. In 1993, Arora *et al.* (1993) observed a reduction in the K_d and B_{max} for ^{3}H-PA binding in PTSD relative to normal controls in a population of Vietnam veterans. K_d represents an inverse measure of affinity for paroxetine binding to the uptake site, while B_{max} represents the maximum number of binding sites. Thus, there are reduced sites with an increased affinity. No difference was observed in patients with PTSD and comorbid major depression as compared to PTSD alone. Thus, the results could not be explained by a diagnosis of depressive disorder. The authors noted, moreover, that the B_{max} was negatively correlated with state anxiety, whereas the K_d was positively correlated with combat-related PTSD symptoms. The authors draw a distinction in the paroxetine binding profile of PTSD as compared with major depression, suggesting a difference between the disorders in this respect. Their patients did have considerable comorbidity, numbers were relatively small and they mention these as complicating factors which limit the interpretation of their findings. Nonetheless, these findings are of much interest and also provide a theoretical underpinning for the use of 5-HT reuptake inhibitors in treating PTSD. Their correlation between paroxetine binding and symptoms of anxiety and PTSD are also relevant.

In a second study, the same group (Fichtner *et al.*, 1994) noted a relationship between pretreatment paroxetine binding and response to fluoxetine. Clinical global improvement ratings, conducted blind to the biochemical data, were used to separate patients into responders and partial responders. Best response occurred in subjects who had lower pretreatment K_d values and also a trend to lower B_{max} values. Again, the limitations of this study relate to the small numbers and comorbidity, as well as the use of some other medications. However, these are important leads which need to be taken further.

A recent set of results by Southwick *et al.* (1995) found that a challenge with *m*CPP, a 5-HT$_2$ agonist, provoked symptoms of PTSD in a substantial number of patients with the diagnosis, whereas administration of placebo did not do so. The authors point out that individuals who deteriorated upon exposure to *m*CPP were different from those patients with PTSD, who got worse in response to yohimbine, a noradrenergic challenge, strongly suggesting that there may be different neurochemical subtypes of PTSD.

Lastly, evidence to support the involvement of serotonin in PTSD comes from the numerous clinical trials to be reviewed below, wherein the great majority of drugs have either selective or very conspicuous serotonin effects.

TREATMENT OF PTSD

Despite the fact that PTSD was introduced as a diagnosis in 1980, there have been remarkably few clinical trials of pharmacotherapy in the disorder. Those that have been completed and published are reviewed below.

General indications for treatment of PTSD include the presence of clinically distressing symptoms, which may even be diagnostically subthreshold. One does not have to wait for the diagnosis in order to decide upon treatment. Obviously, as the symptom picture becomes increasingly severe, distressing or disabling, then the need for treatment becomes more compelling. The risks of PTSD include severe damage to interpersonal relationships, loss of job, violence, suicide, abuse of alcohol, drugs, other comorbidity or law breaking. All of these are situations which, as far as possible, should be prevented by treatment.

In addition to deciding on the appropriate medication, the physician needs to be attentive to the many other relevant issues seen in PTSD, including stigmatization, ambivalence toward treatment, shame, lack of information, counter-therapeutic attitudes and behaviors in the family, presence or absence of social supports, and whether or not litigation is under way or even being contemplated. These and other issues should definitely be taken into account in assessment and treatment planning.

Main goals of pharmacotherapy are as follows:

1. To control the core of PTSD symptoms of intrusiveness, avoidance, numbing and hyperarousal.

2. To help reduce the associated disability and stress vulnerability.
3. To treat associated comorbidity.
4. To facilitate or potentate non-pharmacologic therapies.

The main drug groups will be described and their experience to date in clinical trials.

TREATMENT CONSIDERATION: OPEN-LABEL STUDIES

Sertraline

Rothbaum and colleagues (1996) studied five rape victims, all women, using doses of sertraline as follows: 50, 75, 100, 150, 150 mg/day. Response was good in four patients using both observer and self-ratings for PTSD. Tolerance of the drug was good, although the following side effects were noted: tremor, sweating, dry mouth, nausea ($N = 1$ each), and drowsiness and dizziness ($N = 2$ each).

In the study by Kline and colleagues (1994), 10 male Vietnam veterans at a mean age of 44 years, all of whom had PTSD and comorbid major depression, received treatment at a mean dose of 98.5 mg/day (range 5–150 mg/day) over a 12-month minimum period. Sixty-three per cent of veterans were responders, based upon several scales. Of note was the fact that all subjects had been poor responders to other treatments either due to efficacy or excessive side effects. The authors noted that insomnia persisted despite general improvement, and that it was often necessary to augment sertraline with low doses of sedative drugs. They observed that the drug seemed to assist with the subject's behavioral responses to extremely stressful life events.

Fluoxetine

Several open-label studies have been conducted with fluoxetine. Shay (1992) noted that 13 of 18 depressed Vietnam veterans with combat-induced PTSD developed less explosiveness when treated with fluoxetine, pointing out an increased ability to think through things rather than acting impulsively. Response occurred as early as 1 week, although the modal response occurred between 3 and 6 weeks after initiating treatment. Their series is a retrospective report, based upon the use of fluoxetine for between 12 and 27 months, at a range of 20–80 mg/day in 28 depressed combat veterans with PTSD. Systematic ratings were not conducted, but Shay observed side effects in 16 of 28 subjects who developed insomnia, a problem which was rectified by addition of trazodone or doxepin at night. Diarrhea was noted in the morning, causing discontinuation or dose reduction in several instances. Mild nausea was also seen, leading to treatment discontinuation in one case. Three of 28 subjects reported marked diminishment of sexual interest, leading to discontinuation in one case.

In another study of combat veterans with PTSD, Nagy and colleagues (1933) treated 27 combat veterans with PTSD at doses ranging from 20 to 80 mg/day over a

10-week period. Nineteen subjects completed at least 3 weeks, and the total CAPS scores decreased from a mean of 64 down to 42 at endpoint, a statistically significant, albeit modest reduction in score. Improvement was observed on re-experiencing, a avoidance/numbing and hyperarousal dimensions. Improvement in social and occupational functioning was minimal. Generally, improvement occurred after 6 weeks of treatment, suggesting that higher doses of drug and longer-term therapy were called for. The authors noted reduction in frequency of panic attacks in 75% of patients who had problems with this symptom. Side effects, persisting anxiety symptoms, external stressors and proneness to substance abuse led to a comparatively high dropout rate.

McDougle and colleagues (1991) further treated 20 male combat veterans from Vietnam with PTSD at fluoxetine doses ranging from 20 to 80 mg/day for a mean duration of 26 weeks. The authors included a clinical global impression scale adapted for the study, defining a 50% symptom reduction as being equivalent to much improvement. Very much improvement was judged to have occurred when almost complete symptom remission had taken place. Of 23 entered patients, 20 completed at least 4 weeks, dropouts having been due to non-compliance and gastrointestinal upset. The mean dose was 35 mg/day for the 20 completers, 65% of whom were judged to have responded on the Clinical Global Impressions Scale (CGI). Comparing responders with non-responders, the authors found that a longer duration of treatment characterized responders. The presence of comorbid major depression was not associated with any particular outcome.

Davidson and colleagues (1991) treated five civilian patients with fluoxetine. Mean doses ranged from 20 to 80 mg/day, treatment being given at a minimum of 8 and maximum of 32 weeks. Inciting traumas consisted of burns ($N = 1$), motor vehicle accident ($N = 1$), incest ($N = 2$) and rape ($N = 1$). Fluoxetine was associated with marked improvement on both intrusive and avoidant symptoms, and a facilitative effect of the drug was noted on trauma-focused psychotherapy in the two adult victims of childhood sexual trauma.

Fluvoxamine

A study with fluvoxamine has been conducted in 24 Dutch World War II resistance fighters with chronic PTSD (de Boer *et al.*, 1991). Twenty-four subjects entered treatment, with fluvoxamine being administered up to 300 mg/day for 12 weeks. Conventionally accepted ratings were used, to include the CGI, the Zung Depression Scale (ZDS), the Spielberg or State Trait Anxiety Inventory (STAI), and a purpose-developed PTSD rating scale. Nine of the 24 subjects stopped treatment because of gastrointestinal side effects, one subject reported deterioration in sleep, and three more discontinued the study for unspecified physical complaints. Eleven subjects (46%) thus completed the entire study, leaving a possibly somewhat unrepresentative sample of completers. However, 17 completed at least 4 weeks of treatment. The author could not demonstrate any differences on baseline symptom measures between the completers and the early dropouts. Statistically significant reductions in score were noted on the PTSD scale, the Trait Anxiety measure, and non-significant trends for improvement were noted on the State Anxiety scale. Significant change was observed on the CGI at 4 weeks, but at the end of the study, more subjects showed worsening or lack of change on the CGI than did those who improved. At the end of treatment, five subjects expressed a preference to continue on fluvoxamine. The results of this study may therefore be taken as generally negative. The authors suggest that it could possibly be related to the characteristics of the sample, as well as poor tolerance of the drug.

In a second open-label trial of fluvoxamine, Marmar and colleagues (1996) noted improvement in combat veterans with chronic PTSD. Eleven subjects entered treatment, 10 completing the entire 10-week study period. One subject complained of side effects and dropped out three-quarters of the way through. In all other patients, however, the medication was well tolerated and side effects were minor, comprising largely of sedation, headache, nausea and insomnia. Using the self-rated Revised Impact of Events Scale, fluvoxamine was associated with major improvement on intrusion, avoidance and hyperarousal symptoms. The same was true for the clinician-rated Stress Response Rating Scale (SRRS). Good effects were noted on depression, anxiety, hostility and global symptom severity of the SCL-90R. Most improvement was noted to have taken place by the sixth week of treatment, except for hostility which took somewhat longer. In this often treatment-refractory population, these results may be seen as incurred.

Paroxetine

An open-label 12-week trial with paroxetine has been conducted in 17 patients with non-combat-related, chronic PTSD (Marshall *et al.*, 1998). Outcome was assessed using established rating scales for the symptom clusters of depression, anxiety, general symptoms, and PTSD core symptoms. Significant improvement was observed in all three symptom clusters, with 65% of patients rated as "much" or "very much" improved, and a mean reduction of 48% in PTSD symptom scores was also recorded. Significant variation in the time course of response across the symptom clusters suggested that multiple mechanisms of response might have been involved.

Buspirone

Another selective serotonergic drug, buspirone, a 5-HT$_{1A}$ receptor partial agonist, has been studied in PTSD. Ten patients were treated by Fichtner and Crayton (1994). The dose was titrated from 10 mg/day up to a maximum of 90 mg/day as needed. Patients also participated in group and individual therapy programs. Participants had a mean age of 44 years, treatment was given for 2–9 months, and improvement measured by the CGI. The mean dose of buspirone was 46 mg (range 15–90 mg). At the end of treatment, 40% of subjects were judged to have had a good outcome, 30% an equivocal outcome and 30% poor outcome. All seven patients who showed some degree of improvement exhibited reduction in hyperarousal symptoms, with a weak effect of the drug for re-experiencing, and almost no effect on avoidance. The authors noted that best responses occurred at doses of 60 mg/day or higher.

Cyproheptadine

An interesting report of cyproheptadine, a 5-HT antagonist, noted that nightmares improved in a sample of patients who received the drug along with antidepressants (Brophy, 1991). The author specifically describes four subjects, three of whom benefited from the addition of cyproheptadine at doses of 2, 4 or 6 mg/day, and treatment failure in a subject who received up to 28 mg. Visual hallucinations and worsening of flashbacks, along with sedation and some confusion, were observed in one subject.

Trazodone

Hertzberg *et al.* (1996) noted modest benefits for trazodone in combat veterans with PTSD. Treatment was initiated at 50 mg/day and increased to 400 mg/day in six patients, in whom CAPS scores were reduced from 92 at baseline to 79 at endpoint. On the self-rated DTS, scores dropped from 102 to 88. Minimal improvement occurred in social and occupational functioning, as well as in depression. Sleep did improve, and the drug was well tolerated. However, overall these findings represent only modest efficacy, and need to be extended to civilian populations, as well as include a placebo control, before we can better evaluate the role of trazodone.

Nefazodone

Findings from two open-label studies of nefazodone in combat-related PTSD have been reported. In the first study, Hertzberg *et al.* (1998) treated 10 combat veterans with DSM-IV PTSD with nefazodone for 12 weeks, starting at 100 mg/day and increasing up to 600 mg/day. Following treatment, all patients were rated as much improved using the CGI-I scale. Significant improvement was observed in all PTSD symptoms (except self-ratings of re-experiencing), sleep, anger and clinician-rated depression at week 12. At a 4-week follow-up, these gains were all maintained and significant improvement was found. Treatment was well tolerated and there was no evidence of sexual side effects.

In a second open-label study (Davis *et al.*, 2000), 36 veterans with chronic PTSD were treated with nefazodone for 8 weeks. Thirty-one subjects completed at least 4 weeks of treatment, with 26 completing the 8-week study. Significant improvement was observed in overall PTSD and in the individual symptom clusters, with the greatest gains in the first 4 weeks of treatment, as measured by changes on the CAPS. Comparable changes were also found on the HAM-D and HAM-A scales. The treatment was well tolerated, with only four patients discontinuing the medication due to adverse effects.

DOUBLE-BLIND STUDIES OF SELECTIVE SEROTONIN REUPTAKE INHIBITORS

Fluoxetine

The first study to evaluate an SSRI vs. placebo was the comparison of van der Kolk *et al.* (1994). In this 5-week study, fluoxetine was given up to a maximum dose of 60 mg/day to 31 combat veterans and 33 civilian patients with PTSD. Relatively few patients completed the study, but overall there was an effect greater for fluoxetine than placebo. The predominantly female civilian group showed the greatest drug vs. placebo differences, while in the male combat veterans fluoxetine was equivalent to placebo, with neither treatment producing very much improvement. In the civilians, fluoxetine was particularly related to improvement in re-experiencing and numbing as well as depression, labile affect and impaired interpersonal relationships. The combat veteran group responded to fluoxetine in terms of their depression, but not in respect of PTSD. Hyper-arousal in both populations failed to respond well to fluoxetine and, unlike the study of Marmar *et al.* (1996) with fluvoxamine, there was little improvement in hostility. In their group, 54.8% met comorbid major depression, although the authors did not further discuss the implications of this for their results. The average dose of fluoxetine was 40 mg/day, and side effects were noted in respect of diarrhea, sweating and headaches, all found more frequently with fluoxetine than with placebo.

In a second randomized, double-blind study Connor *et al.* (1999), demonstrated that fluoxetine (up to 60 mg/day) was more effective than placebo in civilian PTSD patients ($N = 53$), over a 12-week treatment period. At week 12, compared to placebo, fluoxetine was shown to be superior for measures of PTSD severity, disability, stress vulnerability, and high end-state function. Specific symptom-responses were described by Meltzer-Brody *et al.* (2000), who noted benefits on intrusive recollections, avoidance, anhedonia, estrangement, foreshortened future and poor concentration in particular. Less benefit was found for nightmares.

In a third trial using an identical protocol, Hertzberg *et al.* (2000) found no difference between drug and placebo in combat veterans. These results suggest that patient type is an important variable in trials of PTSD.

Paroxetine

Recently, overall data from three short-term 12-week double-blind placebo-controlled multicenter studies, conducted on approximately 1200 patients, have shown that paroxetine is an effective, safe and well-tolerated treatment for PTSD (Stein, 2000).

The studies consisted of a fixed dose trial (20 or 40 mg paroxetine/day) and two flexible dose trials (starting on 20 mg paroxetine daily and titrating up to a maximum of 50 mg paroxetine, according to clinical response). All three studies used CAPS-2 as one of the primary outcome measures. CAPS-2 scores were significantly reduced following 20 mg and 40 mg paroxetine treatment in the fixed dose study and following a mean dose of 32.5 mg/day for the flexible dose studies (mean dose at study endpoint 32.5 mg/day for study 648; 31.3 mg/day for study 637), with a highly significant improvement appearing within 4 weeks after the start of treatment and continuing through to study end (it should be noted that CAPS-2 was only assessed at weeks 4, 8 and 12 in two of the studies). Paroxetine was also effective compared with placebo for the CAPS-2 PTSD symptom cluster areas, re-experiencing/intrusion ($p < 0.001$), avoidance/numbing ($p < 0.001$) and increased arousal ($p < 0.001$); note that p values are based on combined data pooled across the three studies. Paroxetine was well tolerated with an adverse event profile similar to that in other anxiety disorders. Treatment benefit was observed across all trauma types and in both male ($p < 0.001$) and female ($p < 0.001$) patients.

Sertraline

Sertraline was shown to be a safe, well-tolerated and effective treatment for PTSD in two 12-week multicenter double-blind, placebo-controlled trials. In the study by Brady *et al.* (2000), patients were randomized to sertraline (50–200 mg/day flexible dosage) following one week at 25 mg/day ($N = 94$) or placebo ($N = 93$). Significantly greater improvement was noted in the sertraline treatment group compared to the placebo group on three of the four primary outcome measures—CAPS-2 total severity score, CGI-S and CGI-I. The fourth measure, Impact of Event Scale total score, tended towards significance. The responder rate (defined as > 30% reduction from baseline in CAPS-2 total severity score and a CGI-I score of I or 2) for sertraline was 53% compared to 32% for placebo at the end of the study. Furthermore, sertraline was significantly effective from week 2 on the CAPS-2 total severity score, and displayed significant efficacy vs. placebo on the CAPS-2 PTSD symptom clusters of avoidance/numbing and increased arousal, but not in relation to re-experiencing/intrusion. In the second study by Davidson *et al.* (2001), comparable results were obtained favoring sertraline across a wide range of symptoms.

OTHER DOUBLE-BLIND CONTROLLED TRIALS WITH SEROTONERGIC DRUGS

Additional clinical studies have evaluated tricyclic and MAO inhibitors which, while not selective in their actions upon serotonin, nevertheless have conspicuously pre-serotonergic properties. These include amitriptyline, imipramine, phenelzine and brofaromine.

Amitriptyline

In the first trial, which evaluated amitriptyline and placebo in combat veterans from World War II, Korea and Vietnam, Davidson *et al.* (1990) found that, over an 8-week period, subjects who received amitriptyline responded better than those on placebo on general measures of depression and anxiety, global severity for PTSD and the self-rated Impact of Event Scale, which measures PTSD symptoms. On structured interview for PTSD, no drug–placebo differences emerged. A high proportion of patients still retained diagnostic criteria for PTSD at the end of treatment, and comorbid major depression, panic disorder and alcohol abuse were regarded as negative predictors for good response to the drug. Nevertheless, amitriptyline did perform better than placebo when some degree of comorbidity was present, as compared to those who had only simple PTSD. In fact, it is rare for chronic PTSD to exist in isolation, and finding this to be the case in a person is atypical of clinical reality. In the absence of another comorbid disorder, the placebo response rate increased, while the drug response rate remained essentially the same. A slight, statistically significant, tendency was noted for amitriptyline to be more effective on avoidant symptoms than on intrusive symptoms, although the magnitude of the effect was small.

A subsequent report by the same group (Davidson *et al.*, 1993) evaluated predictors of response to amitriptyline in 62 patients. Bivariate statistical approaches were used and it was found that response to amitriptyline was best when original trauma exposure was less severe, when intensity of depression, anxiety and PTSD were less severe, and in the absence of neuroticism. Specific symptoms which predicted poorer outcome were: impaired concentration, somatic symptoms, feelings of guilt, and several avoidant symptoms from the Impact of Event Scale. When multivariate analyses were used to control for the effect of each variable upon each other, the following emerged as contributing the most to outcome. Using the CGI response status as outcome measure, logistic regression analysis revealed that a low baseline Hamilton score was the most powerful single predictor of good outcome. Using the Impact of Event Scale score as final outcome measure, linear regression analysis revealed that level of combat intensity was the single most powerful predictor. This is particularly interesting in light of the fact that between 20 and 40 years had elapsed between original trauma and entry into the protocol, and indicates the potent effects and influences of trauma exposure in underlying psychobiology and later treatment response.

Imipramine/phenelzine

A study evaluating imipramine and phenelzine vs. placebo was undertaken by Kosten and colleagues (1991). Imipramine was used up to a maximum of 300 mg/day, and phenelzine up to a maximum of 75 mg/day for a total of 8 weeks. In this combat veteran population, at least 8 years had elapsed since original exposure to trauma. Phenelzine produced by far the most marked improvement, with a high rate of global response (68%), and considerable reduction in intrusive and avoidant symptoms. Imipramine was associated with a clinical response of 65, and some degree of improvement on intrusive and avoidant symptoms, although less than that associated with phenelzine.

Brofaromine

Brofaromine is a reversible inhibitor of monoamine (RIMA) oxidase type A and, as such, a drug with considerable serotonergic effects. In a European study (Katz *et al.*, 1995) it was more effective than placebo in 45 subjects, most of whom were civilians. The mean length of treatment was 11–13 weeks. In the entire group, brofaromine was favored relative to placebo on the CAPS at significance level of $p = 0.08$, but in the more chronic PTSD groups, with symptoms lasting greater than 1 year, the difference was significant at $p < 0.05$. Fifty-five per cent of the brofaromine group were relieved of their diagnosis by the end of treatment, as compared to only 26% of the placebo group. The dose was started at 50 mg/day, and titrated up to a maximum of 150 mg/day, with the modal dose ending up as 100 mg/day. The drug produced some insomnia and agitation, along with headaches, nausea, dry mouth and 'flu-like symptoms, as the most common side effects. Insomnia was mentioned as the one side effect which imposed some limitation on clinical treatment.

In a larger US trial of brofaromine (Baker *et al.*, 1996), 118 patients were randomized to double-blind treatment, 113 of whom were eligible for an intent-to-treat analysis. While significant reductions in PTSD symptoms as measured by the CAPS were noted in both groups, no significant brofaromine–placebo differences were observed. The same was true of all other rating scales, except for the CGI which did show a 60% response rate for brofaromine, compared to 39% on drug, a difference which was statistically significant at $p < 0.05$. This raises the important question of just what is being rated in the CGI, and the need to include a composite of scales as representing a more comprehensive clinical picture. Unfortunately, brofaromine has been discontinued and at this point there is no concerted effort to explore the place of RIMAs in PTSD. However, both of the completed studies do suggest some promise for this class of drugs in the disorder.

SUMMARY

There seems no question that serotonergic drugs are effective in PTSD, a statement that can be supported on the basis of both theoretical considerations and direct practical application. There have been two positive placebo-controlled trials of fluoxetine in civilians with PTSD, and two negative trials in combat veterans with PTSD. On the other hand, there have been two positive placebo-controlled trials of tricyclic drugs and one of phenelzine in combat veterans with the disorder, so it would be premature to conclude that such patients are inherently treatment-resistant. The reversible inhibitor of MAO-A, brofaromine, did show promise, but in each study there were some qualifications as to the drug's efficacy: in the US study benefit was limited to a CGI rating, while in the European study efficacy was strongest in a subpopulation, namely the more chronic cases of PTSD. This in itself seems somewhat counterintuitive but raises the question of whether drug therapy is more effective once a clear set of pathogenic changes has become established. Somewhat related is the suggestion that comorbid PTSD responds better to antidepressant drug relative to placebo than does non-comorbid PTSD. Both studies by the author of this chapter (the amitriptyline study and the unpublished fluoxetine study) indicate that the drug–placebo differences are greatest in the presence of comorbidity. In part, this is thought to be related to the higher placebo response rate of non-comorbid PTSD. One important unanswered question is whether the efficacy of an antidepressant relative to placebo is sustained for a longer period of time, and what happens upon drug discontinuation. No data are available with respect to the last-mentioned point, but this author has unpublished data suggesting that continued treatment of fluoxetine or placebo for up to 6 months results in continued benefits of the drug, with no decline in efficacy, but relatively little further gain as compared to those who have initially responded to placebo and continued on the same. Some evidence has been provided for further improvement in disability measures beyond 12 weeks while taking fluoxetine. Long-term discontinuation design studies are important to consider in PTSD.

REFERENCES

American Psychiatric Association (1994) *Diagnostic and Statistical Manual of Mental Disorders*, 4th edn. Washington, DC: American Psychiatric Association.

American Psychiatric Association (1987) *Diagnostic and Statistical Manual of Mental Disorders*, 3rd edn (revised). Washington, DC: American Psychiatric Association.

Arora RC, Fichtner CG, O'Connor F, Crayton JW (1993) Paroxetine binding in the blood platelets of post-traumatic stress disorder patients. *Life Sciences*, **53**, 919–928.

Baker DG, Diamond BI, Gillette G, Hamner M, Katzelnick D, Keller T, Mellman TA, Pontius E, Rosenthal M, Tucker P, van der Kolk BA, Katz RJ, Lott MH (1996) A double-blind randomized, placebo-controlled, multi-center study of brofaromine in the treatment of post-traumatic stress disorder. *Psychopharmacology*, **122**, 386–389.

Blank AS (1993) The longitudinal course of post-traumatic stress disorder. In: JRT Davidson, EB Poa (eds) *Post-traumatic Stress Disorder: DSM-IV and Beyond*. Washington, DC: American Psychiatric Press, 3–22.

Brady K, Pearlstein T, Asnis GM, Baker D *et al.* (2000) Efficacy and safety of sertraline treatment of posttraumatic stress disorder: a randomized controlled trial. *JAMA*, **283**, 1837–1844.

Breslau N, Davis GC, Andreski P, Peterson E (1991) Traumatic events and post-traumatic stress disorder in an urban population of young adults. *Arch Gen Psychiat*, **48**, 216–222.

Brophy MH (1991) Cyproheptadine for combat nightmares in post-traumatic stress disorder and dream anxiety disorder. *Military Med*, **156**, 100–101.

Connor KM, Sutherland SM, Tupler LA, Malik ML *et al.* (1999). Fluoxetine in post-traumatic stress disorder. Randomised, double-blind study. *Br J Psychiat*, **175**, 17–22.

Davidson J, Roth S, Newman E (1991) Fluoxetine in post-traumatic stress disorder. *J Traum Stress*, **4**, 419–423.

Davidson JRT, Kudler H, Smith R, Mahorney SL, Lipper S, Hammett E, Saunders WB, Cavenar JO (1990) Treatment of post-traumatic stress disorder with amitriptyline and placebo. *Arch Gen Psychiat*, **47**, 259–266.

Davidson JRT, Kudler HS, Saunders WB, Erickson L, Smith RD, Stein RM, Lipper S, Hammett EGB, Mahorney SL, Cavenar JO (1993) Predicting response to amitriptyline in post-traumatic stress disorder. *Am J Psychiat*, **150**, 1024–1029.

Davidson JRT, Rothbaum BO, van der Kolk BA, Sikes CR, Farfel GM (2001) Multicenter, double-blind comparison of sertraline and placebo in the treatment of posttraumatic stress disorder. *Arch Gen Psychiat*, in press.

Davis LL, Nugent AL, Murray J, Kramer GL, Perry F (2000) Nefazodone treatment for chronic posttraumatic stress disorder: an open trial. *J Clin Psychopharmacol*, **20**, 159–164.

Deakin JFW (1988) 5-HT$_2$ receptors, depression and anxiety. *Pharmacol Biochem Behav*, **29**, 819–820.

de Boer M, Op der Velde W, Falger RJR, Hoveas JE, deGroen JHM, van Duijn H (1991) Fluvoxamine treatment for chronic PTSD. *Psychother Psychosomat*, **57**, 158–163.

Fichtner CG, Crayton JW (1994) Buspirone in combat-related post-traumatic stress disorder. *J Clin Psychopharmacol*, **14**, 79–81.

Fichtner CG, Arora RC, O'Connor FL, Crayton JW (1994) Platelet paroxetine binding and fluoxetine pharmacotherapy in post-traumatic stress disorder: preliminary observations on a possible predictor of clinical treatment response. *Life Sciences*, **54**, 39–44.

Friedman MJ, Schnurr PP (1995) The relationship between trauma, post-traumatic stress disorder, and physical health. In: MJ Friedman, DS Charney, AY Deutsch (eds) *Neurobiological and Clinical Consequences of Stress: From Normal Adaptation to Post-traumatic Stress Disorder*. New York: Lippicroft-Raven, 507–526.

Golding JM (1994) Sexual assault history and physical health in randomly selected Los Angeles women. *Health Psychol*, **13**, 130–138.

Hensman R, Guimaraes FS, Wang M, Deakin JFW (1991) Effects of ritanserin on aversive classical conditioning in humans. *Psychopharmacol*, **104**, 220–224.

Hertzberg MA, Feldman ME, Beckham JC, Davidson JRT (1996) Trial of trazodone for post-traumatic stress disorder using a multiple baseline group design. *J Clin Psychopharmacol*, **16**, 294–298.

Hertzberg MA, Feldman ME, Beckham, JC, Moore SD, Davidson JRT (1998) Open trial of nefazodone for combat-related posttraumatic stress disorder. *J Clin Psychiat*, **59**, 460–464.

Hertzberg MA, Feldman ME, Beckham JC, Hudler HA, Davidson JRT (2000) Lack of efficacy for fluoxetine in PTSD: a placebo-controlled trial in combat veterans. *Ann Clin Psychiat*, **12**, 101–105.

Joseph MH, Kennett GA (1983) Corticosteroid response to stress depends upon increased tryptophan availability. *Psychopharmacol*, **79**, 79–81.

Katz RJ, Lott MH, Arbus P, Crocq L, Harlobsen P, Lingjaerde O, Lopez G, Loughery GC, MacFarlane DJ, McIvor R, Mehlum L, Nugent D, Turner SW, Weisaeth L, Yule W (1995) Pharmacotherapy of post-traumatic stress disorder with a novel psychotropic. *Anxiety*, **1**, 169–174.

Kennett GA, Dickinson SL, Curzon G (1988) Enhancement of some 5-HT-dependent behavioral responses following repeated immobilization in rats. *Brain Res*, **330**, 253–263.

Kessler R, Sonnega A, Bromet E, Hughes M, Nelson CB (1995) Post-traumatic stress disorder in the National Comorbidity Survey. *Arch Gen Psychiat*, **52**, 1048–1060.

Kimerling R, Calhoun KS (1994) Somatic symptoms, social support and treatment seeking among sexual assault victims. *J Consult Clin Psychol,* **2**, 333–340.

Kline NA, Dow BM, Brown SA, Matloff JA (1994) Sertraline efficacy in depressed combat veterans with post-traumatic stress disorder. *Am J Psychiat,* **151**, 621.

Koss MP, Woodruff WJ, Koss PG (1990) Criminal victimization among primary care medical patients: prevalence, incidence and physician usage. *Behav Sci Law,* **9**, 85–96.

Kosten TR, Frank JB, Dan E, McDougle CJ, Giller EL Jr (1991) Pharmacotherapy for post-traumatic stress disorder using phenelzine or imipramine. *J Nerv Men Dis,* **1179**, 366–370.

Marmar CR, Schoenfeld F, Weiss DS, Metzler T, Zatzick D, Wu R *et al.* (1996) Open trial of fluvoxamine treatment for combat-rated posttraumatic stress disorder. *J Clin Psychiat,* **57** (suppl 8), 66–72.

Marshall RD, Schneier FR, Fallon BA, Knight CB *et al.* (1998) An open trial of paroxetine in patients with noncombat-related, chronic posttraumatic stress disorder. *J Clin Psychopharmacol,* **18**, 10–18.

McDougle CJ, Southwick SM, Charney DS, St. James RL (1991) An open clinical trial of fluoxetine in the treatment of post-traumatic stress disorder. *J Clin Psychopharmacol,* **11**, 325–327.

McFarlane AC (1989) The aetiology of post-traumatic morbidity: predisposing, precipitating and perpetuating factors. *Br J Psychiat,* **154**, 221–228.

Meltzer-Brody S, Connor KM, Churchill LE, Davidson JRT (2000) Symptom-specific effects of fluoxetine in post-traumatic stress disorder. *Int Clin Psychopharmacol,* **15**, 227–231.

Miller TR, Cohen MA, Rossman SB (1993) Victim costs of violent crime and resulting injuries. *Health Affairs,* **Winter**, 186–197.

Miller TR, Cohen MA, Wiessman B (1996) *Victim Costs and Consequences: A New Look.* Washington DC: United States Department of Justice, National Institute of Justice, Research Report.

Nagy LM, Morgan CA, Southwick SM, Charney DS (1993) Open prospective trial of fluoxetine for post-traumatic stress disorder. *J Clin Psychopharmacol,* **13**, 107–114.

Resnick PJ (1995) Guidelines for the evaluation of malingering in post-traumatic stress disorder. In: RL Simon (ed) *Post-traumatic Stress Disorder in Litigation.* Washington, DC: American Psychiatric Press, 117–136.

Rothbaum BD, Ninan PT, Thomas L (1996) Sertraline in the treatment of rape victims with post-traumatic stress disorder. *J Traum Stress,* **9**, 865 471.

Rothbaum BO, Foa EB, Riggs DS, Murdock T, Walsh W (1992) A prospective examination of post-traumatic stress disorder in rape victims. *J Traum Stress,* **5**, 455–475.

Shay J (1992) Fluoxetine reduces explosiveness and elevates mood of Vietnam combat veterans with PTSD. *J Traum Stress,* **5**, 97–101.

Solomon SD, Davidson JRT (1997) Trauma, prevalence, impairment, service use, and cost. *J Clin Psychiat,* **58** (suppl 9), 5–11.

Southwick SM, Yehuda R, Morgan CA III (1995) Clinical studies of neurotransmitter alterations in post-traumatic stress disorder. In: MJ Friedman, DS Charney, AY Deutsch (eds) *Neurobiological and Clinical Consequences of Stress: From National Adaptation to Post-Traumatic Stress Disorder.* New York: Lippicroft-Raven, 335–349.

Stein DJ (2000) Improving treatment options—new clinical data on paroxetine. CINP 2000.

van der Kolk BA, Dreyfuss D, Michaels M, Shera D, Berkowitz B, Fisher R, Saxe G (1994) Fluoxetine in post-traumatic stress disorder. *J Clin Psychiat,* **55**, 517–522.

Weissman A, Herbert CA (1972) Recent developments relating serotonin and behavior. *Ann Rep Med Chem,* **7**, 47–58.

Wolfe J, Schnurr PP, Brown PJ *et al.* (1994) Post-traumatic stress disorder and war-zone exposure as correlates of perceived health in female Vietnam War veterans. *J Consult Clin Psychol,* **62**, 1235–1240.

9

SSRIs in the treatment of generalized anxiety disorder

David S. Baldwin

INTRODUCTION

Generalized anxiety disorder (GAD) is a common and usually long-standing medical condition which often requires long-term treatment (Mahe and Balogh, 2000). The lifetime prevalence of GAD in the general population is estimated to be around 5–6% (Wittchen *et al.*, in press). The 12-month prevalence for GAD varies according to which diagnostic criteria are used—from 1.5% according to DSM-IV (Wittchen *et al.*, in press) to 3.1% with DSM-III-R criteria (Wittchen *et al.*, 1994). GAD is amongst the most common psychiatric disorders seen in primary health care (Sartorius *et al.*, 1996). The point prevalence of ICD-10 defined GAD in five European primary care settings was 4.8% for GAD without other depressive or anxiety disorders, and 3.7% for GAD with depression; a further 4.1% of patients had "sub-threshold" GAD (Weiller *et al.*, 1998).

The core features of GAD are uncontrollable worrying, somatic anxiety and tension. Other common symptoms include insomnia and headache. The DSM-IV criteria for GAD (American Psychiatric Association, 1994) are shown in Table 9.1, and the ICD-10 criteria in Table 9.2 (World Health Organization, 1993). Like other anxiety disorders, GAD is often comorbid with other mental disorders, most commonly with major depression (Wittchen *et al.*, 1994; Kessler *et al.*, 1997; Wittchen *et al.*, 1998). Comorbidity, especially with major depressive disorder, has been shown to increase the disability and impairment associated with GAD (Wittchen *et al.*, 2000).

SSRIs in Depression and Anxiety, Second Edition. Edited by S.A. Montgomery and J.A. den Boer.
© 2001 John Wiley & Sons Ltd.

Table 9.1. Simplified DSM-IV diagnostic criteria for generalized anxiety disorder.

A	Excessive anxiety and worry (apprehensive expectation), occurring more days than not for at least 6 months, about a number of events or activities.
B	The person finds it difficult to control the worry.
C	The anxiety and worry are associated with three or more of the following six symptoms: 1 Restlessness or feeling keyed up or on edge 2 Being easily fatigued 3 Difficulty concentrating or mind going blank 4 Irritability 5 Muscle tension 6 Sleep disturbance
D	The focus of the anxiety and worry is not confined to features of another axis I disorder
E	Symptoms cause clinically significant distress or impairment in social, occupational or other important areas of functioning
F	The disturbance is not due to the direct physiological effects of a substance or a general medical condition, and does not occur exclusively during a mood disorder, psychotic disorder or pervasive developmental disorder

Modified from American Psychiatric Association (1994), by permission.

Effective treatment of patients with GAD can be achieved with pharmacological and psychological approaches. Approximately 50% of patients make a significant response to cognitive behavioural therapy (Nathan and Gorman, 1998). Pharmacological treatments which have been used successfully in the treatment of GAD include various antidepressant drugs, benzodiazepines and azapirones (Gale and Oakley-Browne, 2000).

In view of the potential of benzodiazepines to lead to dependence and impairment of cognitive and psychomotor functions, their long-term use should usually be avoided (Lydiard, 2000). Although initial findings generally showed that buspirone was effective in patients with GAD (Strand et al., 1990; Enkelman, 1991), other studies have reported conflicting results (Ansseau et al., 1990; Rickels and Schweizer, 1998). In 1986, the tricyclic antidepressant imipramine was found to be efficacious in patients with mixed anxiety and depressive disorders (Kahn et al. 1986). The beneficial properties of imipramine in relieving psychic anxiety were confirmed shortly thereafter (Hoehn-Saric et al., 1988). In 1993, Rickels demonstrated the efficacy of antidepressants (imipramine) in GAD, even in patients without depressive features or panic attacks (Rickels et al., 1993). The first evidence for the efficacy of selective serotonin reuptake inhibitors in the treatment of GAD came from a comparative study in which paroxetine and imipramine showed greater efficacy than a benzodiazepine (Rocca et al., 1997): this is now supported by the findings of larger placebo-controlled treatment studies with paroxetine.

Table 9.2. Simplified research diagnostic criteria for ICD-10 generalized anxiety disorder.

A	At least 6 months with prominent tension, worry and feelings of apprehension about everyday events and problems.

B At least four of the following symptoms (at least one from items 1–4):

Autonomic arousal symptoms
1   Palpitations or pounding heart or accelerated heart rate
2   Sweating
3   Trembling or shaking
4   Dry mouth (not due to medication or dehydration)

Symptoms involving chest and abdomen
5   Difficulty in breathing
6   Feeling of choking
7   Chest pain or discomfort
8   Nausea or abdominal distress

Symptoms involving mental state
9   Feeling dizzy, unsteady, faint or light-headed
10 Feeling that objects are unreal (derealization) or that the self is distant or "not really here" (depersonalization)
11 Fear of losing control, "going crazy" or passing out
12 Fear of dying

General symptoms
13 Hot flushes or cold chills
14 Numbness or tingling sensations

Symptoms of tension
15 Muscle tension or aches and pains
16 Restlessness and inability to relax
17 Feeling keyed up, on edge or mentally tense
18 A sensation of a lump in the throat, or difficulty in swallowing

Other non-specific symptoms
19 Exaggerated responses to minor surprises or being startled
20 Difficulty in concentrating, or mind "going blank"
21 Persistent irritability
22 Difficulty in getting to sleep because of worry

C   The disorder does not meet the criteria for another anxiety disorder.

D   The disorder is not due to a physical disorder, organic mental disorder or a psychoactive substance-related disorder

Modified from World Health Organization (1993), with permission.

DIAGNOSIS OF GENERALIZED ANXIETY DISORDER

Like most depressive and anxiety disorders, GAD is under-diagnosed and under-treated. The DSM-IV diagnostic criteria for GAD have greatly clarified the diagnosis, but recognition is often complicated by the presence of comorbid psychiatric disorders such as depression or other anxiety disorders (Wittchen *et al.*, 1994). However, a recent study (Kessler *et al.*, 1999) has shown that a substantial amount of GAD occurs independently of major depression, indicating that GAD is neither a prodromal condition for, nor a consequence of, depression. Comorbid depressive symptoms do appear to improve the chances of a patient's being recognized as suffering from a psychological problem, though not necessarily from GAD (Weiller *et al.*, 1998).

The characteristic features of GAD are unrealistic or excessive anxiety and worrying about a number of events or activities, which is persistent (more than 6 months) and not restricted to particular circumstances. Common features include apprehension, with worries about future misfortune, inner tension and difficulty in concentrating; motor tension, with restlessness, tremor and headache; and autonomic anxiety, with excessive perspiration, dry mouth and epigastric discomfort.

The diagnosis of GAD may be made in individuals who have multiple chronic worries, including finance, family, work and health amongst other issues. There is excessive worrying, most of the day, most days for 6 months. Patients are usually aware that they are worrying excessively, but are unable to stop (American Psychiatric Association, 1994; Andrews and Garrity, 2000). The anxiety is "free-floating", i.e. is not confined to any particular thing or event, as is the case with the other anxiety disorders. A minimum of three physical symptoms such as fatigue, irritability, tension, insomnia or restlessness are also required to meet the DSM-IV diagnosis of GAD (American Psychiatric Association, 1994).

Many patients with GAD present with some accompanying depressive symptoms, although, where they occur together, anxiety usually precedes depression (Andrews and Garrity, 2000; Breslau *et al.*, 1995; Wittchen *et al.*, 1998; Kessler *et al.*, in press). General somatic presentations such as headaches, fatigue, muscular tension and sleeping problems may also delay diagnosis. In primary care, patients usually present with mainly somatic symptoms or sleeping problems.

BURDEN OF THE DISORDER

GAD is associated with significant disability (Weiller *et al.*, 1998; Kessler *et al.*, 1999), the functional impairment being similar in magnitude to that of major depression (Kessler *et al.*, 1999; Wittchen *et al.*, 2000). When comorbidity does exist, patients have more severe symptoms and greater functional impairment, and are more likely to have a prolonged course of illness (Wittchen *et al.*, 1995; Weiller *et al.*, 1998; Kessler *et al.*, 1999).

Community and primary care surveys consistently demonstrate a high degree of comorbidity between depression and anxiety disorders (Kessler *et al.*, 1994; Wittchen *et al.*, 1994; Stein *et al.*, 1995; Kessler *et al.*, 1997; Judd *et al.*, 1998; Wittchen *et al.*, 1998). The burden of comorbid GAD and depression includes decreased productivity (Wittchen *et al.*, in press; Carter *et al.*, in press) and high levels of healthcare utilization (Brown *et al.*, 1990; Maier and Falkai; 1999; Carter and Maddock, 1992; Logue *et al.*, 1993; Lydiard *et al.*, 1993; Greenberg *et al.*, 1999).

COURSE OF ILLNESS

The age of onset of GAD differs from that usually seen with the other anxiety disorders. Although some cases can occur before the age of 25, the majority of patients present somewhat later in life, typically around 35–45 years old (Carter *et al.*, in press; Wittchen *et al.*, in press; Yonkers *et al.*, 2000). GAD is probably the most common anxiety disorder among the elderly population (55–85 years) (Beekman *et al.*, 1998).

Typically GAD is a chronic and fluctuating disorder with a waxing and waning course, which is frequently associated with other psychiatric disorders (Wittchen *et al.*, 1994; Carter *et al.*, in press). Although the symptoms of GAD may fluctuate over time, it is usually a chronic anxiety disorder (Weiller *et al.*, 1998). The duration of the key symptom of excessive worrying increases with age: from around 1 month for younger patients to up to 6 months or more in elderly patients. GAD is particularly associated with adverse life events and environmental stress, and there is a strong association with physical illness. It is often present in patients with "medically unexplained physical symptoms".

EFFICACY OF SSRIs IN GENERALIZED ANXIETY DISORDER

The efficacy of SSRIs has been demonstrated in placebo-controlled studies in anxiety disorders such as obsessive compulsive disorder, panic disorder and social phobia (Lydiard *et al.*, 1996; Davidson, 1998; Baldwin and Birtwistle, 2000). More recently, SSRIs have shown efficacy in post-traumatic stress disorder (Davidson, 2000) and generalised anxiety disorder.

Paroxetine

The efficacy of paroxetine in patients with GAD has been evaluated in four randomized double-blind controlled studies. One study compared paroxetine to imipramine and a benzodiazepine; the other three compared paroxetine to placebo.

The first evaluation of paroxetine was through a comparator-controlled trial involving 81 patients with a DSM-IV diagnosis of GAD, in which paroxetine was compared with imipramine and 2′-chlorodesmethyldiazepam over an 8-week treatment period (Rocca *et al.*, 1997). Paroxetine showed superior efficacy to 2'-chlorodesmethyldiazepam and similar efficacy to imipramine. The efficacy of paroxetine differed significantly ($p < 0.05$) from that of 2'-chlorodesmethyldiazepam from week 4 onwards, while imipramine did so only at week 8.

The second investigation was an 8-week dose-finding study of 566 patients with GAD, performed in the United States. In this, paroxetine (20 or 40 mg/day) was significantly superior to placebo ($p < 0.001$) in the reduction of both the HAM-A total score (see Figure 9.1) and the scores on HAM-A items 1 and 2, key items in patients with GAD (Bellew *et al.*, 2000a). In addition, 68% and 81% of patients treated with paroxetine 20 mg and 40 mg/day, respectively, were considered responders to treatment, compared with 52% of patients in the placebo group (observed case data). Furthermore, a health-related quality of life questionnaire (EuroQol-5D) and a visual analogue scale (VAS), administered at baseline and at the end of treatment, showed that patients had significantly impaired quality of life at baseline compared with the general population. By the end of the study, the mean change from baseline in the EuroQol-5D and VAS was significantly greater for both paroxetine treatment groups (vs. placebo), indicating a significant improvement in quality of life (Bellew *et al.*, 2000b).

Similarly, in an 8-week flexible-dose study conducted in 326 patients with GAD in the United States, paroxetine (20–50 mg/day) was also significantly superior to placebo ($p < 0.05$) in the reduction of the HAM-A total score and HAM-A Items 1 and 2 (McCafferty *et al.*, 2000) (see Figures 9.2 and 9.3). In addition, paroxetine was well tolerated in the dose range 20–50 mg/day. Finally, a study of the same design was conducted in 372 patients in Europe, and similar reductions in HAM-A total score and HAM-A Items 1 and 2 were observed (Baldwin, 2000).

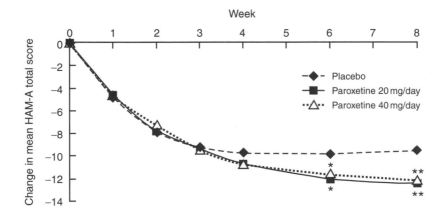

Figure 9.1. Fixed dose study: HAM-A total score. * $p < 0.027$ vs. placebo (adjusted for pairwise comparisons), ** $p < 0.001$ vs. placebo

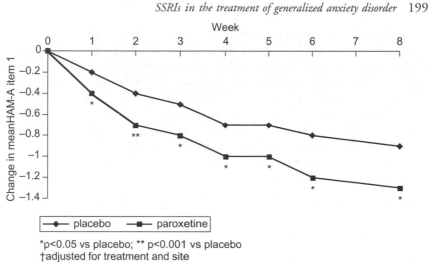

*p<0.05 vs placebo; ** p<0.001 vs placebo
†adjusted for treatment and site
Mean dose at endpoint = 34.3mg/day

Figure 9.2. Flexible dose study: HAM-A item 1 (anxious meed). $^*p < 0.05$ vs. placebo, $^{**}p < 0.001$ vs. placebo. Mean dose at endpoint = 34.3 mg/day

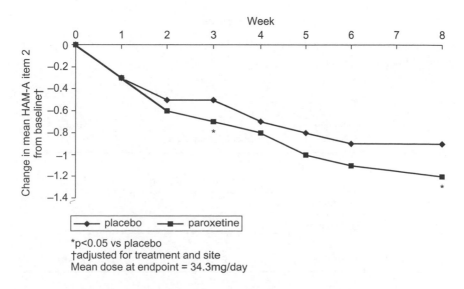

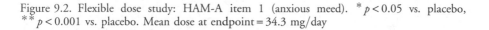

*p<0.05 vs placebo
†adjusted for treatment and site
Mean dose at endpoint = 34.3mg/day

Figure 9.3. Flexible dose study: HAM-A items 2 (tension). $^*p < 0.05$ vs. placebo, † adjusted for treatment and site. Mean dose at endpoint = 34.4 mg/day

The beneficial effects of paroxetine in GAD may extend beyond symptom reduction and improved quality of life. In a small, uncontrolled pilot study of volunteers with GAD ($n = 29$), treatment with paroxetine for between 4 and 6 months was associated with a reduction in maladaptive personality traits (Allgulander *et al.*, 1998). Following assessment with the Temperament and Character Inventory (Cloninger *et al.*, 1994), patients showed a significant decrease in harm avoidance ($p = 0.0001$) and novelty seeking ($p = 0.006$), and a significant increase in self-directedness ($p = 0.0004$). These intriguing findings require confirmation in a controlled study.

Recently, paroxetine has been found efficacious in the long-term treatment of GAD, there being fewer relapses with paroxetine (11%) than with placebo (40%) in a six month relapse-prevention study (Montgomery, 2000) (Figure 4.4).

Fluoxetine

There are no published studies of fluoxetine in the treatment of adults with DSM-IV GAD. An open pilot treatment study in 16 children and adolescents (9–18 years) with mixed anxiety disorders showed that fluoxetine might be of some benefit. In this investigation, mean doses of fluoxetine of 24 mg/day in children and 40 mg/day in adolescents produced clinical improvement in 10 of 10 patients with current separation anxiety disorder, 8 of 10 with social phobia, 4 of 6 with specific phobia, 3 of 5 with panic disorder, and 1 of 7 with GAD, the mean time to improvement being 5 weeks (Fairbanks *et al.*, 1997).

Citalopram

No controlled trials with citalopram in the treatment of GAD have yet been presented or published.

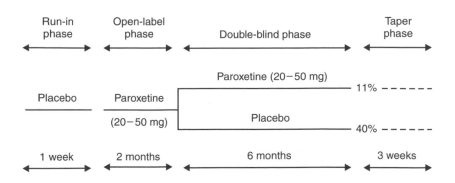

Figure 9.4. Paroxetine. GAD relapse prevention study.

Fluvoxamine

The efficacy of fluvoxamine as a treatment for GAD has not been established. However, in a small open study of patients with comorbid major depression and GAD ($n = 30$), fluvoxamine treatment led to significant improvement in both anxiety and depressive symptoms (Sonawalla *et al.*, 1999). Understandably, this finding requires replication in patients with GAD before the efficacy of fluvoxamine can be assumed.

Sertraline

No clinical trials of sertraline in the treatment of GAD have been reported.

EFFICACY OF OTHER SEROTONERGIC ANTIDEPRESSANT DRUGS IN GENERALIZED ANXIETY DISORDER

Nefazodone

Nefazodone inhibits the reuptake of both serotonin and noradrenaline, although its strongest action is antagonism of the 5-HT_{2A} receptor (Taylor *et al.*, 1995). Studies in patients with major depression and associated anxiety indicate that nefazodone can significantly reduce anxiety symptoms (Fontaine *et al.*, 1994), and a small open-label evaluation suggests that it can improve the symptoms of GAD (Hedges *et al.*, 1996).

Venlafaxine

Venlafaxine is a serotonin–noradrenaline reuptake inhibitor (SNRI), with proven efficacy in the treatment of depression and GAD. A preliminary study (Feighner *et al.*, 1998) in depressed outpatients indicated that once-daily venlafaxine was efficacious in relieving anxiety symptoms, and suggested it might therefore have a role in the management of patients with GAD. This supposition was confirmed by the findings of two studies of short-term treatment of GAD with venlafaxine (Davidson *et al.*, 1999; Rickels *et al.*, 2000). In one study, venlafaxine was significantly superior to the active comparator buspirone in reducing anxiety symptoms, and there was some evidence that venlafaxine had an earlier onset of action (Davidson *et al.*, 1999). Three other placebo-controlled studies of venlafaxine in the short-term treatment of GAS have been presented (Salinas, 1999; Hackett *et al.*, 2000). Efficacy is reported in two of the three studies of venlaflaxine compared to placebo, but until these studies are published fully it is difficult to make a detailed assessment. The long-term efficacy of venlafaxine extended-release capsules has been shown through the results of a 6-month randomized, double-blind, placebo-controlled, parallel-group study (Gelenberg *et al.*, 2000). These six-month results were replicated in a second placebo-controlled study, as yet unpublished (Allgulander *et al.*, in press). The single relapse prevention study, over a period of four months, did not show efficacy for venlafaxine, compared to placebo. Evidence supporting a dose-response relationship for venlafaxine is reported in the six-month studies, with higher doses associated with a better response.

Mirtazapine

The primary mechanism of action of mirtazapine is through antagonism of presynaptic α_2-receptors and heteroceptors. No studies of mirtazapine in GAD have been reported, although a small placebo-controlled study of outpatients with primary anxiety disorders indicated that it could reduce anxiety symptoms and improve overall functioning (Sitsen *et al.*, 1994). A meta-analysis of eight double-blind, controlled treatment studies in patients with major depression suggests that mirtazapine is efficacious in reducing anxiety-related items of the Hamilton Rating Scale for Depression (Fawcett and Barkin, 1998).

RECOMMENDATIONS FOR TREATMENT

Pharmacological approaches

Although many patients with GAD are not recognized as suffering from a potentially treatable medical condition, it seems probable that most recognized patients receive some form of treatment. The results from the five European centres in the World Health Organization study on Psychological Problems in General Health Care indicate psychotropic drug treatment rates of 64.3% for subthreshold GAD, 44.7% for GAD itself, and 51.9% for GAD with depression (Weiller *et al.*, 1998). However, it is unclear whether GAD patients receive drugs of proven efficacy at the right dosage or for sufficient duration to have symptoms relieved effectively.

It is common practice in the United Kingdom for general practitioners and psychiatrists to prescribe either β-blockers, or even conventional antipsychotic drugs to patients with anxiety symptoms (El-Khayat and Baldwin, 1999): this cannot be considered "evidence-based" practice in patients with GAD (Gale and Oakley-Browne, 2000), as no double-blind, placebo-controlled studies of β-blockers have been published, and the evidence regarding trifluoperazine is based on one short-term randomized, controlled trial in which it was found to be efficacious but poorly tolerated (Mendels *et al.*, 1986). Furthermore, treatment with antipsychotics carries a significant risk of extrapyramidal symptoms including tardive dyskinesia, and cannot be recommended (El-Khayat and Baldwin, 1998).

Recommendations for the treatment of anxiety disorders changed considerably between 1992 and 1997: more recently, tricyclic antidepressants are advocated noticeably less often and SSRIs are recommended considerably more frequently, whereas the use of benzodiazepines is mentioned at a similar frequency (Uhlenhuth *et al.*, 1999). A systematic review of randomized controlled trials has established that benzodiazepines are an effective and rapid treatment for many patients with GAD (Gould *et al.*, 1997).

However, the benzodiazepines are far from ideal anxiolytic drugs. The untoward effects of benzodiazepines include sedation, memory disruption and psychomotor impairment, with an associated increased risk of traffic accidents. Other problems include the development of tolerance, abuse and dependence, and withdrawal symptoms on stopping the drug. This being so, many authorities counsel that benzodiazepines should be reserved for short-term use (up to 4 weeks), and prescribed at low dosage (Lader, 1999). Others have argued that benzodiazepines are clearly efficacious, and that withholding treatment on the basis of a potential risk of dependence may be unjustified and detrimental to overall well-being (Argyropoulos and Nutt, 1999). The comparative efficacy and tolerability of benzodiazepines, buspirone, tricyclic antidepressants and SSRIs are compared in Table 9.3).

Buspirone is a azapirone anxiolytic drug, with partial agonist properties at 5-HT_{1A} receptors, which has proven efficacy in the treatment of patients with GAD (Goa and Ward, 1986). An early study (Goldberg and Finnerty, 1979) established that buspirone had comparable efficacy to diazepam in patients with generalized anxiety, and a meta-analysis of eight controlled treatment studies indicates that buspirone has comparable efficacy to benzodiazepines in the management of GAD (Gammans *et al.*, 1992). It also appears efficacious in reducing associated depressive symptoms in patients with GAD, but is not an accepted treatment for patients with major depression (Sramek *et al.*, 1996). However, not all studies with buspirone have been positive (Ansseau *et al.*, 1990; Rickels and Schweizer, 1998).

Table 9.3. Comparison of anxiolytic properties of differing drugs.

Property	Benzodiazepines	Buspirone	Tricyclic antidepressants	SSRIs
Onset of action	Fast	Slow	Slow	Slow
Initial exacerbation	No	Sometimes	Sometimes	Sometimes
Tolerance	Rare	No	No	No
Acute withdrawal	~30%	No	~10%	~10%
Chronic withdrawal	~10%	No	No	No
Abuse liability	Moderate	Zero	Zero	Zero
Ethanol interaction	Marked	Slight	Some	None
Sedation	Yes	No	Yes	No
Amnesia	Marked	No	Moderate	No
Cardiovascular effects	No	No	Marked	No
Depression	Sometimes	No	No	No
Gastrointestinal effects	No	Yes	Some	Yes
Dizziness	No	Yes	Yes	Yes
Insomnia	No	Rare	No	Yes

Based on Argyropoulos and Nutt (1999), by permission.

Flesinoxan is a related drug, which acts as a full agonist at somatodendritic 5-HT$_{1A}$ receptors: it too has been found efficacious in the treatment of GAD. A five-arm study comparing three doses of flesinoxan, alprazolam and placebo found that both the highest dose of flesinoxan and alprazolam were significantly more efficacious than placebo in reducing anxiety symptoms, rated by the HAM-A (Bradford and Stevens, 1994), but there is little further information on the efficacy of the drug.

Other potential future approaches to the management of patients with GAD include treatment with subtype-selective benzodiazepines, and cholecystokinin (CCK) antagonists. There is good evidence for the efficacy of the β-carboline abercarnil, which acts as an agonist (full or partial, depending on site) at the benzodiazepine–GABA complex (Aufdembrinke, 1998). Four placebo-controlled studies (Ballenger *et al.*, 1991; Lydiard *et al.*, 1997; Pollack *et al.*, 1997; Small and Bystritsky, 1997) have provided evidence for the efficacy of abercarnil in the management of patients with GAD. So far, trials with CCK antagonists have produced disappointing results: a 4-week multi-centre double-blind, placebo-controlled, parallel-group study with the CCK-B antagonist CI-988 failed to reveal efficacy, although interpretation of the study findings is difficult because of a significant treatment-by-centre interaction (Adams *et al.*, 1995).

At present, only the SSRI paroxetine and the SNRI venlafaxine are licensed for the treatment of DSM-IV GAD. A consensus statement on the treatment of GAD, which considers the evidence for efficacy of different management options, has been prepared by the International Consensus Group on Depression and Anxiety and is to be published shortly. At present, the evidence for efficacy of drug treatment in GAD is strongest for paroxetine and venlafaxine, being based upon the results of randomized, double-blind, placebo-controlled studies in short- and long-term treatment.

Psychological approaches

A systematic review of 35 randomized, controlled trials has found that cognitive therapy, using a combination of interventions such as anxiety management training, relaxation, cognitive restructuring and exposure, is more effective than remaining on a waiting list, anxiety management alone, or non-directive therapy (Gould *et al.*, 1997). Furthermore, a 1-year follow-up found that cognitive therapy was associated with better outcomes than either analytic psychotherapy or anxiety management training (Durham *et al.*, 1999).

It is unclear whether there is a clear advantage for combining pharmacological and psychological treatment approaches in the management of patients with GAD, over using single approaches alone (Lader and Bond, 1998). In a comparative study of behaviour therapy and cognitive therapy in 40 patients with GAD (Durham and Turvey, 1987), concomitant treatment with benzodiazepines significantly reduced the proportion of patients with a good outcome (8% with benzodiazepines, 86% without) (Wardle, 1990). By contrast, a 10-week treatment study in general practice patients with GAD found that the combination of diazepam and cognitive-behaviour therapy was more effective than either treatment given alone, in terms of the onset of improvement and clinical response at the end of the study (Power *et al.*, 1990).

CONCLUSIONS

GAD is a common and disabling anxiety disorder: epidemiological studies indicate that the lifetime prevalence of GAD is approximately 5%, and that it is associated with a degree of social and occupational impairment which is comparable to that with major depression. GAD has considerable comorbidity, with depression, other anxiety disorders and physical illness. Many patients with GAD are not recognized as suffering from a potentially treatable anxiety disorder; many others are recognized, but are either not treated or receive treatment with drugs of unproven efficacy. Whilst some tricyclic antidepressants and benzodiazepines have been found efficacious in GAD, tolerability problems and other risks limit their use in clinical practice. By contrast, buspirone, the selective SSRI paroxetine and the SNRI venlafaxine have all established their efficacy in placebo-controlled trials. There is a need for a comparative trial of venlafaxine and paroxetine, to establish which drug has the better benefit-to-risk profile in routine practice.

REFERENCES

Adams JB, Pyke RE, Costa J, *et al.* (1995) A double-blind, placebo-controlled study of a CCK-B antagonist, CI-988, in patients with generalised anxiety disorder. *J Clin Psychopharmacol,* **15**, 428–434.

Allgulander C, Cloninger CR, Przybeck TR, Brandt L (1998) Changes on the temperament and character inventory after paroxetine treatment in volunteers with generalized anxiety disorder. *Psychopharmacol Bull,* **34**, 165–166.

Allgulander C, Hackett D, Salinas E. Venlafaxine ER in the treatment of generalised anxiety disorder: a 24-week placebo-controlled dose-ranging study. *Br J Psychiatry,* in press.

American Psychiatric Association (1994) *Diagnostic and Statistical Manual of Mental Disorders,* 4th edn. Washington, DC: American Psychiatric Association.

Andrews G, Garrity A (2000) Anxiety disorders: recognition and management. *Aust Fam Physician,* **29**, 337–341.

Ansseau M, Papart P, Gerard MA, von Frenckell R, Franck G (1990) Controlled comparison of buspirone and oxazepam in generalized anxiety. *Neuropsychobiology,* **24**, 74–78.

Argyropoulos SV, Nutt DJ (1999) The use of benzodiazepines in anxiety and other disorders. *Eur Neuropsychopharmacol,* **9**(suppl 6), S407–S412.

Aufembrinke B (1998) Abercarnil, a new beta-carboline, in the treatment of anxiety disorders. *Br J Psychiatry,* **173**(suppl. 34), 55–63.

Baldwin DS (2000) SSRIs in the treatment of Generalised anxiety disorder. SB satellite symposium during European College of Neuropsychopharmacology, Munich, September 10.

Baldwin DS, Birtwistle J (2000) Selective serotonin re-uptake inhibitors in anxiety disorders: room for improvement. In: M Briley, D Nutt (eds) *Anxiolytics.* Basel: Birkhäuser, 55–75.

Ballenger JC, McDonald S, Noyes R, *et al.* (1991) The first double-blind placebo-controlled trial of a partial BZD agonist abercarnil (ZK-112-119) in generalised anxiety disorder. *Psychopharmacol Bull,* **27**, 171–179.

Beekman AT, Bremmer MA, Deeg DJ, van Balkom AJ, Smit JH, de Beurs E, van Dyck R, van Tilburg W (1998) Anxiety disorders in later life: a report from the Longitudinal Aging Study Amsterdam. *Int J Geriatr Psychiat,* **13**, 717–726.

Bellew KM, McCafferty JP, Lyengar M, *et al.* (2000a) Short-term efficacy of paroxetine in generalized anxiety disorder: a double-blind placebo controlled trial. Presented at the 153th Annual Meeting of the American Psychiatric Association, Chicago, May 13–18 (NR253).

Bellew KM, McCafferty JP, Zaninelli R (2000b) Paroxetine improves quality of life in patients with generalized anxiety disorder. *Int J Neuropsychopharmacol,* **3**(suppl 1), S226–227.

Bradford LD, Stevens G (1994) Double-blind, placebo-controlled fixed dose study of flesinoxan in generalized anxiety disorder. *Am Coll Neuropsychopharmacol,* **167**.

Breslau N, Schultz L, Peterson E (1995) Sex differences in depression: a role for preexisting anxiety. *Psychiat Res,* **58**, 1–12.

Brown FW, Golding JM, Smith GR Jr (1990) Psychiatric comorbidity in primary care somatization disorder. *Psychosom Med,* **52**, 445–451.

Carter CS, Maddock RJ (1992) Chest pain in generalized anxiety disorder. *Int J Psychiat Med,* **22**, 291–298.

Carter RM, Wittchen H-U, Pfister H, Kessler RC One-year prevalence of subthreshold and threshold DSM-IV generalised anxiety disorder in a nationally representative sample. *Depress Anxiety,* in press.

Cloninger CR, Przybeck TR, Svrakic DM *et al.* (1994) The temperament and character inventory (TCI): a guide to its development and use. St Louis, Mo: Center for Psychobiology of Personality, Washington University.

Davidson JRT (2000) Pharmacotherapy of social anxiety disorder. *J Clin Psychiat,* **59**(suppl 17), 47–51.

Davidson JRT (2000) Pharmacotherapy of posttraumatic stress disorder: treatment options, long-term follow-up, and predictors of outcome. *J Clin Psychiat,* **61**, 52–59.

Davidson JRT, DuPont RL, Hedges D, *et al.* (1999) Efficacy, safety, and tolerability of venlafaxine extended release and buspirone in outpatients with generalized anxiety disorder. *J Clin Psychiat,* **60**, 528–530.

Durham RC, Turvey AA (1987) Cognitive therapy versus behaviour therapy in the treatment of chronic generalised anxiety. *Behav Res Ther,* **25**, 229–234.

Durham RC, Fisher PL, Trevling LR *et al.* (1999) One year follow-up of cognitive therapy, analytic psychotherapy and anxiety management training for generalised anxiety disorder: symptom change, medication usage and attitudes to treatment. *Behav Consult Psychother,* **27**, 19–35.

El-Khayat R, Baldwin DS (1998) Antipsychotic drugs for non-psychotic patients: assessment of the benefit/risk ratio in generalized anxiety disorder. *J Psychopharmacol,* **12**, 323–329.

El-Khayat R, Baldwin DS (1999) Antipsychotic drugs for non-psychotic patients. Results of a questionnaire survey of prescribing practices among Wessex psychiatrists. *Psychiatr Bull,* **23**, 416–418.

Enkelman R (1991) Alprazolam versus buspirone in the treatment of outpatients with generalized anxiety disorder. *Psychopharmacology,* **105**, 428–432.

Fairbanks JM, Pine DS, Tancer NK, Dummit ES III, *et al.* (1997) Open fluoxetine treatment of mixed anxiety disorders in children and adolescents. *J Child Adolesc Psychopharmacol,* **7**, 17–29.

Fawcett J, Barkin RL (1998) Meta-analysis of eight randomized, double-blind, controlled trials of nefazodone, a novel antidepressant drug. *J Clin Psychiat,* **59**, 123–127.

Feighner JP, Entsuah AR, McPherson MK (1998) Efficacy of once-daily venlafaxine extended release (XR) for symptoms of anxiety in depressed outpatients. *J Affect Disord*, **47**, 55–62.

Fontaine R, Ontiveros A, Elie R, *et al.* (1994) Double-blind comparison of nefazodone, imipramine, and placebo in major depression. *J Clin Psychiat*, **55**, 234–241.

Gale C, Oakley-Browne M (2000) Anxiety disorder. Extracts from "Clinical Evidence". *Br Med J*, **321**, 1204–1207.

Gammans RE, Stringfellow JC, Hvizdos AJ, *et al.* (1992) Use of buspirone in patients with generalized anxiety disorder and coexisting depressive symptoms: a meta-analysis of eight randomized controlled trials. *Neuropsychobiol*, **25**, 193–201.

Gelenberg AJ, Lydiard RB, Rudolph RL, *et al.* (2000) Efficacy of venlafaxine extended-release capsules in nondepressed outpatients with generalized anxiety disorder. *JAMA*, **283**, 3082–3088.

Goa KL, Ward A (1986) Buspirone: a preliminary review of its pharmacological properties and therapeutic efficacy as an anxiolytic. *Drugs*, **32**, 114–129.

Goldberg HL, Finnerty RJ (1979) The comparative efficacy of buspirone and diazepam in the treatment of anxiety. *Am J Psychiatr*, **136**, 1184–1187.

Gould RA, Otto MW, Pollack MH, Yap L (1997) Cognitive behavioural and pharmacological treatment of generalised anxiety disorder: a preliminary meta-analysis. *Behav Ther*, **28**, 285–305.

Greenberg PE, Sisitsky T, Kessler RC, *et al.* (1999) The economic burden of anxiety disorders in the 1990s. *J Clin Psychiat*, **60**, 427–435.

Hackett D, Meoni P, White C, Rasmussen J (2000) Efficacy of short and long-term venlafaxine ER treatment as somatic and psychic symptoms of GAD. *Eur Neuropsychopharmacol*, **10**(suppl. 10), 337.

Hedges DW, Reimherr FW, Strong RE, *et al.* (1996) An open trial of nefazodone in adult patients with generalized anxiety disorder. *Psychopharmacol Bull*, **32**, 671–676.

Hoehn-Saric R, McLeod DR, Zimmerli WD (1988) Differential effects of alprazolam and imipramine in generalized anxiety disorder: somatic versus psychic symptoms. *J Clin Psychiat*, **49**, 293–301.

Judd LL, Kessler RC, Paulus MP *et al.* (1998) Comorbidity as a fundamental feature of generalised anxiety disorders; results from the National Comorbidity Study (NCS). *Acta Psychiat Scand Suppl*, **393**, 6–11.

Kahn RJ, McNair DM, Lipman RS, *et al.* (1986) Imipramine and chlordiazepoxide in depressive and anxiety disorders. II. Efficacy in anxious outpatients. *Arch Gen Psychiat*, **43**, 79–85.

Kessler RC The epidemiology of pure and comorbid generalized anxiety disorder: a review and evaluation of recent research. *Acta Psychiatr Scand*, in press.

Kessler RC, McGonagle KA, Zhao S, *et al.* (1994) Lifetime and 12-month prevalence of DSM-III-R psychiatric disorders in the United States. *Arch Gen Psychiat*, **51**, 8–19.

Kessler RC, Berglund PA, Foster CL, Saunders WB, Stang PE, Walters EE (1997) Social consequences of psychiatric disorders, II: Teenage parenthood. *Am J Psychiat*, **154**, 1405–1411.

Kessler RC, DuPont RL, Berglund P, Wittchen HU (1999) Impairment in pure and comorbid generalized anxiety disorder and major depression at 12 months in two national surveys. *Am J Psychiatry*, **156**, 1915–1923.

Lader MH (1999) Limitations on the use of benzodiazepines in anxiety and insomnia: are they justified? *Eur Psychopharmacol*, **9**(suppl 9), S399–S405.

Lader MH, Bond AJ (1998) Interaction of pharmacological and psychological treatments of anxiety. *Br J Psychiat*, **173**(suppl 34), 42–48.

Logue MB, Thomas AM, Barbee JG, *et al.* (1993) Generalized anxiety disorder patients seek evaluation for cardiac symptoms at the same frequency as patients with panic disorder. *J Psychiatr Res*, **27**, 55–59.

Lydiard RB (2000) An overview of generalised anxiety disorder: disease state—appropriate therapy. *Clin Ther*, **22**(a), A3-A19.

Lydiard RB, Fossey MD, Marsh W, *et al.* (1993) Prevalence of psychiatric disorders in patients with irritable bowel syndrome. *Psychosomatics*, **34**, 229–234.

Lydiard RB, Brawman-Mintzer O, Ballenger JC (1996) Recent developments in the psychopharmacology of anxiety disorders. *J Consult Clin Psychol*, **64**, 660–668.

Lydiard RB, Ballenger JC, Rickels K (1997) A double-blind evaluation of the safety and efficacy of abercarnil, alprazolam, and placebo in outpatients with generalized anxiety disorder. *J Clin Psychiat*, **58**(suppl 11), 11–19.

Mahe V, Balogh A (2000) Long-term pharmacological treatment of generalized anxiety disorder. *Int Clin Psychopharmacol* **15**, 99–105

Maier W, Falkai P (1999) The epidemiology of comorbidity between depression, anxiety disorders and somatic diseases. *Int Clin Psychopharmacol*, **14**(suppl 2), 51–56.

McCafferty J *et al.* (2000) Paroxetine is effective in the treatment of generalised anxiety disorder: Results from a randomised placebo-controlled flexible dose study. *Eur Neuropsychopharmacol*, **10**(suppl 3), S348.

Mendels J, Krajewski TF, Huffer V *et al.* (1986) Effective short-term treatment of generalised anxiety with trifluoperazine. *J Clin Psychiat*, **47**, 170–174.

Montgomery SA (2000) Long-term treatment of GAD. First International Forum on Mood and Anxiety Disorders, Monte Carlo, 2 December, 2000.

Nathan PE, Gorman JM (1998) (eds) A guide to treatments that work. Oxford: Oxford University Press.

Pollack MH, Worthington JH, Manfro GG, *et al.* (1997) Abercarnil for the treatment of generalised anxiety disorder: a placebo-controlled comparison of two dose ranges of abercarnil and buspirone. *J Clin Psychiat*, **58**(suppl 11), 19–23.

Power KG, Simpson RJ, Swanson V, *et al.* (1990) A controlled cognitive-behaviour therapy, diazepam and placebo, alone and in combination, for the treatment of generalised anxiety disorder. *J Anxiety Disord*, **4**, 267–292.

Rickels K, Schweizer E (1998) The spectrum of generalized anxiety in clinical practice: the role of short-term, intermittent treatment. *Br J Psychiat*, **173**(suppl 34), 49–54.

Rickels K, Downing R, Schweizer E, Hassman H (1993) Antidepressants for the treatment of generalized anxiety disorder. A placebo-controlled comparison of imipramine, trazodone, and diazepam. *Arch Gen Psychiat*, **50**, 884–895.

Rickels K, Pollack M, Sheehan D, *et al.* (2000) Efficacy of venlafaxine extended-release (XR) capsules in nondepressed outpatients with generalized anxiety disorder. *Am J Psychiat*, **157**, 968–974.

Rocca P, Fonzo V, Scotta M, Zanalda E, Ravizza L (1997) Paroxetine efficacy in the treatment of generalized anxiety disorder. *Acta Psychiatrica Scand*, **95**, 444–450.

Salinas E (1999) Placebo-controlled evidence for the use of antidepressants in generalised anxiety disorder. *Eur Neuropsychopharmacol*, **9**(suppl. 5), 176.

Sartorius N, Üstün TB, Lecrubier Y, Wittchen HU (1996) Depression comorbid with anxiety: results from the WHO study on psychological disorders in primary health care. *Br J Psychiat*, **30**, 38–43.

Sitsen JMA, Moors J (1994) Mirtazapine, a novel antidepressant, in the treatment of anxiety symptoms: results from a placebo-controlled trial. *Drug Invest*, **8**, 339–344.

Small GW, Bystritsky A (1997) Double-blind, placebo-controlled trial of two doses of abercarnil for geriatric anxiety. *J Clin Psychiat*, **58**(suppl 11), 24–29.

Sonawalla SB, Spillmann MK, Kolsky AR, Alpert JE, Nierenberg AA, Rosenbaum JF, Fava M (1999) Efficacy of fluvoxamine in the treatment of major depression with comorbid anxiety disorders. *J Clin Psychiatry*, **60**, 580–583.

Sramek JJ, Tansman M, Suri A, *et al.* (1996) Efficacy of buspirone in generalized anxiety disorder with coexisting mild depressive symptoms. *J Clin Psychiat*, **57**, 287–291.

Strand M, Hetta J, Rosen A, *et al.* (1990) A double-blind, controlled trial in primary care patients with generalized anxiety: a comparison between buspirone and oxazepam. *J Clin Psychiat*, **51**(suppl), 40–45.

Stein MB, Kirk P, Prabhu V, Grott M, Terepa M (1995) Mixed anxiety-depression in a primary-care clinic. *J Affect Disord*, **34**, 79–84.

Uhlenhuth EH, Balter MB, Ban TA, Yang K (1999) Trends in recommendations for the pharmacotherapy of anxiety disorders by an international expert panel, 1992–1997. *Eur Neuropsychopharmacol*, **9**(suppl 6), S393–S398.

Taylor DP, Carter RB, Eison AS, *et al.* (1995) Pharmacology and neurochemistry of nefazodone, a novel antidepressant drug. *J Clin Psychiat*, **56**(suppl 6), 3–11.

Wardle J (1990) Behaviour therapy and benzodiazepines: allies or antagonists? *Br J Psychiat*, **156**, 163–168.

Weiller E, Bisserbe JC, Maier W, Lecrubier Y (1998) Prevalence and recognition of anxiety syndromes in five European primary care settings. A report from the WHO study on Psychological Problems in General Health Care. *Br J Psychiat*, **173**(suppl 34), 18–23.

Wittchen HU, Zhao S, Kessler RC, *et al.* (1994) DSM-III-R generalized anxiety disorder in the National Comorbidity Survey. *Arch Gen Psychiat*, **51**, 355–364.

Wittchen HU, Kessler RC, Zhao S, Abelson J (1995) Reliability and clinical validity of UM-CIDI DSM-III-R generalized anxiety disorder. *J Psychiatr Res*, **29**, 95–110.

Wittchen HU, Nelson CB, Lachner G (1998) Prevalence of mental disorders and psychosocial impairments in adolescents and young adults. *Psychol Med*, **28**, 109–126.

Wittchen HU, Carter RM, Pfister H *et al.* (2000) Disabilities and quality of life in pure and comorbid generalized anxiety disorder and major depression in a national survey. *Int Clin Psychopharmacol*, **15**, 319–328.

Wittchen HU, Carter RM, Pfisster H (2001) Epidemiology of generalised anxiety disorder in the community and in primary care. *Neuropsychiatry*, in press.

World Health Organization (1993) *The ICD-10 Classification of Mental and Behavioural Disorders. Diagnostic criteria for research*. Geneva: World Health Organization.

Yonkers KA, Dyck IR, Warshaw M, Keller MB (2000) Factors predicting the clinical course of generalised anxiety disorder. *Br J Psychiat*,**176** 544–549.

Index

Note: Page references in *italics* refer to Figures; those in **bold** refer to Tables. Abbreviations used in index are: GAD, generalized anxiety disorder; OCD, obsessive compulsive disorder; PTSD, post-traumatic stress disorder.

abercarnil in GAD   204
α-adrenoceptors
  challenge in OCD   29
  challenge in panic disorder   27
  challenge in social phobia   29–31
  platelet studies in panic disorder   28
β-adrenoceptors, challenge in panic disorder
  27–8
adrenocorticotrophic hormone (ACNI) 31
agoraphobia
  comorbidity   **12**
  comorbidity with panic disorder   10, **10**
  mean age at onset   13
  prevalence   12–13
alcohol abuse/dependence, comorbidity
  with major depression   4
  with panic disorder   11
  with social anxiety disorder   134–5
alprazolam in panic disorder   119, 120
Alzheimer's disease   58
amitriptyline   110, 111
  depression and   166
  double-blind studies in PTSD   187
  in OCD   152
anxious depression   107–16
azapirones   45
  GAD and   194

behaviour therapy
  fluvoxamine and, in OCD   169
  in long-term treatment of OCD   163
benign essential tremor, comorbidity with
  social anxiety disorder   136
benzodiazepines   110
  efficacy and tolerability   **203**
  GAD and   194, 202, 203
  in panic disorder   28, 119

side effects   203
  in social anxiety disorder   145
β-blockers in anxiety   202
bipolar disorder
  comorbidity with social anxiety disorder
    135
  gender differences   5
  mean ages at onset   5
  prevalence   5, **6**
blood platelet studies in depression and
  anxiety   42–3
body dysmorphic disorder, comorbidity with
  social anxiety disorder   135
brofaromine, double-blind studies in PTSD
  188, 189
buspirone
  in combination in OCD   168
  efficacy and tolerability   **203**
  GAD and   194, 203
  in OCD   153
  in PTSD   183–4
  in social phobia   40, 41, 45

carbidopa   34
2'chlorodesmethyldiazepam, GAD and
  197–8
cholecystokinin (CKK)
  in anxiety   49–55, **52–3**
  challenge as human panic model   49–50
  distribution of CKK and CKK receptors
    in brain   49
  In OCD and social phobia   54–5
  In GAD   204
cholecystokinin$_B$ (CCK$_B$) receptor
  antagonists,
  effect on CCK$_4$-induced panic   50–4
cholecystokinin-4 (CCK-4) 46

CI-988   54
  in GAD   204
citalopram   46, 48
  anxious depression   115
  in combination in OCD   168
  drug comparisons   125
  GAD and   200
  in OCD   156
  in panic disorders   119, 120, 122
  in social anxiety disorder   144
clonazepam   38, 39
  in adolescents   167
  in combination in OCD   167
  comparisons of SSRIs with   **158**
  depression and   165–6
  dosage in OCD   159, 160
  drug comparisons   125–6
  long-term treatment   162–3, 165
  in OCD   152, 153, 157–9
  in panic disorders   119, 120–1
  safety   161
  side effects   160–1
  in social phobia   41
clonidine   27, 29
  in obsessive-compulsive disorder   29
clorgyline in OCD   153
cognitive behavioural therapy
  GAD and   194
  in panic disorder   28, 126
comorbidity, patterns of   88–102, **90,**
      129
  comorbidity and severity   96–7, **97**
  effects of comorbidity on disorder
      persistence   95–6, **96**
  effects of earlier anxiety on risk of
      secondary MDD   92–5
  temporally primary and secondary
      disorders   89–92, **91**
corticotrophin-releasing hormone (CRH)
      40
cortisol   31, 34
CSF studies in depression and anxiety
      42–3
  in OCD   44
  in panic disorder   43–4
CT studies in depression   56
cyproheptadine in PTSD   184

D2-dopamine receptors as challenge in social
      phobia   29–31
desensitization hypothesis   31, 46–7

desipramine   26, 111
  depression and   166
  in OCD   152
  in panic disorder   121
d-fenfluramine   32
dopaminergic function in social phobia
      29–31
drug abuse/dependence, comorbidity
  with major depression   4
  with panic disorder   11
  with social anxiety disorder   134–5
DSM diagnostic system, controversies in
      87–8
dysthymic disorder, prevalence   6

eating disorders, comorbidity with social
      anxiety disorder   135
β-endorphin   31

familial pure depressive disease   58
fenfluramine   31, 42
  5-H_{1D} receptors in OCD and   40–1
  in combination in OCD   168
  in depression   32
  in OCD   39–40
  in panic disorder   32–4, **33**
  in social phobia   41
flesinoxan in GAD   204
flumazenil, panic disorder and   51
fluoxetine   32, 38, 40
  in anxious depression   111–12
  in combination in OCD   168
  development of depression and   125
  dose in OCD   159
  double-blind studies in PTSD   185
  GAD and   200
  long-term treatment   162–3
  in OCD   154–5, 158, 161, 162
  in panic disorders   119, 120, 124–5
  in PTSD   180, 181–2
  in social anxiety disorder   144
fluvoxamine   39, 48
  in anxious depression   110, 111, 114–15
  behaviour therapy and, in OCD   169
  depression and   166
  development of depression and   125
  drug comparisons   125
  GAD and   201
  in long-term treatment of OCD   163,
      165
  in OCD   152, 153–4, 158, 161

in panic disorders 51, 119, 120, 121–2
in PTSD 182–3
in social anxiety disorder 138, 144
functional MRI in OCD 62, **63**, 65

gabapentin in social anxiety disorder 135,
145
generalized anxiety disorder
comorbidity
with panic disorder 10
with social anxiety disorder 135
course of illness 197
diagnostic criteria 193, **194, 195**, 196
impairment in 196–7
pharmacological recommendations
202–4
prevalence 15–16, **15**, 193
psychological approaches 204–5
serotonergic antidepressants in 201–2
SSRIs in 197–201
gepirone 42
Gilles de la Tourette's syndrome 168

homovanillic acid (HVA) 27
Huntington's disease 58
5-hydroxyindole-acetic acid (5-HIAA)
in depression 43
in panic disorder 43–4
5-hydroxytryptophan (5-HTP) 31
in OCD 38–9
hypometabolism in depression 56–8

ImICPP in OCD 64
imipramine 111
in agoraphobia 120
double-blind studies in PTSD 187–8
GAD and 194, 197–8
in OCD 152
in panic disorder 28, 50–1, 121
[^{3}H]-imipramine binding 42–3
ipsapirone 40, 41, 42
irritable bowel syndrome, comorbidity with
social anxiety disorder 136

jitteriness syndrome 124–5

L-365, 260, panic disorder and 51–4
levodopa in social phobia 29–1
lithium therapy 45
in combination in OCD 168
lorazepam in anxious depression 115

magnetic resonance imaging (MRI) studies
in depression 55–6
in panic disorder 61
major depression
comorbidity 4–5, **5**
with panic disorder **11**
with social anxiety disorder 132
gender differences 3
historical trends 4
marital status 4
mean age at onset 4
prevalence rates 2–3, **2**, 88
public health impact 5
risk factors 3–4
type of residence 4
work status 4
major depressive episode (MSE), prevalence
88
maprotiline 111
m-chlorophenylpiperazine (*m*CPP) 31, 42
5-HT$_{1D}$ receptors in OCD and 40–1
in obsessive-compulsive disorder 35–8,
36–7
in panic disorders 35, 50
in PTSD 180
metergoline 38
3-methoxy-4-hydroxy-phenylethyleneglycol
(MHPG) 27
α-methyl-*p*-tyrosine (αMPT) 26–7
mianserin 109
minor depressive disorder, prevalence 6
mirtazapine 48
GAD and 202
mixed anxiety depression 107
anxiety systems in depression 109
definition 108
prevalence 6
research criteria 108–9, **108**
treatment of anxiety symptoms
109–15
MK-212 40
5-HT$_{1D}$ receptors in OCD and
40–1
monoamine function
monoamine hypothesis 26
noradrenergic function in depression
26–7
monoamine oxidase inhibitors (MAOIs) in
panic disorder 28, 110, 119
morbidity, patterns of 88–97
multiple sclerosis 58

nefazodone 111
  GAD and 201
  in PTSD 184–5
  in social anxiety disorder 144, 145
neuroendocrine strategy 31
neuroimaging
  in depression 55–9, **57**
  in obsessive-compulsive disorder 61–5,
    63–4
  in panic disorder 59–61, **60**
noradrenaline depletion paradigm 26
noradrenaline hypothesis, critique of 28
noradrenergic function
  obsessive-compulsive disorder 29, **30**
  in panic disorder 27–8
  in social phobia 29–31
nortriptyline
  depression and 166
  in OCD 152

obsessive-compulsive disorder
  age and 167
  combination treatments 167–9
  comorbidity
    with major depression 4
    with panic disorder 10
    with social anxiety disorder 135
  depression and 165–7
  differences between SSRIs 161–2
  dosage of SSRIs in 159–60
  long-term treatment 162–5, **164**
  pharmacology vs behaviour therapy in
    169–70
  prevalence 16, 151
  response to SSDIs 152–3
  safety 161
  side effects and tolerability 160–1
ondansetron 41
  in social phobia 41
oxaprotiline 111

panic disorder
  age at onset 9
  comorbidity 9–10
    with major depression 4
    with social anxiety disorder
      132–3
  cultural differences 9
  educational level 9
  gender differences 9
  life events 9

marital status 9
  physical/sexual abuse 9
  prevalence 7–12, **7**, **8**
  residence location 9
  risk factors 9
  suicidality 11–12, **11**
Parkinson's disease 58
paroxetine 48
  in anxious depression 110, 112–14
  depression and 143
  dosage
    in OCD 159–60
    in social anxiety disorder 143
  double-blind studies in PTSD 185–6
  drug comparisons 125
  early termination and dropouts 144
  efficacy in 141–2
  fixed dose studies in social anxiety
    disorder 139
  flexible dose studies in social anxiety
    disorder 139
  GAD and 194, 197–200, **200**, 204
  in long-term treatment of OCD 165
  in OCD 155, 158, 161
  in paediatric patients 167
  in panic disorders 119, 120, 122–4
  patient characteristics in studies for social
    anxiety disorders **140**
  in PTSD 180, 183
  secondary efficacy measures 142, **143**
  severity of SAD and treatment
    response 144
  in social anxiety disorder 138, 141–2,
    145
  tolerability 143–5, **144**
p-chlorophenylalanine 45
PCPA 179
pentagastrin 50, 54–5
personality disorder, 5-HIAA, suicidality
    and 43
PET studies in depression 56, 58
  in panic disorder 59, 60
  in OCD 62, **63**
phenelzine
  double-blind studies in PTSD
    187–8
  in OCD 153
  in panic disorder 119
  in social anxiety disorder 135
pindolol 31, 32, 48
  augmentation strategies 46–8

post-traumatic stress disorder
  comorbidity
    with panic disorder   10
    with social anxiety disorder   133–4
  cost   178–9
  definition   175
  diagnostic criteria   176, **177**
  double-blind studies
    with serotonergic drugs   186–8
    with SSRIs   185–6
  impairment   178–9
  open-label studies   181–5
  prevalence   16–18, 176–8
  serotonin in   179–80
  treatment   180–1
prolactin   31, 32, 34, 35

recurrent brief depressive disorder,
    prevalence   6
regional cerebral blood flow (r-CBF)
  in depression   56
  in panic disorder   59–61
reserpine, monoamine hypothesis and   26
ritanserin   32, 35, 42, 111

schizophrenia, 5-HIAA, suicidality and
    43
serotonin
  challenge studies   31
  in depression and anxiety   31–49
  in PTSD   179–80
serotonin (5-HT) depletion paradigms   26
serotonin precursors
  in OCD   38–9
  in panic disorder   32–4, **33**
serotonin receptor subtypes
  in depression and anxiety   44–5
  5-HT$_{1A}$ receptors in depression and
    anxiety   45–6
    postsynaptic   48–9
  5-HT$_{1D}$ receptors in OCD   40–1
sertraline
  in adolescents   167
  in anxious depression   110, 111, 114
  dose in OCD   159
  double-blind studies in PTSD   186
  GAD and   201
  in long-term treatment of OCD   163,
    165
  in OCD   155–6, 158, 161
  in panic disorders   119, 120, 124

in PTSD   181
in social anxiety disorder   138, 144
simple phobia
  comorbidity with social anxiety disorder
    135
  prevalence   14–15
social phobia/social anxiety disorder
    129–45
  assessment instruments/frequency of
    assessment   140
  diagnostic features   129, **130**
  differential diagnosis   137–8, **137**
  fixed dose studies   139
  flexible-dose studies   139
  inclusion and exclusion criteria   139–40
  medical comorbidity   136
  prevalence   13–14, **13**
  psychiatric comorbidity   131–5
    alcohol/substance abuse   134–5
    with major depression   132
    with panic disorder   10, 132–3
    with post-traumatic stress disorder
      133–4
  SSRIs as first line treatment for   138–45,
    138
  treatment implications of comorbidity
    136–7
sodium lactate infusion, panic attacks and
    50
SPECT studies in depression   56, 58
  in OCD   62, **64**, 65
  on panic disorder   59, 60–1
stressor-precipitated cortisol-induced
    5-HT-related anxiety/aggression-driven
    depression   43
stuttering, comorbidity with social anxiety
    disorder   136
subcortical hyperintensities   55
substance abuse *see* drug abuse
suicidality
  5-HIAA and   43
  in panic disorder   11–12, **11**
sumatriptan   40–1

trazodone   35, 111
  in OCD   152
  in PTSD   184
trichotillomania   38
tricyclic antidepressants (TCAs)   110
  comparison with SSRIs in panic
    disorder   126

tricyclic antidepressants (TCAs) (*continued*)
  efficacy and tolerability   **203**
  in GAD   202
  in panic disorder   28, 119
tryptophan   31, 34
  in combination in OCD   168
tryptophan depletion   26, 45–6
  in depression   56

vascular depression hypothesis   55
venlafaxine
  GAD and   201–2, 204
  in OCD   156
  in social anxiety disorder   144, 145

ventricle-to-brain (VBR) ratio   61
ventricular enlargement   56

WAY 100635   48

yohimbine   27, 29, 45
  panic attacks and   28, 50
  in PTSD   180

zimelidine   110, 111
  in panic disorder   120
zolmitriptan   41

Index compiled by Annette Musker